THE CITY & GUILDS TEXTBOOK

LEVEL 3 VRQ DIPLOMA IN
BEAUTY THERAPY

INCLUDES SPA UNITS

DEE GERRARD
HELEN BECKMANN
PLUS EXPERT CONTRIBUTORS

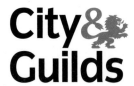

About City & Guilds

City & Guilds is the UK's leading provider of vocational qualifications, offering over 500 awards across a wide range of industries, and progressing from entry level to the highest levels of professional achievement. With over 8500 centres in 100 countries, City & Guilds is recognised by employers worldwide for providing qualifications that offer proof of the skills they need to get the job done.

Equal opportunities

City & Guilds fully supports the principle of equal opportunities and we are committed to satisfying this principle in all our activities and published material. A copy of our equal opportunities policy statement is available on the City & Guilds website.

First edition 2013

ISBN 978 0 85193 234 7

Publisher Louise Le Bas
Commissioning Editor Fiona McGlade
Development Editor James Hobbs
Production Editor Natalie Griffith

Cover design by Select Typesetters Ltd
Typeset by GreenGate Publishing Services
Printed in the UK by Cambrian Printers Ltd

Publications

For information about or to order City & Guilds support materials, contact 0844 534 0000 or centresupport@cityandguilds.com. You can find more information about the materials we have available at www.cityandguilds.com/publications.

Every effort has been made to ensure that the information contained in this publication is true and correct at the time of going to press. However, City & Guilds' products and services are subject to continuous development and improvement and the right is reserved to change products and services from time to time. City & Guilds cannot accept liability for loss or damage arising from the use of information in this publication.

City & Guilds
1 Giltspur Street
London EC1A 9DD

T 0844 543 0033
www.cityandguilds.com
publishingfeedback@cityandguilds.com

CONTENTS

ACKNOWLEDGEMENTS

Much love and thanks to my parents who have always encouraged me to follow my dreams. Thanks to my brilliant family Steve, Callum and Keira for all their patience, love and support during the writing of this book. Lastly to my dear friends Helen and Nathalie for making me laugh and to Jo Lord for inspiring me.

Dee Gerrard

Thanks to all those who have given me time, advice and support during the writing of this book. Thanks in particular to my family: Howard, Connor, Alex and Hazel for their love and understanding. Lastly to my wonderful team at Hebe, in particular Hannah, Julie and Kathy.

Helen Beckmann

City & Guilds would like to sincerely thank the following.

For invaluable beauty therapy expertise and editing
Anita Crosland, Tracey Bennett and Melissa Peacock

For taking college photos
Andrew Buckle, Pierre Marcar and Jules Selmes

For supplying the front cover photo
Larysa Dodz (photographer)

For their help with photoshoots
To all the tutors and learners at Cambridge Regional College, Canterbury College, Kent Beauty Academy, London School of Beauty Therapy and Warwickshire College.

Thanks also to Carolyn Claypole at Sterex Electrolysis International Ltd

For supplying additional photos
Kirsten McNeill and Natalie Campbell at Fake Bake UK Ltd, Janice Brown at HOF Beauty, Lucy Hunt and Jannette Cook at Lash FX, Lash Perfect and The Eyelash Design Company, Laura Fisher at The Carlton Beauty and Spa Group and Elaine Stoddart at Sterex Electrolysis International Ltd

For their photo research work
Emma Whyte

Picture credits
Every effort has been made to acknowledge all copyright holders as below and the publishers will, if notified, correct any errors in future editions.

Alamy: © Peter S Noyce p141; **Andover College:** pp146, 147, 151, 158, 159, 176, 192, 194, 200, 209, 218, 235, 391, 400; **Anti-Aging Clinic & Dispensary:** p473; **Bedford College**: pp142, 145, 155, 171, 177, 178, 185, 189, 190, 211, 237; **Central Sussex College:** p189; **Cambridge Community College:** pp7, 164, 165, 168, 207, 210, 212, 213, 220, 222, 226, 229, 231, 391, 392, 393, 394, 396, 397, 398, 399, 401, 402, 403, 409, 410, 418, 419, 420, 421, 422, 423, 426, 438, 439, 440, 481, 486, 495, 496; **Canterbury College:** pp9, 138, 148, 161, 166, 169, 172, 173, 175, 187, 193, 217, 225, 233, 242, 247, 257, 269, 270, 276, 277, 280, 285, 287, 290, 299, 300, 310, 311, 319, 324, 329; **The Carlton Beauty and Spa Group:** pp277, 296, 297, 303, 304, 320, 427, 428; **DermaCo Skincare:** p441; **Di Vapor:** p484; **Epping Forest College:** p12; **FakeBake:** pp398, 399, 404; **Fotolia:** © Alan Stockdale p196; **Germaine de Capuccini:** p390; **Glowimages:** © Imagesource p33; © Superstock p150; **Goddess International**: p434; **Goldwell:** p196; **Havering College:** p193;

Disclaimer

Please note that all of the equipment and products shown in this book are to illustrate what you may use in your learning centre and/or salon. We recommend that you use equipment and products from one brand only when carrying out treatments. In most instances, these items have been constructed and formulated specifically to work in harmony with other equipment and products of the same brand and we cannot guarantee compatibility or end results with other brands. If you are unsure as to whether certain equipment or a product of one brand can be used in conjunction with another, please consult your supervisor or contact the brand's company directly for further advice.

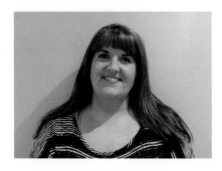

DEE GERRARD

LEAD AUTHOR

After training as a beauty and holistic therapist I have worked in salons, freelance, in my own salon and then in education. I love working with people and even after 20 years I still get a buzz from learning new treatments and techniques. I became a college lecturer as I needed a new challenge; it has been a very rewarding career and I've been lucky enough to work with some great teams and people especially at The Manchester College. My aim has always been to improve the standards and professionalism of therapists joining our industry today and I'm very fortunate to have a career where I can do that.

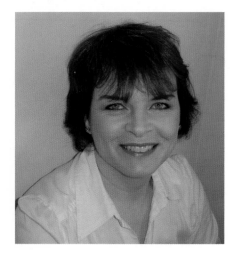

HELEN BECKMANN

ANATOMY AND PHYSIOLOGY AND MASSAGE

I have worked in the beauty therapy industry since I left college – 30 years ago! During this time I have worked for several salons and I have also been an international examiner. For the last ten years I have owned my own beauty and holistic therapies salon where I still practise. I have taught in further education but currently teach in higher education lecturing on a foundation degree in complementary therapies and I am at present studying for my second degree.

JANICE BROWN

MICRODERMABRASION

From providing treatments to managing salons and working in sales, Janice has had a diverse and fulfilling career in the beauty industry. She has been involved in teaching, training, giving demonstrations, helping set standards, writing and research and development. She currently owns and runs Hof Beauty Ltd alongside her husband Robert.

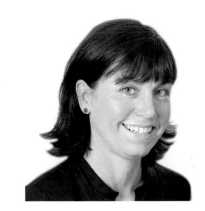

PENNY HALLWORTH

PROMOTE AND SELL PRODUCTS AND SERVICES

Penny has over 30 years' experience in the beauty industry. Her career has covered salon therapy, teaching in further education and various roles in the cruise ship spa sector, from therapist to supervisor overseeing spa standards and business and latterly becoming Head of Training at the Steiner Training Academy. Penny loves to use her experience in beauty to teach and inspire others to deliver the best customer experience and develop great business skills. She currently teaches at Harrow College, Middlesex.

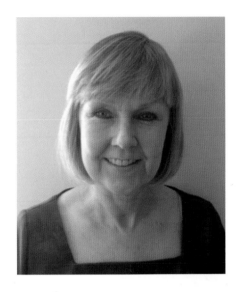

LOUISE HOCKINGS

HEALTH AND SAFETY

Louise's career began at the age of 14 as a Saturday girl in a local salon. She then began a three-year hairdressing apprenticeship on the day after she left school. After completing her apprenticeship she moved to a large chain of salons and became the salon trainer, beginning her career move into training and education. She has enjoyed a fulfilling and varied career for 30 years in the industry and believes that hard work, dedication and a passion to succeed are all you need to achieve your dreams.

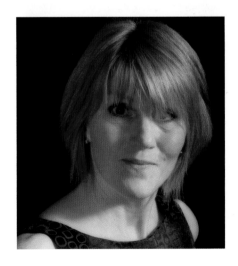

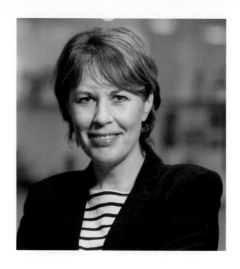

ANDREA PLIMMER

SPA THERAPY

Andrea has been Head of Department at Trafford College for 13 years and has developed an extensive knowledge and experience of the beauty and spa industry over the past 20 years including working in the UK, overseas and on cruise ships. She currently teaches on a foundation degree in spa management and is the co-author of several beauty resource packs and a Level 2 and 3 spa book. She has combined her passion for the spa industry and travel into inspiring students through education and training.

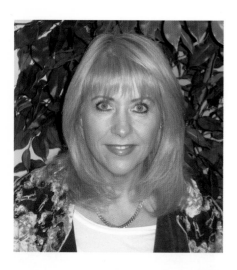

ELAINE STODDART

ELECTRICAL EPILATION

Elaine is Director of Education for Sterex Electrolysis International Limited and is a highly qualified and experienced specialist electrolysist. She is the most prolific trainer in Advanced Electrolysis/Advanced Cosmetic Procedures in the UK as well as running busy private practices in Harley Street, London and Buckinghamshire. She is a published author, teacher and international speaker and has appeared on educational programmes for the BBC and created the first ever transgender electrolysis course in the UK.

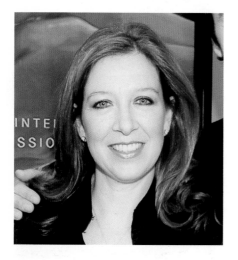

HELLEN WARD

WORKING IN THE BEAUTY INDUSTRY

Hellen trained as a hairdresser upon leaving school at 16. She progressed up the ranks of the company from Salon Manager, then Regional Manager to General Manager of Harrods Hair & Beauty Salon before opening her own business with her husband Richard nearly 20 years ago. She now runs one of the largest independent hair and beauty salons and brands in the country and continues to lecture at business seminars, educate salon owners, write a monthly column for a beauty magazine and she has written three books for City & Guilds.

FOREWORD

I have been in this industry for over 30 years and my initial beauty therapy training has allowed me to have a truly exciting and varied career. I have been on a fantastic journey and have met some inspirational people from working in salons, spas and health farms. I went on to work within the beauty education sector at a large FE college and also with City & Guilds as an External Quality Assurer and Chief International Examiner. I am a published author of a beauty textbook and now I work as a Portfolio Manager within City & Guilds and look after all the beauty, nails, spa and complementary therapies qualifications both nationally and internationally.

City & Guilds has produced this fantastic textbook to help support you with your chosen qualification. A career in beauty or spa therapy is an incredible industry to be in and our qualifications are recognised across the world. This textbook has a number of inspirational sections and will give you a broad insight into the practical and underpinning knowledge required to complete your qualification. It's also a great reference tool once you are qualified. The images, step-by-steps and end-of-unit 'Test your knowledge' sections all work really well together to give you a comprehensive support resource. The authors and contributors have fantastic breadth and depth of knowledge between them and are well thought of in the educational and beauty industries.

The beauty and spa industries are diverse and exciting ones, from working in salons, spas, hotels or cruise ships; whichever you choose to work in will be inspirational, challenging and exciting. It's a wonderful and global industry to work in! I want to take this opportunity to wish all who are studying the City & Guilds Level 3 Beauty Therapy or Body and Spa Therapy the best of luck throughout their chosen careers.

Anita Crosland

Beauty Therapy Portfolio Manager, City & Guilds

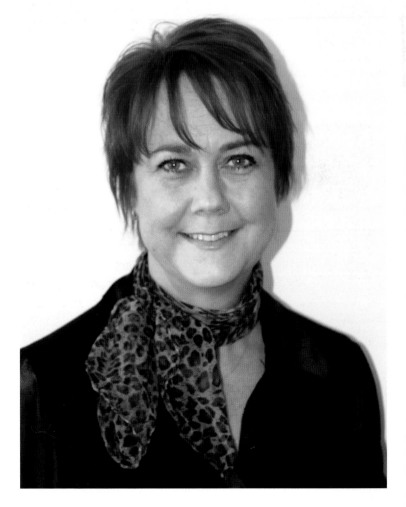

HOW TO USE THIS TEXTBOOK

You will find that your City & Guilds VRQ Level 3 Beauty Therapy is laid out in the same way as your City & Guilds VRQ Level 2 Beauty Therapy logbook to aid your navigation and understanding of both.

Each chapter in your textbook covers everything you will need to understand in order to complete your written or online tests and practical assessments.

Throughout this textbook you will see the following features:

HANDY HINTS

Toner is also available as a spray which is ideal for male clients as it eliminates the risk of getting cotton wool caught in facial hair. It is also more cost-effective to use toner in a spray format.

Handy hints are particularly useful tips that can assist you in your revision or help you remember something important.

Strip lashes

Very dramatic artificial lashes that are applied to the length of the eye

Words in bold in the text are explained in the margin to aid your understanding.

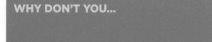

WHY DON'T YOU...

Why don't you – These hints suggest activities for you to try to help you practise and learn.

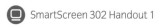

ACTIVITY

Activities – The activities help to test your understanding and learn from your colleagues' experiences.

SmartScreen 302 Handout 1

SmartScreen – These icons refer to the City & Guilds SmartScreen resources and activities. Ask your tutor for your log-in details.

At the end of each chapter are some 'Test your knowledge' questions. These are multiple-choice questions, designed to prepare you for your written or online tests and to identify any areas where you might need further training or revision.

Some units are followed by a case study on an industry expert, who explains the background to their career, and offers helpful advice in their specialist area.

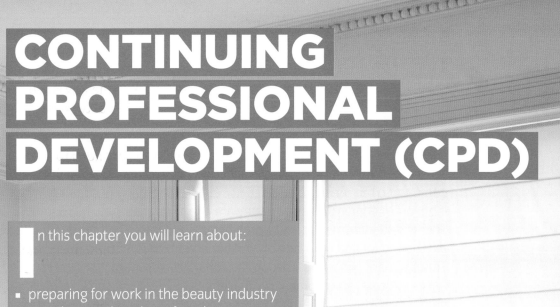

CONTINUING PROFESSIONAL DEVELOPMENT (CPD)

In this chapter you will learn about:

- preparing for work in the beauty industry
- searching and applying for jobs
- interviews
- employment rights and practices
- continuing professional development (CPD)
- career opportunities and planning
- fitting into the workplace.

PREPARING FOR WORK IN THE BEAUTY INDUSTRY

Starting work in a salon means that you have to put what you have learnt into practice. In a practical salon environment you are faced with the commercial realities of the everyday world, including problems and time pressures. Working on models in a learning environment can never really compare to the pressure of pleasing real, paying clients, especially when it becomes your job to ensure they are happy so that they will rebook. The transition from student to professional can mean an introduction to different ways and methods of working and this will naturally take time. This invaluable phase of your professional development is critical to your future success, so embrace the challenges ahead. Even the very best students still have to learn to 'cut the mustard' in the real environment.

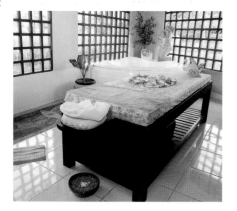

Preparing for work involves many stages. In this chapter we are going to look at some of the stages and elements you will need to consider as you make the transition from learner into seasoned professional. Every employer is different and will operate in different ways. As a new employee, part of the challenge is to work out how the knowledge and skills that you have learned can be adapted to fit with the salon's practices and ethos. What is really important is to learn how to integrate into an established team and to develop the skills to fit in easily. It is important to feel comfortable in your surroundings. Any feelings of unease will be picked up on by your customers.

SEARCHING AND APPLYING FOR JOBS

Before you start looking for a job, it is worth considering what options are available to you. There are several things you need to think about:

- The type of salon you want to work in and why: a department store salon, a beauty salon, a spa resort, a hotel spa, a cruise ship. Why do you want to work there? What is it that appeals to you? What skill sets do you have that make this salon a 'natural fit' for you?
- Location: Are you willing to travel for work? Is commuting an option (cost, travel time)? Is moving closer an option?
- The benefits to your career: There will be pros and cons to every opportunity or job role. Some examples follow:

  - Some spas are overnight retreats and building up regular, repeat business is difficult and you might also carry out the same treatments on a regular basis (eg massage).
  - A larger organisation may have a more defined structure making it easier to progress up the ladder if becoming a supervisor is part of your long-term career plan.
  - In larger beauty salons, spas and cruise ships, it is often possible to carve out a specific role to use the skills that you enjoy and excel at (eg if you are confident and have excelled at massage treatments and body treatments, there might be a specialist body therapist role).

DOING YOUR RESEARCH

Once you have established the type of salon or spa that you would like to work in, you need to do your homework. Find out as much as you can about salons or spas that you are interested in working for. Use the Internet to find out about them as most salons have a website. The website will allow you to get a feel for:

- their clientele
- the services or treatments they offer
- the type of work they do.

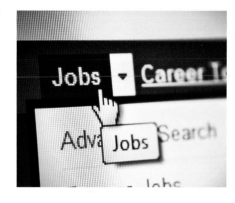

WHERE TO FIND VACANCIES

- Further education colleges often advertise local vacancies on their noticeboards and websites.
- The local job centre will also have details of local vacancies.
- Trade publications often contain job adverts.
- Industry-specific recruitment websites.

HANDY HINT

Figuring out at the start where you want to get to is pretty vital so you can make the right decisions to take you to your chosen destination.

APPLYING FOR JOBS

Most websites will also have a recruitment or careers section on their website so you can see whether they have any vacancies and apply online.

If the salon/spa you are interested in working for is close by, drop by in person to see if they have any vacancies or to deliver your CV by hand.

Even if there aren't any positions available, it is still worth emailing or posting your CV to employers you are interested in working for. Good employers will keep these on file and look at them even if they aren't actively recruiting.

When sending your CV be sure to include:

- a recent, appropriate picture of yourself
- up-to-date contact details
- a brief one- to two-page summary (including dates) of your qualifications and training.

HANDY HINT

Be sure to look at all the different sources of vacancies.

INDUSTRY TIP

Make sure that any photos you send are suitable. Don't send pictures taken from your Facebook page that may not show you in a professional light.

HANDY HINT

There is no substitute for doing proper research, so be sure to find out plenty of information about the salons or spas you are applying to. This not only makes sure you aren't wasting your time (or the salon's time) but it will also be beneficial in an interview. It will show that you have a good understanding of the role you are applying for and will help demonstrate your keenness for the position.

INTERVIEWS

Being a good interviewee is a skill you develop over time. However, even the most inexperienced interviewees can follow some basic rules.

PUNCTUALITY

- Be on time or early – it's never acceptable to be late.
- If you know you are going to be unable to make the interview, phone the company that is interviewing you first thing on the day of the interview and apologise for any inconvenience. Ask if you can rearrange the interview.

LOOK THE PART

- Dressing smartly gives the right first impression. Make sure that:
  - your hair is clean
  - your make-up has been applied professionallly and appropriately
  - your hands look moisturised, your nails are filed and a suitable length, with no chipped varnish
  - your clothes are ironed
  - you look clean and professional
  - your shoes are clean and appropriate
  - you have high standards of personal hygiene.
- Don't be scruffy. Being well-presented is vital in the hair and beauty industry – a potential employer won't have much confidence that you can promote and sell treatments if you aren't well-groomed yourself.

BE PREPARED

Most salons will require a **trade test**, so be prepared. This may be part of the first interview or you may be called back to carry out a trade test separately. Make sure you ask about this as you will need to take a clean pressed uniform, have your hair secured appropriately, remove all jewellery and have short varnish-free nails.

- Make sure you've done your research and can answer basic questions that the interviewer may have (eg 'What do you know about our salon/company?').
- Take anything with you that might help your application (eg portfolios, certificates, photographic work, marketing or media work you have been involved with).
- Take with you another copy of your CV to leave with the interviewer (even if you have already emailed it) or so that you can use it to refer to.

CREATE A POSITIVE IMPRESSION

- Use positive body language (eg nodding, smiling, eye contact) and use a firm handshake when meeting the interviewer and at the end of the interview.
- Sit forward (avoid slouching) and make sure you are giving the interviewer your full attention.
- Take notes and don't be afraid to ask questions.
- Look enthusiastic, interested and keen.
- Don't make negative comments about former employers or salons where you have worked. It won't look good in the eyes of a potential employer.
- Provide explanations for leaving and changing jobs.
- Be prepared for some random questions – if you're not sure how to answer them, jot the questions down and come back to them.

INTERVIEW QUESTIONS

The interviewer is likely to ask you open questions (who, what, why, when, how, tell me) that you cannot answer 'yes' or 'no' to.

Trade test

A test, often carried out after a first interview, to demonstrate your practical skills and techniques to a potential employer

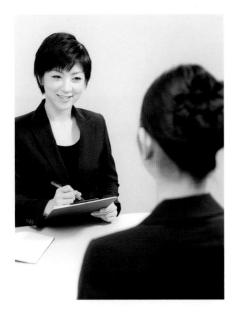

WHY DON'T YOU...
practise answering open questions with a friend and do some role plays of interviews.

FINISHING THE INTERVIEW

Finish the interview by thanking the interviewer for their time. You should have already established what the next steps will be or when you may hear back but if not, ask before you leave.

EMPLOYMENT RIGHTS AND PRACTICES

Once you are lucky enough to become an employee, it is worth familiarising yourself with some standard workplace employment rights and practices.

TERMS AND CONDITIONS OF EMPLOYMENT (CONTRACT OF EMPLOYMENT)

Within two months of starting work, all employees must be given a written document outlining their terms and conditions of employment. You may initially receive a letter detailing your basic terms (salary, hours of work, number of days holiday, supervisor/manager etc) but the terms and conditions of employment/a contract is the main document given to all employees.

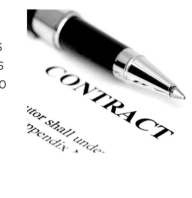

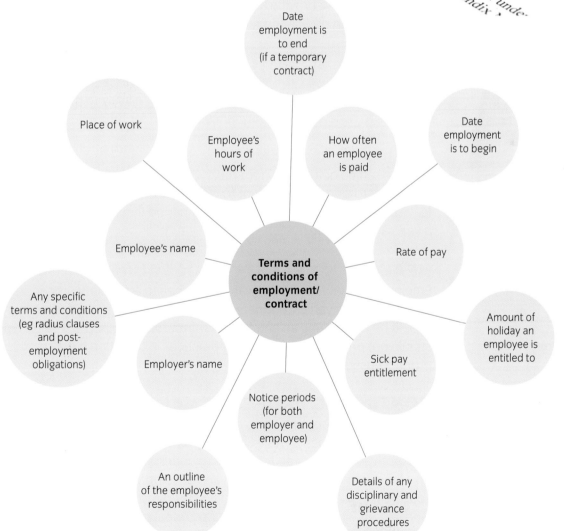

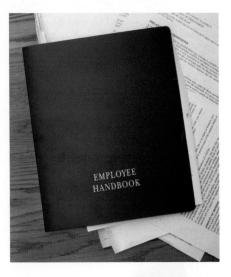

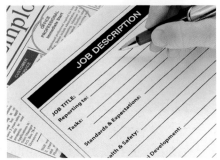

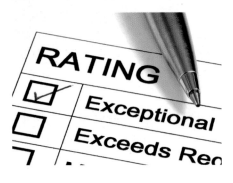

Interpersonal skills

Communication skills

GRIEVANCE AND DISCIPLINARY PROCEDURES

These will give details about the company's procedures for dealing with a grievance or disciplinary matters. They will outline the process for raising a grievance and the procedures (eg verbal and written warnings) for taking disciplinary action against an employee. They will also contain details of how an employee can appeal against any action.

EMPLOYEE HANDBOOK/RULES AND REGULATIONS

Some salons will have their own employee handbook. An employee handbook should include information on rules and regulations (eg appearance, sickness, reporting procedures, reporting absences from work, booking holidays). If a salon doesn't have a handbook, the same information that is included in the handbook (ie rules and regulations) might be issued verbally or put on the staff noticeboard. Other relevant information (eg on reporting lines and management or supervisory structure) may be given verbally.

JOB DESCRIPTION

It's always helpful to know exactly what is expected of you. A job description should provide a short summary of the job role you are undertaking and outline the requirements of the job from the company's perspective.

APPRAISAL AND REVIEW SYSTEM

As part of your development and training you are likely to have an appraisal to review your performance and plan for future development.

TRAINING AGREEMENTS

Training can be quite costly for employers. On starting a job, it may be necessary to sign an agreement to repay any training costs should you leave the company within a certain time period (normally six months to a year) after starting the job.

HEALTH AND SAFETY PROCEDURES

Employees should be made aware of any health and safety procedures and should be given appropriate training. Any health and safety training should be held during an employee's normal working hours. The training should not only cover safe working practices in the salon but also products used in the salon.

CONTINUING PROFESSIONAL DEVELOPMENT

Wherever you choose to work, make sure they have a programme of ongoing development. This is vital for your professional development and motivation. You need to be able to undertake training and education on a long-term basis to strengthen and develop your skills and improve your weaker areas. As a newly qualified therapist, you will still be working out what are your strengths and weaknesses (both in terms of your technical and **interpersonal skills**). As you gain more experience you will become aware of areas that you could improve on. It is therefore important to develop a healthy attitude towards professional development and learning from the start.

Depending on the type of salon you start off in, it may be necessary to undergo some further on-the-job training straight away. Some salons will want to refine your skills so you can deliver services to their required level. Any further training needs may be established during the skills test or trade test after a successful first interview or it may come to light during a performance review or appraisal.

On-the-job training might involve further training in-house during working hours from colleagues who specialise in the areas that you need to develop. Alternatively, it may be necessary to attend off-the-job training with specific manufacturers and suppliers whose products you are using within the salon. Off-the-job training isn't always **subsidised** or paid for by your employer.

Subsidised
Where part of something has been paid

AREAS FOR IMPROVEMENT

From a salon owner's perspective, there are traditionally some areas where college leavers' skills need attention and further development when it comes to working in a productive, commercial salon. Aside from the technical skills which need further development over time to become more slick, professional and speedy, interpersonal skills need to be developed further. Learning how to manage relationships with clients successfully comes with time and experience. You need to become an expert at making people feel good and learn to trust your judgement and ability.

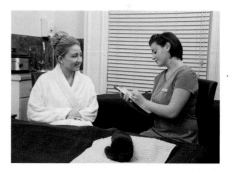

As a newly qualified therapist it is often consultation and customer service skills that need further development. Learning to interpret body language and non-verbal communication signals and using open questions (to probe) and closed questions (to clarify) to establish clients' expectations will help you develop good relationships with clients and create a meaningful treatment plan for future bookings.

Carrying out a detailed consultation is essential to understanding and confirming the client's expectations. It will be your job to establish, meet and exceed these expectations and a repeat booking will only be guaranteed if you are able to do this.

Initially, newly qualified therapists may also struggle with the time pressures of a commercial salon.

CAREER OPPORTUNITIES AND PLANNING

The hair and beauty industries are so broad and provide a diverse range of career opportunities. The sector continues to grow and now employs 1% of the UK's working population. The variety of opportunities and experiences available to you will depend on the type of salon you work in. Most salons in the UK will carry out day-to-day treatments rather than undertaking treatments for celebrities or being involved in media work. However, some salons may be involved in seminars, shows and photographic work. There are opportunities to work all over the world if you are in the right place at the right time or take the right career path for you.

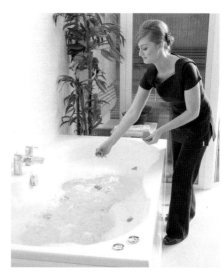

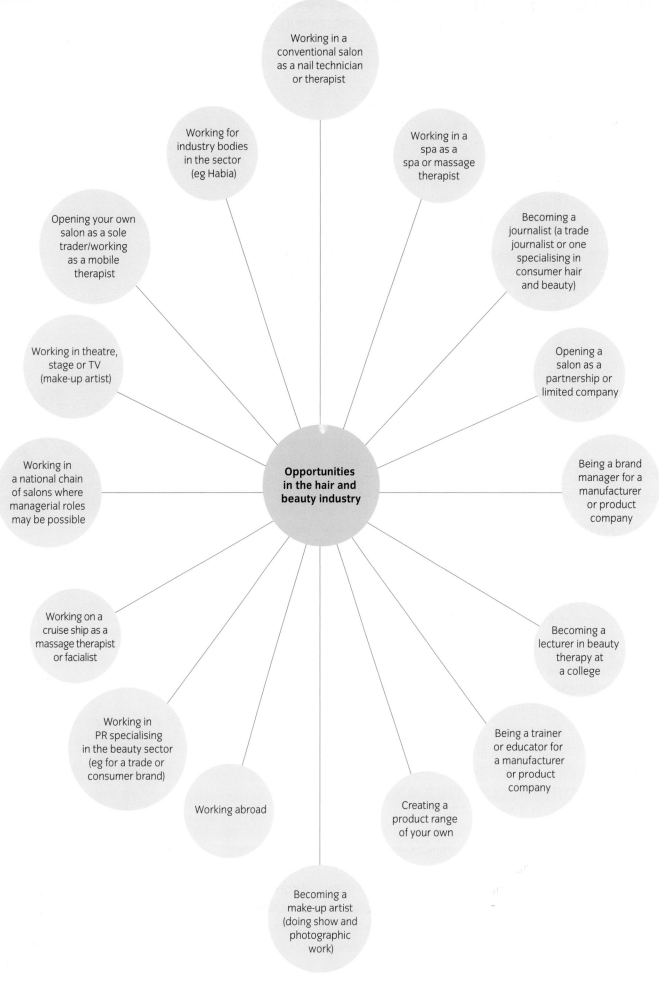

Working in a conventional salon as a nail technician or therapist

Working for industry bodies in the sector (eg Habia)

Working in a spa as a spa or massage therapist

Becoming a journalist (a trade journalist or one specialising in consumer hair and beauty)

Opening your own salon as a sole trader/working as a mobile therapist

Working in theatre, stage or TV (make-up artist)

Opening a salon as a partnership or limited company

Opportunities in the hair and beauty industry

Working in a national chain of salons where managerial roles may be possible

Being a brand manager for a manufacturer or product company

Working on a cruise ship as a massage therapist or facialist

Becoming a lecturer in beauty therapy at a college

Working in PR specialising in the beauty sector (eg for a trade or consumer brand)

Being a trainer or educator for a manufacturer or product company

Working abroad

Creating a product range of your own

Becoming a make-up artist (doing show and photographic work)

Whatever you end up doing, all jobs will have a common starting point – on-the-job training (eg an apprenticeship) or a qualification in beauty, nails, spa or media make-up.

WHAT NEXT?

Keeping your skills and training up to date is vital. Whichever career route you choose, it is essential to ensure your skill set is up to date. Many stylists or therapists at the highest level take a **proactive** approach to ensuring they are fully up to speed with new innovations and that they keep up to date with new techniques and treatments. It is important as a newly qualified therapist to:

- watch and learn from colleagues who are at a more senior level – make sure you benefit from their knowledge and expertise
- attend any out-of-hours training that you can and any sessions where other members of the team share knowledge and skills that they have gained from training
- attend update sessions, seminars and courses run by product companies and manufacturers
- take an active role in your own professional development and training by attending everything that is on offer
- go to trade exhibitions and shows where you can see industry names in action, watch practical demonstrations and keep in touch with industry developments and innovations.

Proactive
Taking control of a situation

FITTING INTO THE WORKPLACE

Working in a salon is all about teamwork so demonstrating that you are a good team player is vital. As the saying goes, 'there's no 'i' in team'. Make sure you 'buddy up' with an existing team member who can help show you the ropes. Knowing the ins and outs of the salon's working practice and salon etiquette will help you understand the unwritten rules of the salon.

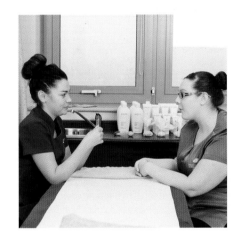

Dos and don'ts of fitting into the salon team
Dos

- Follow the examples of other team members, even if it isn't what you are used to. Every salon operates differently, so for example if people in your workplace clear up after each other, follow their lead.
- Make a real effort to fit in. Take up any social invitations and try to get to know your new colleagues.
- Be sure to take part in any further education opportunities the salon is offering. Think of yourself as a sponge soaking up information about your new workplace.
- Keep up with the pace and speed of the team. Get used to the timings of treatments.
- Fit in with the way the team works. Observe and follow the way they work and their conduct in the salon.
- Show a willingness to put yourself out by staying late and coming in early if required – it is all about building respect and relationships.

Don'ts

- Don't alienate yourself by sticking to old routines and regimes. Make sure you are open-minded about new ways of working and understand what is and isn't appropriate salon etiquette.
- Don't expect to fit in straight away. Give yourself time to integrate into the team.
- Don't show off or talk yourself up. Your new team members will be impressed by your standard of work and behaviour so you should let your work speak for itself.
- Don't knock salon procedures that you are unfamiliar with. They may not be a familiar way of working but if they are how your new workplace operates, get used to them.

SUMMARY

Fitting into a salon team is not easy and will certainly take time but by ensuring you follow the dos and don'ts you can make the transition smoother. Following the examples of other team members will certainly make the process more painless and will help you feel comfortable with your new colleagues. Demonstrating your talent and skills on the salon floor to paying clients will seem daunting at first as there is nowhere to hide.

Being a successful therapist in the commercial world means not only becoming technically, creatively and artistically proficient but also proficient at building great relationships with your clients based on trust and mutual understanding. Therefore developing your interpersonal skills is vital; having good communication skills is equally as important as delivering skilful and competent treatments.

As with any service industry, being on 'good form' (ie delivering good conversation, making people feel at ease and ensuring they are comfortable and looked after) is as important as performing the treatment well. An experienced therapist knows when to talk and when to let a client relax so watch and learn from those who have already developed this skill to learn how to recreate the same ambience yourself.

> **HANDY HINT**
>
> Always bear in mind that you are a business within a business. Each and every client you do has the potential to become one of your regulars and help expand your client base through personal recommendation and word of mouth.

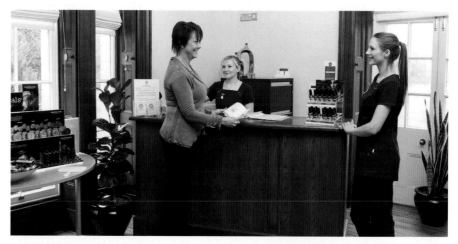

CASE STUDY: GINA CHARALAMBOUS

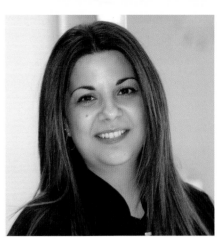

BEAUTY DIRECTOR, METROSPA

The majority of junior therapists I have met have come through the conventional route of going to college to gain their level 1, 2 and 3 qualifications. Although you have passed your exams, transferring your skill base into a spa or beauty salon will often prove scary. For any newly qualified therapist there are five main areas you need to consider when working in a salon:

- personal appearance
- technique
- client satisfaction
- timekeeping
- attention to detail.

PERSONAL APPEARANCE

Many therapists seem to forget that they are the biggest advertisement for their own skills. It is only too obvious when visiting spas and other beauty salons how poor personal appearance can let a therapist down. If you want a client to have confidence in the treatments you are offering, their first point of reference is how you look. Being well-groomed, having clean hair and nails, simple, classic and carefully applied make-up and a properly ironed uniform are a must for any therapist.

TECHNIQUE

Although college will have provided you with the basic techniques for carrying out facials and body treatments, each beauty product company will have its own specialised treatment **protocol**, techniques and facial routines. A newly qualified therapist must always remember that their skills provide a base from which they need to move on and develop further with training. You must adapt your basic knowledge to the beauty brand/salon you are representing.

Protocol
Official procedure

CLIENT SATISFACTION

The clients you will now be looking after may prove much more demanding than the models you have practised on at college. Watch how the other therapists in your workplace deal with their clientele. Ask if a more senior therapist can be your **mentor** and shadow them when they are doing treatments to watch and learn. This will prove invaluable and will give you an insight into the speed you will need to be working at and how to develop good interpersonal relationships with clients.

Mentor
A more experienced person who trains and supports new employees

TIMEKEEPING

Be aware of your treatment list (or **column**) and your timekeeping. You may well be part of a larger team and in order to work well and efficiently in a busy salon you will need to finish your treatments on time so that the salon continues to run smoothly. If you are not busy, use your

Column
A column of appointments (ie the day's appointment schedule)

time constructively. If appropriate, practise on other team members and be proactive in asking more senior members of staff if there are any jobs that need doing. In helping out around the workplace, you will demonstrate you are a team player and develop an awareness of all the elements needed in the smooth running of the business.

ATTENTION TO DETAIL

Finally, the biggest area for improvement in newly qualified therapists is attention to detail. Clients will expect the highest standards, so how you finish a manicure (ie how well you apply the polish), for instance, may make all the difference between a client having faith in you to do other treatments or not. Learn to accept nothing less than expert standards. If you have areas of weakness, practise, practise, practise! Doing so in the early stages of your career will give you a massive payback in the long term when you have a good client base and are earning excellent rates of pay and commission.

CASE STUDY: GAVIN HOARE

SALON MANAGER, RICHARD WARD HAIR AND METROSPA

Joining an existing salon team is a daunting experience for any fledgling stylist or therapist but more so if you are making the transition from classroom to salon. The salon is where your practical training really begins. How you respond to this transition will often shape the stylist/therapist you become in years to come.

Start as you mean to go on; look and learn. Watch how your colleagues conduct themselves in the salon and how they interact with their clients and colleagues. You must be ready to adapt your behaviour to fit into this new environment. Forget former salons where you may have worked or any **preconceived** ideas of how a salon works.

You should demonstrate a willingness to work and get involved:

- Make those in charge of making bookings aware that you are willing to come in early for a client or stay late. Being flexible in your approach will pay off in the long run in terms of growth of your client base and will demonstrate to your colleagues that you can be a team player.
- Offer to cover if colleagues call in sick. This will relieve stress on your business owner or manager and it will give you the opportunity to demonstrate you can manage a busy workload and showcase your beauty skills to the wider team.

Always be available for extra training. Accept that your technical skills are always a work in progress and you will go on learning throughout your career. Most of all just enjoy your new work environment. You have worked hard to get to this point so now you need to capitalise on your skills and your new working relationships.

Preconceived
Formed without knowing what something is really like

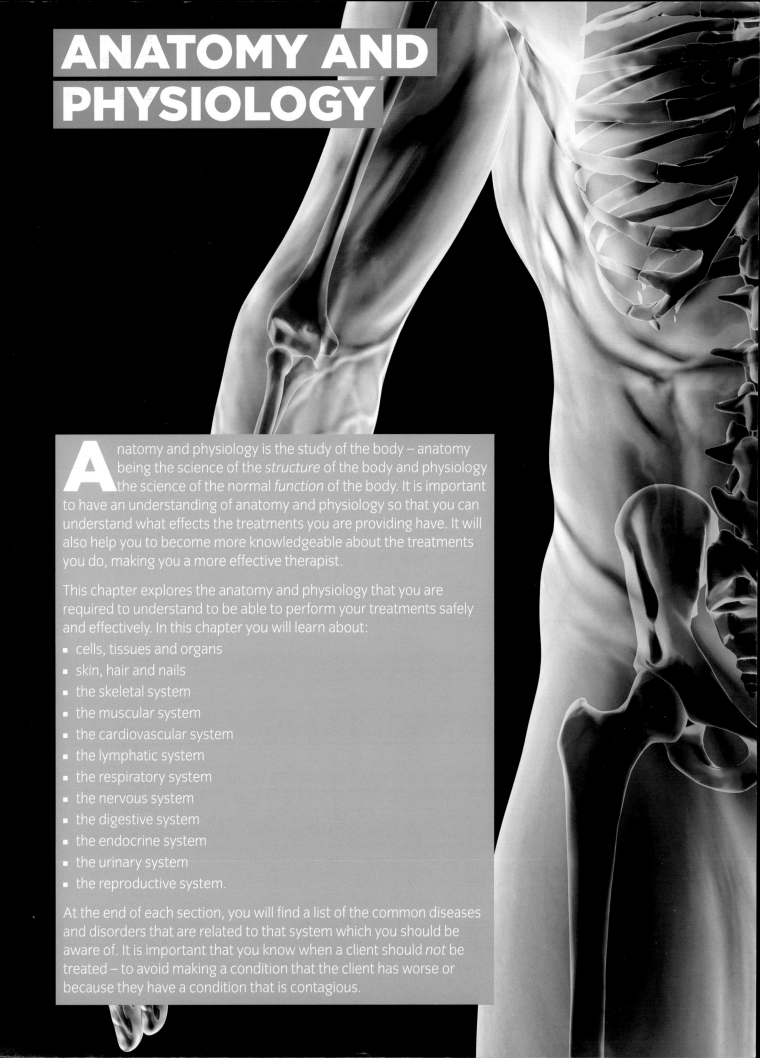

ANATOMY AND PHYSIOLOGY

Anatomy and physiology is the study of the body – anatomy being the science of the *structure* of the body and physiology the science of the normal *function* of the body. It is important to have an understanding of anatomy and physiology so that you can understand what effects the treatments you are providing have. It will also help you to become more knowledgeable about the treatments you do, making you a more effective therapist.

This chapter explores the anatomy and physiology that you are required to understand to be able to perform your treatments safely and effectively. In this chapter you will learn about:

- cells, tissues and organs
- skin, hair and nails
- the skeletal system
- the muscular system
- the cardiovascular system
- the lymphatic system
- the respiratory system
- the nervous system
- the digestive system
- the endocrine system
- the urinary system
- the reproductive system.

At the end of each section, you will find a list of the common diseases and disorders that are related to that system which you should be aware of. It is important that you know when a client should *not* be treated – to avoid making a condition that the client has worse or because they have a condition that is contagious.

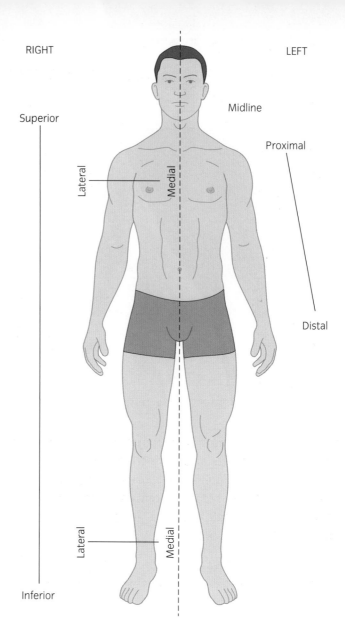

RIGHT

LEFT

Superior

Midline

Proximal

Lateral

Medial

Distal

Lateral

Medial

Inferior

HANDY HINT

Before you begin to learn about anatomy and physiology, there are some anatomical terms you need to know:

- anterior – front of the body
- posterior – back of the body
- lateral – away from the midline of the body
- medial – towards/closest to the midline of the body
- superior – above
- inferior – below
- proximal – close to the body
- distal – furthest from the body.

CELLS, TISSUES AND ORGANS

Before looking at the different systems of the body, it is a good idea to understand about cells and tissues. Cells and tissue are the basic building blocks of each of the body's systems. Cells and tissues form organs which are the main **components** of the body's systems.

In this part of the chapter you will learn about:

- the structure of a cell
- the reason for cellular reproduction
- the process of cellular division
- the four main types of tissue, their function and location
- what an organ is.

Components

Parts

THE STRUCTURE OF A CELL

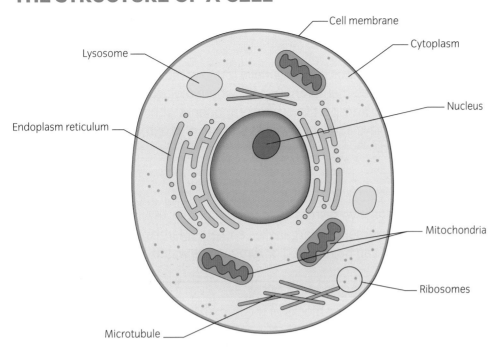

CELL MEMBRANE

This is a double layer, semipermeable membrane that surrounds the cell, keeping the contents together and protecting the cell. It allows certain substances required by the cell (such as oxygen, nutrients, hormones and proteins) to enter the cell through **active transport** but keeps other substances out. Another important function of the cell membrane is to help maintain the shape of the cell.

Special structural proteins help to support the shape of the cell while transport proteins help in active transport by carrying molecules across the cell membrane.

Active transport

The process by which dissolved molecules move across a cell membrane from a lower concentration outside the cell to a higher concentration inside the cell. As the particles are moving from a lower concentration to a higher concentration (ie against the concentration gradient), energy from the cell is needed in the process

CYTOPLASM

Cytoplasm is a clear, gel-like fluid in which all the cell components, excluding the nucleus, exist. It is held in by the cell membrane.

INTRACELLULAR FLUID

The fluid between the cells is intracellular fluid and contains organelles. Organelles all have special functions that allow the cell to function properly.

ORGANELLES

Nucleus

This is the largest organelle. It can be described as the control centre of the cell. It contains the body's genetic material. The nucleus of a cell consists of 46 **chromosomes** which are made up of **DNA** – deoxyribonucleic acid.

Chromosomes

Thread-like strands of DNA

DNA

Deoxyribonucleic acid

Mitochondria

These organelles have a sausage-shaped structure and are known as the 'powerhouse' of the cells. They convert energy into forms that can be used by the cell for processes such as movement and cell division.

Synthesise
Manufacture or create

Ribosomes

Ribosomes are tiny organelles. They **synthesise** proteins and other materials that the cell needs.

Golgi apparatus

The Golgi apparatus is an organelle found in most cells. These are stacks of closely folded membranous sacs where molecules are sorted and packaged for transport to other components within the cell. The Golgi apparatus plays a role in the cell's storage of enzymes and the cell's metabolism.

Lysosome

These are cellular organelles formed in the Golgi apparatus that act as the cell's digestive system. Lysosomes contain enzymes which break down the fragments of organelles and other large molecules in the cell so that they can be recycled or removed as waste.

CELL REPRODUCTION

Cells are the building blocks of the human body. Cells are microscopic and have a slightly different structure and shape depending on their location and the function they have to perform in the body. Our body is always renewing cells to replace worn-out cells or cells that have done their job.

Cells are produced through cellular division which is occurring constantly throughout our bodies. There are two types of cell division – mitosis and meiosis.

MITOSIS

During mitosis a cell goes through a process of change before dividing and producing two exact replicas or daughters of the original cell. There are four stages to the process:

1 Prophase – the cell begins to double in size. The chromosomes replicate to form two identical copies of DNA. The chromosomes are now called chromatids and are connected by a spindle of fibres called a centromere. The nuclear membrane dissolves.

2 Metaphase – the centromere divides pulling the chromatids apart. These line up along the centre of the cell.

3 Anaphase – the centromeres separate and one pair of chromatids (now 46 chromosomes again) move to opposite ends of the cell.

4 Telophase – a new membrane forms to surround each new set of chromosomes. The contents of the cytoplasm divide and two new daughter cells are produced.

Interphase		46 chromosomes
Prophase		Chromosomes doubled to 92
Prometaphase		Nucleus dissolves and microtubules attach to centromeres
Metaphase		Chromosomes align at middle of cell
Anaphase		Separated chromosomes pulled apart
Telophase	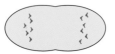	Microtubules disappear, cell division begins
Cytokinesis		Two daughter cells form each with 46 chromosomes

TISSUES

Cells are grouped together in specialised groups to become tissues. There are different types of tissues and each has a very specialised function. Tissues are classified by their shape, size and function. There are four main types of tissue in the body:

- epithelial tissue
- connective tissue
- muscle tissue
- nervous tissue.

Each of these four groups can be broken down into more specialised tissues.

EPITHELIAL TISSUE

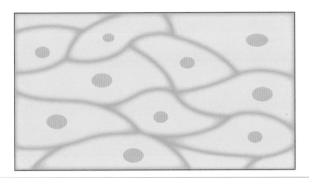

Epithelial tissue

This tissue covers the body (the skin) and lines the cavities, hollow organs, glands and tubes within the body. There are two types of epithelial tissue:

- simple
- stratified.

Simple epithelial tissue

Simple epithelial tissue is made up of *one* layer of epithelial cells. There are three main types of simple epithelial tissue that are named according to their shape:

- *Squamous or pavement* **epithelium** has a flattened appearance and forms a paving-stone pattern. Squamous epithelium lines the heart and blood vessels.
- *Cuboidal epithelium* is made up of cube-shaped cells and is found in some glands. Cuboidal epithelium is involved in secretion, excretion and absorption.
- *Columnar epithelium* has a more rectangular appearance and lines many organs (eg the stomach).

Epithelium
(Singular) refers to a single layer of cells

Epithelia
(Plural) refers to two or more layers of cells

Stratified epithelial tissue

Stratified (or compound) epithelium is made up of *several* layers of epithelial cells. There are four types of stratified epithelium:

- *Stratified squamous epithelium* has many layers of cells which are mainly column shaped. As they grow towards the surface they become flattened and shed.

Keratinisated

Describing cells that have become hard, flat and dead. This is caused by the production of a protein called keratin and the **degeneration** of the nucleus of the cell

Degeneration

Deterioration

- **Keratinised** *stratified epithelium* is found in dry areas, such as the skin, hair and nails, and is designed to withstand wear and tear. The surface layer of keratinised stratified epithelium is made up of dead epithelial cells that produce a tough, protective, semi-waterproof layer protecting the living layers underneath.
- *Non-keratinised stratified epithelium* is found where surfaces need to be kept moist (eg the eye and mouth).
- *Transitional epithelium* varies in appearance. It is similar to stratified squamous epithelium except the surface cells are not flattened. Transitional epithelium lines organs that need to be waterproof and those that need to expand (eg the bladder and the ureters).

CONNECTIVE TISSUE

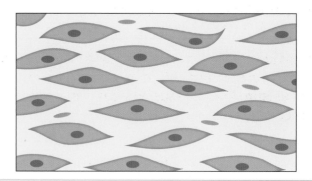

Connective tissue

Connective tissue is the most common tissue in the body. The function of connective tissue is to:

- protect
- transport
- insulate
- support.

The cells in connective tissue are more widely spaced than in epithelial tissue. In between the cells in connective tissue is a special substance called the **matrix**. This is a gel-like substance that contains fibres which provide support and protection. Types of connective tissue include:

- lymphoid tissue
- blood
- bone
- fibrous tissue
- elastic tissue
- areolar tissue
- adipose tissue.

Matrix

The material (tissue) between cells in which more specialised structures are embedded

Lymphoid tissue

This tissue is found in the lymphatic system (eg tonsils, appendix and lymph nodes). It is an important part of the body's **immune system** and helps protect it from infection and foreign bodies. For more information on lymphoid, please see pages 95–96.

Immune system

The system that protects the body against disease

Blood

For more information on blood, please see pages 83–86.

Bone

For more information on bone, please see pages 57–60.

Fibrous tissue

Fibrous connective tissue contains loosely packed collagen fibres in a thin matrix. Fibroblasts, which are the main active cells of connective tissue, are found within fibrous tissues. This tissue is found:

- in ligaments
- in the outer protective bone layer
- around some organs for protection (eg the kidneys)
- in muscle fascia which extend to form the muscle tendon.

Elastic tissue

Elastic tissue is found where stretching of various organs occurs (eg in the walls of the arteries and the respiratory tract).

Areolar tissue

Areolar tissue is loose connective tissue. This tissue is semi-solid and contains **fibroblasts**, some fat cells, **mast cells** and **macrophages**, **collagen** and **elastin**. Areolar tissue provides elasticity and connects and supports other tissues.

Adipose tissue

Adipose tissue is a type of areolar tissue containing fat cells.

MUSCLE TISSUE

Muscle tissue has the unique ability to contract and relax producing movement. There are three types of muscle tissue:

- skeletal/voluntary/striated
- smooth, visceral or involuntary
- cardiac.

Further information on muscle tissue can be found in the section on the muscular system (see pages 74–75).

NERVOUS TISSUE

We have two types of nervous tissue cell:

- neurones: a type of cell that carries information or signals to and from the brain and the rest of the body
- glial cells: supportive cells in the central nervous system.

Further information on nervous tissue can be found in the section on the nervous system (see pages 103–104).

ORGANS

The organs of the human body (eg the heart) are groups of specialised tissues. Specific organs are grouped together to form the systems of the body. The organs of the body carry out many functions, such as transporting materials within the body, absorbing food into the blood, helping you move, protecting your body from infection and removing dead cells from your body.

Fibroblasts
A type of cell found in connective tissue that produces collagen

Mast cells
A type of tissue cell of the immune system

Macrophages
White blood cells within tissues. Part of the immune system

Collagen
A type of white protein that gives strength to tissues

Elastin
Yellow protein fibres that are capable of considerable extension

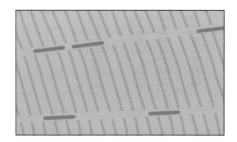

Muscle tissue

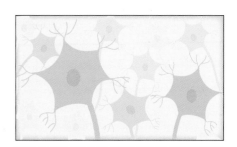

Nervous tissue

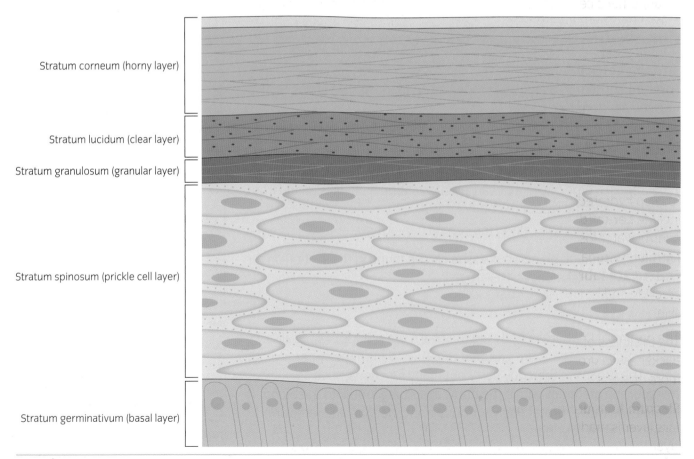

Skin surface

Epidermal–dermal junction

Epidermis

Dermis

Hypodermis

THE SKIN

The skin is the layer of tissue that covers the body and is the largest organ in the human body. The condition of the skin is subject to constant change and can therefore reflect the general health of an individual. The skin has two main layers, the epidermis and the dermis, and a third layer, the hypodermis, beneath.

In this part of the chapter you will learn about:

- the structure of the skin
- the functions of the skin
- the repair of the skin
- the effects of ageing on the skin
- the characteristics of the skin
- common skin diseases and disorders.

STRUCTURE OF THE SKIN

The skin has three layers:

- the epidermis
- the dermis
- the hypodermis or subcutaneous layer.

THE EPIDERMIS

The epidermis is made up of five layers.

Stratum corneum (horny layer)

Stratum lucidum (clear layer)

Stratum granulosum (granular layer)

Stratum spinosum (prickle cell layer)

Stratum germinativum (basal layer)

The five layers of the epidermis

These layers are formed of sheets of cells which are held together by a special adhesive protein. There is still some ability for cellular movement between these tight junctions. Skin cells move upwards from the basal layer to the horny layer.

The average thickness of the epidermis is only about 0.12mm. It is thickest on the soles of the feet (1.5mm) and thinnest on the eyelids (0.5mm).

The surface of the epidermis is covered in complex substances, including:

- an acid mantle (or hydrolipidic layer) – a water-in-oil **emulsion** formed from a mixture of sweat and sebum making the skin's surface slightly acidic
- mineral and organic substances, including urea, lactic acid and amino acids.

Cells of the epidermis

There are different types of cells in the epidermis. Each has an important role to play:

- Keratinocytes – keratinocytes produce keratin. Keratin is an insoluble protein which makes the cell more resilient. The amount of keratin in a cell increases as the cell moves towards the skin's surface.
- Melanocytes – melanocytes are cells of connective tissue. They produce the pigment melanin which gives colour to the skin and hair. The melanin forms in the melanocytes and is injected into the skin through finger-like **projections** (called dendrites).
- Langerhans cells – langerhans cells are specialised white blood cells found circulating in the skin. They are a type of **macrophage** and alert the immune system to **pathogens** in the skin.

Stratum corneum (horny layer)

This is the outermost layer of the skin and its surface is in direct contact with the environment. The skin cells are hard and flat. The skin cells are also dead so they don't have a nucleus. They are very different from how they started out in the basal layer. One major function of the stratum corneum is to prevent dehydration of the skin. This is achieved by the **natural moisturising factor (NMF)**. This allows the stratum corneum to keep hydrated despite exposure to the environment. **Lipids**, which include **ceramides**, cholesterol and fatty acids (sebum), also help control water loss and prevent entry of water-soluble agents and harmful bacteria by providing a waterproof layer on the skin's surface. This surface **lubricant** also keeps the skin supple, preventing it from cracking and breaking which would allow pathogens to enter into the skin and could cause the skin to become infected.

The thickness of the stratum corneum also varies with age. It gets thicker as we grow older. As it thickens, the signs of ageing can become more obvious.

Stratum lucidum (clear layer)

This layer is made up of flat transparent cells, hence the name 'clear' layer. There is no melanin present in this layer. This layer controls the amount of water that can pass through the skin.

Emulsion

A liquid evenly suspended in another so that neither can be detected

INDUSTRY TIP

There are two types of melanin:

- eumelanin: a brown or black pigment
- pheomelanin: a yellow or brown pigment.

Projections

Parts that stick out

Macrophage

A small white blood cell of the immune system which moves through tissues and removes cell debris and pathogens

Pathogen

A collective term used to describe a type of microbe. It includes viruses, bacteria, fungi and parasites. A pathogen has the potential to cause harm

Natural moisturising factor (NMF)

Water-soluble substances that absorb water from the air and combine it with their own water content to keep the stratum corneum hydrated

Lipids

A group of organic molecules that don't like water and prevent water entering the skin. They include fats, oils, waxes and fat-soluble vitamins

Ceramides

Natural lipids (fats) that allow the skin to hold onto moisture keeping it hydrated

Lubricant

A substance (such as oil) that reduces friction

INDUSTRY TIP

If the dendrites that inject melanin into the skin become damaged, **pigmentation** is unevenly distributed causing a patchy skin tone.

Pigmentation

Colouration

Granular

Microscopic particles

Keratinisation

The process by which living cells change into flat dead cells with no nucleus

Keratinisation zone

The zone where cells begin to die and from where they are shed from the skin

Stratum granulosum (granular layer)

As the cells lose their nuclei and begin to die, the cell functions begin to decrease dramatically. The cells take on a distinctive flattened shape and a **granular** appearance as a result of **keratinisation**. This is the start of the **keratinisation zone**. The keratin in this layer helps prevent water loss from the skin.

Stratum spinosum (prickle cell layer)

This layer includes the Langerhans cells (see page 21) which help support our immune system.

Keratin production begins in the stratum spinosum (prickly cell layer) and is injected into the living cells. This layer is several layers deep. The cells have connection threads called fibrils which give the cells a prickly appearance.

Stratum germinativum (basal layer)

This is the deepest layer of the epidermis and forms a junction between the epidermis and the dermis. Skin cells are produced here by mitosis (see page 16) to produce new epithelial cells.

The stratum germinativum also contains keratinocytes and melanocytes. The melanocytes help protect the skin against harmful UV rays. Eighty per cent of the moisture required for maintaining a healthy skin surface is found in this layer.

THE DERMIS

The dermis is a layer of skin that is 3–5mm thick that lies beneath the epidermis. It is made up of tough extra-cellular tissue. The dermis has a high water content. It contains most of the living structures of the skin including blood vessels, sweat glands, and sebaceous glands.

The main functions of the dermis are:

- to provide strength and flexibility
- to provide a system of capillaries to nourish the cells of the lower layers of the epidermis and to remove waste products
- to control temperature and blood pressure.

The dermis has two layers:

- the papillary layer
- the reticular layer.

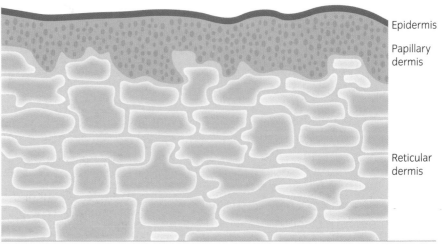

Epidermis

Papillary dermis

Reticular dermis

The dermis

The papillary layer

This papillary layer is made up of loose connective tissue. The surface of the papillary layer is covered with tiny, irregularly shaped projections called dermal papillae. These fit into the underside of the epidermis forming a secure bond (eg like Velcro). They contain intricate networks of blood and lymphatic capillaries and nerve endings. These networks of capillaries nourish the lower layers of the epidermis and hair follicles, carry oxygen to the tissues and remove waste from the tissues. The papillary layer is rich with mast cells and macrophages (see page 85).

The reticular layer

This is made up of thick tough fibrous connective tissue which helps to support the dermis and hold the structures of the dermis in place. It is rich with fibroblasts which form collagen and elastin. The reticular layer connects the dermis to the hypodermis/subcutaneous layer.

CELLS OF THE DERMIS

The main cells of the dermis are fibroblasts, mast cells and phagocytic cells.

Fibroblasts (fibre cells)

Fibroblasts (fibre cells) play an important role in tissue repair following tissue damage. Fibroblasts produce two important proteins – collagen and elastin. Collagen provides strength and elasticity and elastin allows the skin to stretch. The production of collagen and elastin slows down as we age. This reduction, combined with damage caused by ultraviolet (UV) light, causes wrinkles and a loss of skin tone.

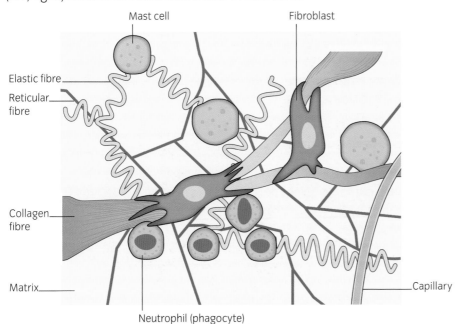

Cells of the dermis

> **INDUSTRY TIP**
>
> If the skin is over-stretched, the elastic fibres break and stretch marks will appear. Elastin makes up 5% of the body's weight.

> **INDUSTRY TIP**
>
> Skin is looser around joints to allow movements without skin damage.

Mast cells

Mast cells release **histamine** in response to damage to local tissues caused by infections. Histamine causes the blood vessels to become dilated and allows fluid and cells of the immune system to leak out of the blood to the site of the infection to help in the healing process. White blood cells are also attracted to histamine, drawing them to the damaged tissue.

> **Histamine**
>
> A chemical which has the effect of vasodilation

> **INDUSTRY TIP**
>
> The direction of collagen fibres can be determined by pinching the skin and seeing which way it folds most easily into wrinkles.

23

INDUSTRY TIP

Hyaluronic acid is a naturally occurring substance in the skin that helps to keep the skin hydrated. It is also found as an ingredient in skincare products to help maintain hydration in the skin.

Tactile

Connected to the sense of touch

INDUSTRY TIP

The most sensitive skin is on your lips.

Phagocytes

Phagocytes are white blood cells that move through the skin's tissues destroying pathogens and other cell debris.

STRUCTURES OF THE DERMIS

Sensory nerve endings

The skin is packed with sensory nerve endings which relay information about **tactile** sensation to the brain. Different nerve receptors respond to different sensations:

Nerve receptor	Sensation
Meissner's corpuscles	Movement and light touch
Ruffini corpuscles	Light pressure
Pacinian corpuscles	Deep pressure and vibrations
Free nerve endings	Pain and temperature

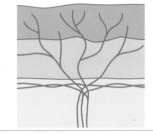
Free nerve endings

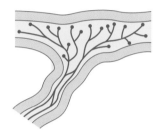
Ruffini corpuscle

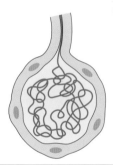
Krause corpuscle

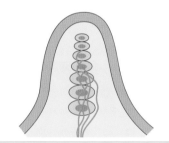
Meissner's corpuscle

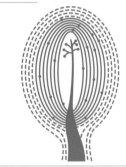
Pacinian corpuscle

Blood vessels

The dermis contains a rich, delicate network of blood vessels. The small blood vessels in the outer areas of the skin are known as the micro-circulation and are prone to **vasodilation** and **vasoconstriction**. Blood circulation brings oxygen and nutrients to the dermis (and epidermis) and removes waste products made during cellular activity.

Vasodilation

Relaxation of the muscles in the walls of the blood vessels, causing the blood vessels to dilate (get wider) and allow the blood to flow more freely

Vasoconstriction

Constriction (shrinking in size) of the muscles in the wall of the blood vessels which restricts blood flow

Lymphatic vessels

A network of lymphatic capillaries nourish the cells in the dermis. These vessels allow lymphatic fluid to leave the network and move around the network of cells as tissue fluid. Tissue fluid moves back in to the lymphatic vessels to take away waste from the extra-cellular tissues. (For more information on the lymphatic system see pages 92–100).

Sweat glands

The two main purposes of sweat glands are:

- to help control or maintain the body's temperature
- to help get rid of waste.

Sweat cools the body down by removing heat from the skin's surface. Sweat is **excreted** as a clear watery fluid. It removes waste substances (eg water, sodium and potassium chloride (salts), ammonia and urea) from the body.

There are two types of sweat glands:
- apocrine glands are found under the arms and around the groin
- eccrine glands are found all over the body.

Sebaceous glands

Sebaceous glands can be found all over the skin (but not on the palms of the hands and soles of the feet)]. Most sebaceous glands open into hair follicles where they secrete sebum but some open directly onto the skin. Sebaceous glands produce sebum (which is a lipid). Sebum is the skin's natural **emollient** and prevents the skin from drying out. It forms a barrier to keep moisture in. Sebum helps prevent the growth of bacteria as long as it does not become excessive. Excessive sebum will cause the skin to become oily and look shiny (particularly around the nose, chin and forehead). Very oily skin attracts surface dirt which may block the pores causing **comedones**, **papules** and **pustules**.

Arrector pili muscle

Arrector pili muscles are tiny muscle fibres that are attached to the hair follicle. When they contract they pull the hair up and away from the skin. The muscles cause goosebumps when we are cold or frightened. The raised hairs trap air next to the skin to keep it warm.

Excreted
Expelled as waste (eg sweat from the skin)

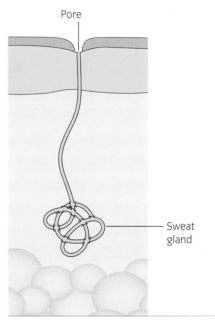

Cross-section of a sweat gland

Emollient
Something that has a softening effect

Comedone
Blackhead

Papule
A small raised solid area of infected unbroken skin, which often develops into a pustule

Pustule
A small collection of pus that is visible through a raised portion of the epidermis

The arrector pili muscle is attached to the hair follicle and the epidermis. When we are cold or scared this muscle contracts and causes the hairs to lift. This helps to trap a warm layer of air between the hairs and protects us from the cold.

Along the hair follicle are sebaceous glands. These produce oil called sebum which naturally protects and conditions the hair. An average hair follicle contains up to three sebaceous glands. Overactive sebaceous glands – or more than three – can cause excessively oily hair.

Above the hair bulb is the hair follicle, where the hair grows from. The follicle stretches from the hair bulb through to the epidermis. The hair seen outside the follicle and above the epidermis is known as the hair shaft; the remainder, below the skin's surface, is the hair root.

Hair shaft

Sweat pore

Epidermis

Dermis

Subcutaneous layer

Sudoriferous glands (sweat glands) travel from the subcutaneous layer through the dermis and up to the epidermis. They contain water which is released as perspiration through sweat pores to cool us down when we are hot.

The matrix, which is wrapped around the dermal papilla, forms the new hair bulb by producing cells called melanocytes. These are made from keratin and are the fastest growing cells in the body.

The dermal papilla nourishes the hair follicles and supplies food and oxygen to the hair and skin from blood cells via capillaries, arteries and veins.

Nerves travel through the subcutaneous layer, into the dermis and attach to the lower layers of the epidermis. When we shed skin it does not hurt, but cutting or bruising ourselves does because we have triggered the nerve endings. Nerves also attach to the hair follicle, causing discomfort if the hair is pulled.

HYPODERMIS (SUBCUTANEOUS LAYER)

The hypodermis forms a link between the structures below the skin and the skin. It is made up of a layer of fat cells. It provides some cushioning from external pressure and some thermal **insulation**. It varies in thickness depending on the person's gender and the area of the body.

Insulation

Protection against heat loss

FUNCTIONS OF THE SKIN

The skin has seven functions:

- sensation
- temperature regulation
- absorption
- protection
- excretion
- secretion
- production of vitamin D.

SENSATION

The skin contains approximately five million tiny sensory cells. These sensory cells enable us to respond to sensations that are applied to the surface of the skin (eg touch, pressure and vibrations). The cells respond to environmental changes and send information to the brain where the sensation is felt. Sensory nerve endings are located mainly in the dermis but some free nerves end in the epidermis.

TEMPERATURE REGULATION

The body needs to be maintained at a constant temperature of about 36.8°C to function correctly.

The skin responds to an increase in temperature by dilating the blood vessels in the dermis (vasodilation) to radiate heat away from the body where it is open to the elements. The skin begins to sweat. As the sweat **evaporates**, it takes the heat away from the skin's surface allowing the body to cool.

Evaporate

To turn into vapour

Essential organs

The organs that are essential to survival

If the body gets too cold, the blood vessels constrict (vasoconstriction) to keep heat nearer to the **essential organs** of the body. Shivering makes the muscle contract. This muscle contraction produces energy to keep warm. Heat loss from the skin is affected by the environment and the amount and type of clothing worn.

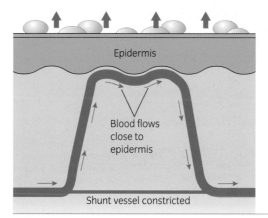

Epidermis

Blood flows close to epidermis

Shunt vessel constricted

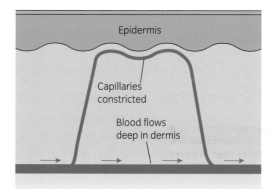

Epidermis

Capillaries constricted

Blood flows deep in dermis

Temperature regulation: vasodilation (left) and vasoconstriction (right)

ABSORPTION

The skin is not totally waterproof. It allows certain substances (eg hormones) to be absorbed only in a limited capacity.

Substances that can enter the skin are absorbed:

- between the cells of the epidermis
- through sweat glands
- through hair shafts.

PROTECTION

The skin forms a water-resistant seal over the body. It is very hard-wearing and acts as a defence against chemicals, micro-organisms, dehydration and damage. Sebum, water and other substances are secreted onto the skin's surface to keep it waterproof, supple and flexible. The surface of skin is slightly acidic (**pH** 4.5–5.5), which prevents harmful bacteria growing. Melanin acts as a chemical filter absorbing and reflecting UV radiation.

The hypodermis (subcutaneous layer) cushions the underlying bones and organs to help prevent damage from external forces and pressure. The hypodermis and dermis together protect the body against temperature changes.

EXCRETION

Excretion is the process that our bodies use to get rid of waste or unwanted substances. The skin is a minor excretory organ. It excretes sweat which contains water, sodium and potassium chlorides (salts), urea and uric acids and an aromatic substance which gives the body its personal odour. If we don't wash our skins or clothes regularly, bacteria break down our sweat causing unpleasant odours.

SECRETION

Secretion is the process that our bodies use to release substances needed by the body. For example, sebum is secreted into the hair follicles and onto the skin. Sebum is an oily substance that keeps the hair and skin soft, supple and flexible. It can also give the skin and hair a shiny appearance.

PRODUCTION OF VITAMIN D

Vitamin D is produced in the skin as a response to exposure to ultraviolet B radiation (UVB). Cholecalciferol is produced when the sun penetrates the skin. Cholecalciferol is taken to the liver where it is made into calcidol and stored as vitamin D.

If you block UVB you will prevent the production of vitamin D. Dark skin needs more exposure to UVB to produce the same amount of vitamin D than light skin as melanin restricts absorption of the UVB rays.

pH

Potential of hydrogen. pH is a measure of the concentration of hydrogen ions in a substance. A low pH is acidic and a high pH is alkaline

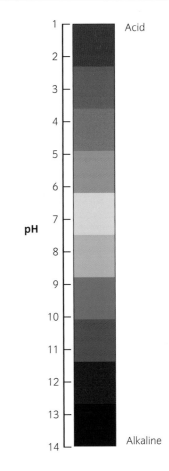

INDUSTRY TIP

We all need to go outside into the sunlight for 20 minutes each day to make sure that we produce enough vitamin D. This does not mean sunbathing but general exposure.

 SmartScreen 305 Worksheet 9

 SmartScreen 306 Worksheet 5

REPAIR OF THE SKIN

The body is excellent at repairing any damage to tissues. However, there will always be some scar tissue.

When the skin is broken, blood cells move into the wound and the blood clotting process starts. A protein in the blood plasma (called fibrinogen) is released and this starts to form a mesh over the surface. This mesh prevents further blood leaking out. The mesh dries out to form a scab.

Histamine is also released which makes the blood vessels dilate. The dilation of the blood vessels allows fluid and cells of the immune system to leak out of the blood to the site of the infection to help in the healing process. The fluid and cells can also attack any unwanted micro-organisms that might have entered in through the open wound. The increased circulation gives the area an inflamed red appearance.

Fibroblast cells begin to produce new collagen cells and a protein called actin. Actin helps to slowly draw the edges of the wound together as it is able to contract. It takes the epidermis about 48 hours to heal but the deeper tissues take much longer and the area may appear red for two to four weeks. Some very deep damage might take even longer to repair fully. Working over scar tissue is contra-indicated as the healing process in the deeper tissues may still be taking place even though the epidermis has healed.

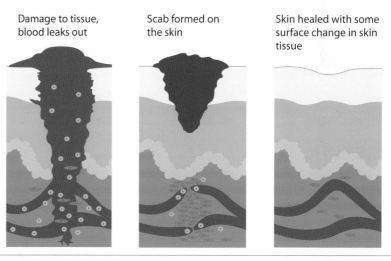

Damage to tissue, blood leaks out

Scab formed on the skin

Skin healed with some surface change in skin tissue

Skin repair

INDUSTRY TIP

The skin repairs and renews itself three times faster at night so it is important to get a good night's sleep. Specialised products to help repair the skin should be used at night.

THE EFFECTS OF AGEING ON THE SKIN

Ageing is dependent on a variety of factors which include internal and external influences. Some ethnic groups have a slower ageing process than others. The large amount of collagen in Afro-Caribbean skin prevents some of the effects of ageing. Caucasian (white) skin tends to be thinner and more prone to damage by the sun and the environment.

Metabolism

The chemical processes that occur within living organisms to maintain life

Contours

Outline shape of the skin

Age	Skin's appearance
Mid twenties 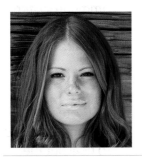	■ The skin's **metabolism** begins to slow down. ■ Skin renewal and repair to damaged cells are decreased. ■ Each cell division passes on genetic information; however as we grow older, minute pieces of genetic information are lost. This means that the next generation of cells produced do not carry the same information as the previous generation of cells.
Mid thirties 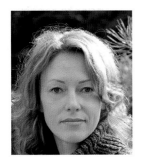	■ The skin **contours** become less defined and the skin starts to sag. ■ The structure of new collagen becomes more uneven. ■ Elastin fibres show signs of cross linking and hardening. ■ The fat cells that plump out the skin begin to reduce causing the skin to sag, thin and become crêpe-like. ■ The skin retains less moisture which means it begins to lose its plump appearance. ■ The blood vessels of the dermis become more fragile and are more easily damaged. ■ The production of sebum from the sebaceous glands declines causing a reduction in the surface lipids and the skin becomes visibly drier.
Forties 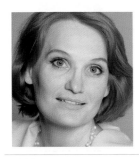	■ Ageing becomes more obvious with lines deepening, particularly along the expression lines (ie lines caused by muscle movement).
Fifties 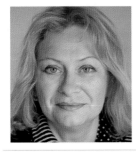	■ The skin is more wrinkled and a loss of elasticity is more noticeable, especially around the contours of the face. ■ Older skins often have a more sallow or yellow tone caused by changes in the skin's brown pigment. ■ Melanin is no longer distributed evenly throughout the skin. Instead melanin becomes patchy leaving the skin with uneven pigmentation and lentigines (see page 33).

INDUSTRY TIP

The hormone oestrogen has water-attracting properties and will influence the amount of moisture held in the skin. Oestrogen levels drop following the menopause. This affects the skin's ability to hold moisture.

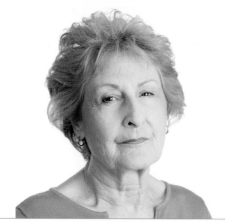
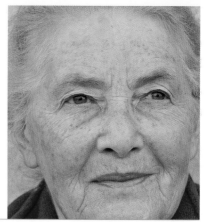

Skin appearance of women in their sixties and seventies

Wrinkles

Whenever we smile, laugh or use our facial expressions, natural expression lines appear on our face. Fine or deep lines are created as a result of muscular movement. Wrinkles are a depression in the skin's surface. Wrinkles occur as result of:

- a loss of skin thickness
- changes in the muscle density
- changes to the structure and position of elastin and collagen
- dehydration
- a decline in hyaluronic acid.

SKIN CHARACTERISTICS

SKIN TONE

All skin has the same number of **melanocytes** but they have a slightly different structure and are more active in darker skins. Melanin, which gives skin its colour, is produced in a specialised area of the melanocytes called a melanosome. There is more melanin in the melanosomes in darker skin. The depth of colour depends on how the melanosomes are distributed in the epidermis. The melanocytes in darker skins have longer and thicker dendrites (see page 21) that distribute melanin differently. In Caucasian skin the melanosomes are smaller, rounder and surrounded by a membrane. The spaces between the cells give the skin a lighter appearance. There are three main skin tones:

- Afro-Caribbean skin
- Caucasian skin
- Asian skin.

The size and quantity of the sebaceous glands also vary between different skin tones. Afro-Caribbean skin has approximately 10% more sebaceous glands than Caucasian skin and they are larger.

Male skin

The male hormone **testosterone** stimulates fibroblasts to produce collagen at puberty which means that male skin has a thicker dermis. On average, male skin has 32% more collagen than female skin. Men have a higher level of **androgen** making the skin secrete more sebum. This makes the skin more oily and the pores more obvious. The two combined give male skin a coarser texture.

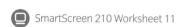
SmartScreen 210 Worksheet 11

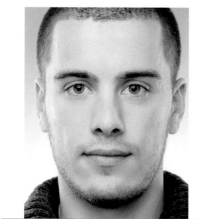
Young male skin appearance

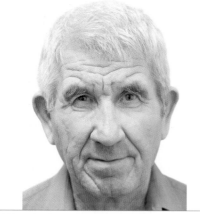
Old male skin appearance

Melanocytes
The cells that produce melanin. Melanocytes contain melanosomes

Androgen and testosterone
Hormones that stimulate male characteristics

ACTIVITY

Create a table to show the differences between the different skin tones based on ethnicity and gender.

Give at least one example of how may this affect your treatments and recommendations.

SKIN TYPES

There are four main skin groups:

- balanced (normal)
- oily
- dry
- combination skin (a mixture of oily and dry).

Balanced (normal) skin

It is very unlikely that you will see a truly balanced skin in an adult. This skin is perfect. It is free from any blemishes or **imperfections**. It is neither dry nor oily as secretion levels are balanced. Pigmentation is even and there are no **abnormalities**. The skin is bright and appears healthy.

Imperfections
Flaws in the skin (eg moles or skin tags)

Abnormalities
Things that are not normal

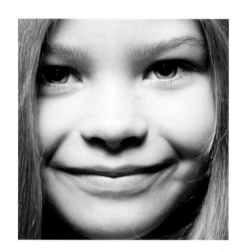

Oily skin

Oily skin suffers from over-secretion of sebum. The skin appears shiny and sallow in appearance from the residue of surface oil. The skin cells do not exfoliate naturally as they stick to the oily surface. Very oily patches can give the skin a rough texture. Pores are relaxed and are more visible on the skin's surface due to the over-activity of the sebaceous glands. The skin can look like orange peel. There are usually comedones present and blocked pores. This skin can feel cool to the touch and have a tacky feel. The excess oil lowers the acidity levels of the skin making it easier for bacteria to multiply so it is prone to blemishes, papules and pustules. A skin with excessive oily secretions is called seborrhoeic.

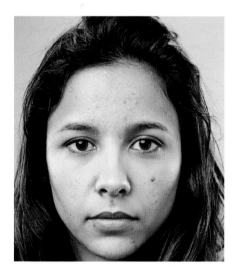

Dry skin

A dry skin lacks the natural lipids (including sebum), which are responsible for keeping the skin lubricated and hydrated. The surface cells appear more flaky and visible to the eye. The skin has a crêpe-like appearance. Dry skin will appear matte and feel warm to the touch. The lack of surface lubrication leaves the skin feeling tight. The skin is often more transparent and this means the circulation is more visible giving it a more rosy appearance.

Combination skin

Typically this skin type has an oily T-zone on the forehead, nose and chin where the sebaceous glands are more concentrated. The cheeks and neck are commonly dry. Around 75% of skin is combination skin.

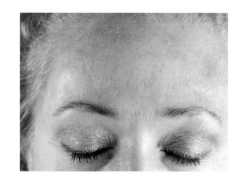

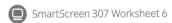
SKIN CONDITION

The skin can also be described by its characteristics or condition which might be:

- mature – showing signs of ageing
- dehydrated – lacking in moisture
- sensitive – reactive to touch or prone to allergic reactions.

Any skin type can have one of more of these characteristics/conditions.

DISEASES AND DISORDERS OF THE SKIN

It is important to be able to recognise common skin diseases and disorders to know whether or not treatments can be carried out (or modified).

DISORDERS AFFECTING PIGMENTATION OF THE SKIN

Several common disorders can affect the pigmentation of the skin. Skin pigment can be lost, causing hypo-pigmentation, or increased, causing hyper-pigmentation. In many cases the changes cannot be reversed. Avoiding sun exposure will help improve hyper-pigmentation. It takes a very long time for pigmentation to even out and, as most clients will not keep affected areas out of the sun completely, their skin won't have a chance to recover.

SPF

Sun protection factor. The number following it, eg 30, indicates the amount of protection the sunscreen will provide when the skin is exposed to UV light

Disorder	Description and cause	Contra-indications and general precautions	Advice for client
Pigmented nevus or mole	A raised, pigmented skin growth. It is caused by a cluster of melanocytes cells between the epidermis and dermis or in the dermis. A mole can vary in size from a pinhead to several centimetres, and in colour from tan to bluish black. Some raised moles have hairs growing from them.	Contra-indicated to microdermabrasion. Adapt treatment to avoid the area. Keep a note on the client's records and be aware of any sudden changes in colour or size or if the mole begins to weep or bleed. Avoid excessive stimulation over and around the mole.	Use sunblock over the mole for protection from UV.
Ephiledes (freckles)	Clusters of melanin. These small areas of pigmentation become more prominent after exposure to UV.	Not contra-indicated.	Use sunblock or a high **SPF** sunscreen to minimise any further changes in pigmentation in the skin. Give advice on camouflage make-up if appropriate.

Disorder	Description and cause	Contra-indications and general precautions	Advice for client
Lentigines (liver spots)	Also called 'age spots'. Areas of darkened pigmentation which are about 1cm in size caused by an abnormality in the production of melanin. Skin is often slightly raised. Changes in the skin can be felt by touching the surface of the lentigines. Commonly found on the back of the hands, face and upper chest of mature clients.	Not contra-indicated.	Use sunblock or a high SPF sunscreen to minimise further pigmentation changes. Give advice on camouflage make-up if appropriate. Recommend a course of microdermabrasion.
Chloasma	A cluster of pigmentation in the skin. Commonly found on the upper cheeks, nose and forehead. Caused by hormonal stimulation (eg pregnancy, contraceptive pill). Sometimes disappears once hormones settle down but might be permanent. Skin can react to perfume and sunlight and cause hyper-pigmentation.	Not contra-indicated.	Use sunblock or a high SPF sunscreen to minimise further pigmentation changes. Spray perfume onto clothing instead of directly on the skin. Give advice on camouflage make-up if appropriate.
Vitiligo	A lack of skin pigmentation where the melanocytes have been destroyed. White patches of skin can be seen. Thought to be an autoimmune disorder (where the body attacks its own tissues) or triggered by stress or severe sunburn. Hair growing in the area will also be white. The skin around the edge of the area may appear darker due to the contrast with the surrounding darker skin.	Be cautious. Some treatments should not be carried out, depending on the severity of the vitiligo. However, most treatments would not be contra-indicated.	Use a total sunblock in the areas affected as there is no melanin to absorb UV radiation and the skin will burn easily. Give advice on camouflage with make-up if appropriate.
Albinism	The near total or total absence of melanin means there is little or no pigmentation. The hair and skin will be white; eye colour may vary but is often pale blue.	Contra-indicated, depending on treatment Tanning treatments would be unsuitable. The skin is often very sensitive so carry out a sensitivity test.	Avoid unnecessary exposure to the sun and use sunblock or high SPF sunscreen.

DISORDERS AFFECTING THE SKIN'S CIRCULATION

There is a wide range of disorders and conditions that affect the skin's circulation. Some of these changes are permanent while others come and go. Some conditions are hereditary and are present at birth (eg birthmarks). Others develop over time and are the result of ageing.

Disorder	Description and cause	Contra-indications and general precautions	Advice for client
Telangiectasis (dilated capillaries)	Permanently dilated capillaries visible through the skin. Repeated changes in temperature both internal (eg hot flushes) and external (eg air conditioning, central heating and extremes of weather) all **aggravate** the condition. Also aggravated by lack of skin care, eating hot spicy food and alcohol.	Not contra-indicated but take care with some treatments (eg steaming and skin warming, exfoliation, vacuum suction treatments and microdermabrasion). Avoid extremes of temperature.	Can be treated and removed using advanced electrolysis techniques. Keep the skin protected with a good moisturiser. Give advice on camouflage make-up if appropriate.
Rosacea	A chronic long-term skin disorder causing redness and swelling, mainly of the face. It can be caused by congestion and enlargement of the **superficial** blood capillaries. It can lead to a permanent mottled appearance. It usually affects the nose, cheeks and centre of the forehead (butterfly pattern). The skin's surface becomes thickened and is superficially dry and flaky in texture. Pustules and papules might be present in more severe cases and are thought to be caused by an immune response. It may also affect the eyes. The cause is often hormonal (affecting women during the menopause). It can also be caused by intestinal disorders, ongoing sinus infections, high blood pressure and certain medication. It can also be hereditary.	Not contra-indicated. Not contagious. Treatment will depend on how severe the condition is. Treat the skin with care and avoid extremes of temperature and **over-stimulation.**	Avoid stress, smoking, spicy foods and alcohol. Use a gentle anti-inflammatory skincare range, with a protective moisturiser and high SPF. Give advice on camouflage make-up and make-up colours to avoid if appropriate.

Aggravate

Make worse

Superficial

On the surface; not deep penetrating

Over-stimulation

Energising and invigorating more than is necessary

Disorder	Description and cause	Contra-indications and general precautions	Advice for client
Vascular **naevi** (singular nervus)	Caused by an abnormality of the capillary blood vessels. These cluster together to form a very red raised area of skin. There are different types and most are **congenital**.	Not contra-indicated. Care should be taken. Avoid excessive stimulation over and around the naevi.	Use sunblock over the area. Give advice on camouflage make-up if appropriate.
Allergies	When an allergic reaction occurs, the immune system produces antibodies in response to **allergens** that most other people would not find harmful. Common allergic conditions include hay fever, allergic asthma, urticaria, dermatitis and eczema. **Anaphylactic shock** is a dangerous allergic reaction.	Contra-indicated depending on the allergy. Include allergies on the client's record card so that allergens can be avoided. Carry out a patch test. You may have to call for medical assistance if the client has an **acute** allergic reaction (eg anaphylactic shock).	Check product labels and make sure you avoid ingredients that you know the client's skin is reactive to.
Urticaria (hives)	Also commonly known as nettle rash. An allergic reaction characterised by red blotchy skin, **wheals** and severe itching. The skin will feel very warm.	Contra-indicated. If the client is already suffering with an allergic reaction, allow the body to heal before treating the client. Carry out a patch/ sensitivity test. If this happens as a contra-action to a product used during a treatment, remove all traces of the products being used from the skin and wash the area with lukewarm water. Do not continue with any further treatment.	Check product labels and make sure you avoid ingredients that you know your client's skin is reactive to. Avoid excessive heat if there is a history of urticaria.

Naevi
Lesions of the skin (eg birthmarks)

Congenital
Present from birth

Allergen
A foreign substance that can trigger an allergic response in the body

Anaphylactic shock
A rare but severe acute allergic reaction

Acute
Sudden and short term

Wheal
A raised fluid-containing area of flesh-coloured or white skin surrounded by a red area. It can look like a cat scratch

INDUSTRY TIP

Anaphylactic shock: symptoms can start within minutes of the client coming into contact with something they are allergic to. Symptoms include sickness, rashes, swelling of the eyes, mouth and skin, difficulty breathing and a rapid pulse. If you think a client is going into anaphylactic shock you should call for an ambulance immediately.

ACTIVITY

Make a list of all the items/products in the salon that could potentially cause an allergic reaction.

SEBACEOUS GLAND DISORDERS

Some of the most common skin disorders and diseases that a therapist will come in contact with will be linked to the sebaceous glands. These glands are very reactive during hormonal changes, particularly during puberty. These conditions are often easily irritated by the use of incorrect products and incorrect skin care. It is important to treat the skin gently and not remove all the natural oils that the skin needs for protection.

Disorder	Description and cause	Contra-indications and general precautions	Advice for client
Milia (whiteheads)	Milia are small cysts. They appear as white pearly lumps of skin and might contain uric acid or sebum. Common around the eye area and on skin which is very dehydrated. Might be caused by inappropriate skincare products.	Not contra-indicated.	Check that their skincare products are appropriate for their skin type and that they are not dehydrating the skin. Skin must be kept moisturised to prevent dehydration. Avoid mineral-based products around the eye. Advise on facial treatments to stimulate and improve the skin's functions and to keep the skin soft. Milia can be removed using advanced electrolysis or a micro lance which gently lifts the skin so the milia can be easily extracted.
Comedone (blackhead)	A grey spot caused by sebum blocking the hair follicle. The change in colour is caused by the **oxidation** of keratin in the sebum as it comes into contact with the air. Further change in colour is also caused by the attraction of surface pollution to the oil.	Not contra-indicated.	Recommend deep cleansing and exfoliating treatments and a suitable home skincare regime.

Oxidation

Interaction between oxygen molecules and other substances

Disorder	Description and cause	Contra-indications and general precautions	Advice for client
Sebaceous cyst	Caused by a plug of hardened sebum in the sebaceous gland blocking the follicle and causing it to expand. There are two types of sebaceous **cyst**: • epidermal cysts that can appear anywhere on the skin • pilar cysts which are commonly found on the scalp.	Not contra-indicated unless the cyst is very large or infected, then the area must be avoided.	Recommend that the client seeks medical advice if the cyst is causing irritation or if they are concerned.
Acne vulgaris	A bacterial infection of the sebaceous glands of the face, neck, chest, shoulders, back, thighs and bottom. It can affect one or more areas. Facial acne normally starts around the nose and spreads out over the face. Usually caused by a hormonal imbalance that can be aggravated by stress and poor diet. It might also be caused by exposure to certain chemicals and the use of certain drugs.	Contra-indicated. Avoid contact with the infected areas to prevent further spread of infection on the client's skin. Only use very limited facial treatment to avoid aggravating the condition.	Seek medical attention early to avoid scarring and to treat any skin infection. Advise on make-up application and the use of matte make-up and oil-free products to protect the skin where appropriate.
Seborrhoea	Excessively oily skin. The skin is very shiny and tacky with a sallow grey tone to the skin caused by the oily surface residue. Lots of comedones. Caused by a hormonal imbalance. Can develop into acne vulgaris.	Not contra-indicated. Do not over-stimulate the skin during treatment.	Recommend deep cleansing and exfoliating treatments and a suitable home skincare regime.

Cyst

A small rounded swelling that might contain fluid, semi-solid or solid material. It extends both above and below the surface of the skin

INDUSTRY TIP

Forty to fifty per cent of adults between the ages of 20 and 40 have persistent oily skin or acne. Acne begins with whiteheads and blackheads and progresses to papules and pustules. Medical treatment may be required if the skin becomes infected and develops cysts to prevent scarring.

DISORDERS OF THE SWEAT (SUDORIFEROUS) GLANDS

Disorder	Description and Cause	Contra-indications and general precautions	Advice for client
Bromidrosis	An unpleasant body odour. Caused by bacteria reacting with sweat.	Not contra-indicated. Might be unpleasant to work on a client who has body odour.	If appropriate, discuss personal hygiene. Recommend a daily shower and washing clothes regularly to remove bacteria.
Anhidrosis	Sweat glands stop working causing a lack of sweating. Caused by a number of factors – damaged nerves, genetic factors, skin damage and certain medication. Can become very serious if it affects large areas.	Contra-indicated.	Seek medical advice.
Hyperhidrosis	Excessive perspiration at normal temperatures.	Not usually contra-indicated. Might be a problem with treatments requiring close contact with the skin.	Seek medical advice.
Miliaria rubra (prickly heat)	Red skin rash which is very itchy. Caused by excessive sweating as the body tries to cool down in hot conditions. Sweat gets blocked into the pores.	Contra-indicated.	Keep the skin cool. Wear light, loose clothing made of natural fabrics (eg cotton).

SKIN DISORDERS INVOLVING ABNORMAL SKIN GROWTH

Therapists commonly see abnormal skin growths (eg thickening of the skin on the soles of the feet to abnormal skin tags) that are a nuisance to the client. A therapist is unable to improve these disorders directly.

Disorder	Description and cause	Contra-indications and general precautions	Advice for client
Keloid scar	A noticeable thickened scar caused by excessive collagen production as the skin heals. The condition is more common in darker skins.	Contra-indicated for any treatment that causes damage to the dermis. Avoid deep scar tissue for six months.	Check with a medical practitioner if concerned about the scar and check with the medical practitioner whether it might be possible to work over scar tissue.
Seborrhoeic keratosis (senile warts)	A brown thickening on the surface of the skin. Range in size from 3mm to 35mm. Exact cause of is unknown. Not caused by exposure to UV.	Not contra-indicated.	Can be removed by a medical practitioner.
Skin tags	Tiny skin extensions. Many have no known cause. Others might be caused by surface stimulation (eg along a neck line or under a bra strap). Made up of loose fibrous tissue.	Not contra-indicated. If there are clusters – avoid stimulation and exfoliation over the area.	If the client is concerned, refer them to an advanced electrolysis practitioner.
Psoriasis	Skin cells are produced very quickly and build up on the surface of the skin leaving scaly, itchy patches. The skin can crack and bleed. The exact cause is unknown. It is linked to stress and can be hereditary.	Not contra-indicated. Not contagious. Can be treated safely. Avoid any affected areas to prevent irritation.	Recommend relaxing treatments that will help to reduce stress. Suggest your client seeks specialist medical treatment from a medical practitioner. Specialist treatments include specialised UV treatment, coal tar treatments and cortisone-based medicines.

Disorder	Description and cause	Contra-indications and general precautions	Advice for client
Hyper-keratosis	A thickening of the skin caused by an excessive amount of keratin. This thickening is often produced to protect the underlying tissue from rubbing, pressure and irritation. Commonly affects the elbow, knees, soles and heels of the feet.	Not contra-indicated.	Exfoliation and a course of microdermabrasion will help improve the skin's texture.
Corns and calluses	An area of hard skin produced by the body to provide additional protection from friction (eg from poorly fitting shoes). Corns are smaller and can be found on the top of toes or between the toe joints. Some people have a corn on the middle finger from holding a pen (writer's lump). Calluses are larger and flatter and occur on the heels, and palms.	Not contra-indicated.	Choose shoes carefully. Regular pedicures and manicures will help soften the skin. Use a pen with a soft cushion design. Refer to a **podiatrist**.
Malignant tumours	A **tumour** may be benign (non-cancerous) or malignant (cancerous). Caused by cells that have lost their normal features and reproduce in an abnormal way. A tumour might be in, or on, the body. It might be contained in an area or it might have spread into the surrounding tissues and organs**.** ■ *Malignant melanoma* – develops in the pigment cells and is associated with excessive exposure to UV radiation. ■ *Basal cell carcinoma* – develops in the epidermis. ■ *Squamous cell carcinoma* (or prickle-cell cancer) – develops within keratinocytes in the epidermis. A thick scab develops over a small area of inflamed skin. As the cancer spreads it looks more like an ulcer and may bleed.	Contra-indicated. The client should not be treated during cancer treatment. It is not contagious.	A client having cancer treatment should seek medical advice before any treatment takes place. Advise clients about excessive exposure to the sun and sun protection.

Podiatrist

A foot specialist

Tumour

A benign or malignant mass of tissues caused by uncontrolled cell growth

SKIN DISORDERS INVOLVING ABNORMAL CELL GROWTH

Therapists will see lots of common skin disorders. It is important that you can recognise these to know whether they are contagious or not. Treatments can then be avoided or modified.

Disorder	Description and cause	Contra-indications?	Advice for client
Eczema	Areas of extreme dryness on the skin. Wet eczema is when there are **vesicles** present. The irritated skin is itchy. Can be caused by an internal irritant (eg a food intolerance) or by contact with an external allergen (eg animal hair or a product). Eczema can be inherited and is often linked to asthma.	Only contra-indicated if severe and the skin is open. Avoid direct contact with any area where the skin is open. Only use gentle products with a natural base. Avoid any abrasive products and over-stimulation.	Seek medical advice as medication can help to relieve the symptoms.
Dermatitis	Symptoms include: ■ redness ■ scaling/flaking ■ blistering ■ weeping ■ cracking ■ swelling. ■ *Irritant contact dermatitis (ICD)* occurs when there is contact with either a strong **irritant** or a weaker irritant over long periods of time. Irritants found in the salon include hand washes, essential oils, dust and wet work (ie constant washing of hands to maintain hygiene). ■ *Allergic contact dermatitis (ACD)* occurs when someone develops an allergy to something that comes into contact with their skin. Any contact with the **allergen** will cause an allergic response. Allergens in the salon include glue adhesives, nail polish and skincare products.	This will depend on symptoms and level of severity.	When washing hands make sure they are dried well. Apply moisturiser regularly. Use specialised creams when recommended by a medical practitioner.

Vesicle

A small, raised blister containing a pale serum

Irritant

A substance, product or chemical that causes inflammation of the skin

Allergen

A substance that causes the immune system to react abnormally

INDUSTRY TIP

Be alert to sores that do not heal. Squamous cell carcinoma (or prickle-cell cancer) is the second most common type of skin cancer. A normal scab should heal in about two weeks. If a wound looks like it is not healing, the client should seek medical advice. This type of cancer is common on the back of the hands, scalp, ears and lip.

VIRAL INFECTIONS OF THE SKIN

Viral infections are very contagious and you should not feel under pressure to treat anyone you feel is unwell or treat any areas that show signs of a viral infection.

Disorder	Description and cause	Contra-indications and general precautions	Advice for client
Herpes simplex (cold sores)	Caused by a **virus**. Starts with itching or irritation in the area where the cold sore is going to occur. It develops into a red patch followed by blisters. These become a moist crusty patch. Tend to develop when the sufferer is run down, under stress or after over-exposure to the sun and wind. The virus remains **dormant** in the skin after the infection has cleared up.	Contra-indicated. Contagious. Can be caught by **direct** or **indirect contact**. Do not treat the area around a cold sore. It is infectious when the blisters are present. If a client is having a facial treatment, ask them to return once the cold sore has gone so they can fully enjoy their treatment.	There is no cure but over-the-counter treatments might help relieve the symptoms.
Human papilloma virus (HPV) wart Verrucae	The virus enters into the skin through a small cut or scratch. It can lie dormant in the skin for many months. Keratin is produced too fast and causes a hard, raised cauliflower-looking growth of skin. The tiny black dots are tiny blood capillaries which get caught as the wart grows. ■ *The common wart:* about 70% of warts are common warts. Can occur singularly or in clusters. ■ *Verrucae (plantar warts):* occur on the soles of the feet. The weight of the body makes them grow inwards. Particularly contagious in damp, warm conditions. Transmitted through direct and indirect contact.	Contra-indicated. Treatment should be modified to avoid putting feet into water or direct contact with the treatment area. Damaged warts are contagious as the viral spores are exposed. Area should be avoided during massage. Precautions should be taken when using spa equipment (ie using equipment such as saunas or steam rooms where footwear might not be permitted or needed). If there are many warts/verrucae treatment is completely contra-indicated.	Most people will develop a wart at some time in their life. Usually the body develops an **immunity** to the virus and the wart disappears within two years.

Disorder	Description and cause	Contra-indications and general precautions	Advice for client
Verrucae filiformis	Small thin tags of skin. Commonly found in clusters around the neck line and bra line.	Contra-indicated as the condition can be easily spread on the client's skin. Avoid any treatment that might irritate the skin (eg body scrubs) and spread the condition further.	Client should seek medical advice before treatment takes place. Can be treated using advanced epilation and specialist medical skin treatments.
Herpes zoster (shingles)	Caused when the chickenpox virus is reactivated after lying dormant in the nervous system. Symptoms include tingling and extreme sensitivity along the nerve pathways followed by pain, itching and blisters. The client may generally feel run down. The pain may last for many months. The physical symptoms disappear after a week.	Contra-indicated. Although shingles is not contagious, you can catch chickenpox from someone who has active shingles if you have not had chickenpox before.	Seek medical advice.

Virus

A micro-organism that multiplies within a living organism

Dormant

Not active

Direct contact

A disease is transmitted by direct contact with a person who has the disease or infection (eg touching)

Indirect contact

A disease is transmitted through another object used by the person with the disease or infection (eg towels, spa bath, etc)

Immunity

Protection from a disease

Bacteria
Tiny single-celled organisms. Some are harmful to us and others are important for our health

BACTERIAL INFECTIONS OF THE SKIN

Our body is covered with millions of tiny **bacteria** at any given moment. Bacteria can be good as well as bad but some bacterial infections are very contagious and can cause nasty infections. You should be able to recognise the following common bacterial infections and you should not feel under pressure to treat any area that is infected with a bacterial infection. If you catch something you will risk passing the disease on and it may also prevent you from working.

Disorder	Description and cause	Contra-indications and general precaution	Advice for client
Furuncles (boils) and carbuncles	A deep bacterial infection of the hair follicle. Starts as an inflamed, tender area which develops into a large painful pustule. Caused by staphylococcus aureus bacteria and linked with poor hygiene and stress. A carbuncle is a collection of boils with several pustule-like heads. A scar is often left once the area has healed.	Contra-indicated. Contagious. Avoid area to prevent cross-infection.	Leave the area alone. Seek medical advice if appropriate.
Impetigo	Caused by staphylococci and streptococci bacteria. Commonly found on the face around the nose and mouth but can occur anywhere with broken skin. Raised red areas of skin which quickly form small blisters, followed by honey-coloured crusts.	Contra-indicated. Contagious. Can be transmitted by direct and indirect contact.	Seek medical advice.
Conjunctivitis	Caused by staphylococci bacteria or occasionally a virus. Inflammation of the mucus membrane lining and covering of the eye. Eyes look red, swollen and will feel itchy and gritty. There might be some sensitivity to light. The discharge might contain pus causing the eyelids to stick together in the mornings.	Contra-indicated. Very contagious. Transmitted by direct contact (eg by sharing make-up brushes).	Seek medical advice.
Hordeolum (stye)	A staphylococcal bacterial infection of one or more follicles of the eyelashes. A small red area on the edge of the eyelid causes irritation. It becomes a small red lump which might contain pus.	Contra-indicated. Contagious. Do not treat the area to avoid cross-infection.	Seek medical advice.

FUNGAL INFECTIONS OF THE SKIN

You should be able to recognise tinea pedis (athlete's foot). It is one of the most common conditions that clients will present to you.

Disorder	Description and cause	Contra-indications and general precaution	Advice for client
Tinea corporis (ringworm of the body)	Initially appears as a pink circular patch, with a defined red outer ring. The skin heals from the centre as the infection spreads outwards.	Contra-indicated. Contagious. Transmitted by direct or indirect contact.	Seek medical advice.
Tinea pedis (athlete's foot)	Symptoms include irritation and sometimes a distinct odour. The **fungus** lives on keratin and likes a moist, warm environment. White spongy looking skin might crack, split and peel. Commonly found between the toes but can also affect larger areas of the foot.	Contra-indicated. Contagious. Transmitted by direct or indirect contact.	Seek medical advice. Wash and dry the feet well, particularly between the toes. Change socks at least once a day. Wear breathable fabrics that keep the feet dry.
Tinea capitis (ringworm of the scalp)	As for tinea corporis but the hair becomes brittle and breaks away leaving short brittle stubs. The scalp becomes patchy, with white or grey scales.	Contra-indicated. Contagious. Transmitted by direct or indirect contact.	Seek medical advice.
Tinea barbae (ringworm of the beard)	Small pustules at the tip of the hair follicle from which broken hair protrudes.	Contra-indicated. Contagious. Transmitted by direct or indirect contact (eg dirty towels or contaminate razors).	See medical advice.

Fungus

A tiny plant micro-organism

Infestation

Invasion by animals that enter the body and survive by feeding off blood and living tissue

INFESTATIONS

You are unlikely to come across many **infestations** in the salon but it is still important that you are familiar with them and are able to recognise them. There is always a possibility that you might be exposed to them.

Disorder	Description and cause	Contra-indications?	Advice for client
Pediculosis corporis (body lice)	Caused by a tiny blood-sucking insect. It lays its eggs on clothing and feeds on the skin. Symptoms include Intense itching at the site of infestation, usually in the skin's creases (eg the elbows).	Contra-indicated. Contagious. Transmitted by direct or indirect contact.	Seek medical advice.
Scabies (sarcoptes scabiei)	Small **parasites** that burrow into the skin and lay eggs. Burrowing mites cause intense itching which is worse at night. They also cause inflammation and irritation of the infected area and a small grey swelling. Commonly found between the fingers and on the wrists but can also be found under the arm and around the groin.	Contra-indicated. Highly contagious. Transmitted by direct or indirect contact.	Seek medical advice.

Parasite

An organism that lives on another organism (a host) causing harm to the host. Parasites include fungi, bacterial and worms

HAIR

INDUSTRY TIP

If you have a Wood's lamp for carrying out a skin analysis/inspection, it can be used to see whether ringworm is present. The fungus glows under the UV light of the Wood's lamp.

INDUSTRY TIP

Clients can often seek medical advice from a pharmacist for minor conditions.

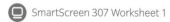

SmartScreen 307 Worksheet 1

SmartScreen 307 Worksheet 6

Hair is 70–80% protein. The protein is in the form of dead keratinised cells which form a thread-like structure. The rest of the hair is made up of a combination of water, minerals, lipids and melanin (the pigment that gives the hairs its colour). Hair grows out from the hair follicle as new cells are produced.

The main function of the hair is protection. Hair covers the head to keep the head warm but also to protect the head from injury and from overexposure to the sun. Eyelashes and eyebrows (supercilia) shield the eyes. They prevent objects from entering into the eyes and catch perspiration.

Hair also provides a larger surface area for sweat to evaporate from to cool the body. When we are cold, the arrector pili muscle, which is attached to the hair follicle, pulls the hair up to trap air next to the skin to keep it warm. Tiny hairs in the ears and nostrils, called cilia, catch and filter out dust particles to prevent them from entering the body.

In this part of the chapter you will learn about:

- the hair follicle
- the structure of the hair shaft
- hair texture
- the hair growth cycle
- hair types
- changes in hair growth
- hair diseases and disorders.

THE HAIR FOLLICLE

The hair follicle is a complex structure that produces hair. It extends deep into the dermis. The follicle has two layers:

- the inner root **sheath**
- the outer root sheath.

INNER ROOT SHEATH

The inner root sheath has three layers:

- the cuticle, which holds the hair in place
- the Huxley layer
- the Henles layer.

OUTER ROOT SHEATH

The outer root sheath is a continuation of the stratum germinativum and surrounds the inner root sheath. This sheath remains static in the skin and does not grow with the hair.

Sheath
A cover around the follicle root

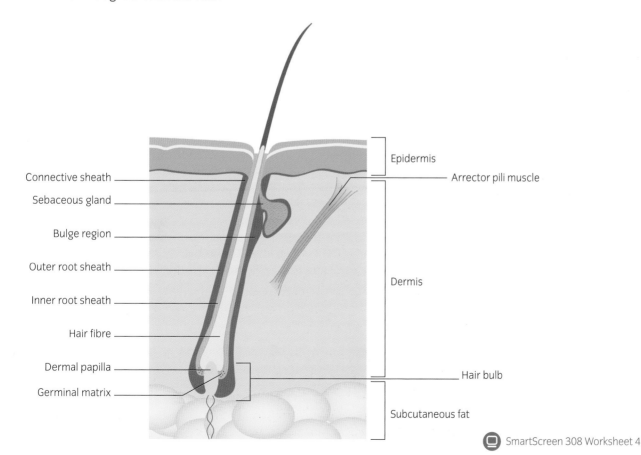

Connective sheath
Sebaceous gland
Bulge region
Outer root sheath
Inner root sheath
Hair fibre
Dermal papilla
Germinal matrix

Epidermis
Arrector pili muscle
Dermis
Hair bulb
Subcutaneous fat

SmartScreen 308 Worksheet 4

CONNECTIVE SHEATH

This sheath surrounds the follicle and the sebaceous gland. It provides the hair with nerve endings and blood vessels.

HAIR BULB

This is the enlarged part of the hair at the base of the hair root. It is surrounded by a mass of loose connective tissue called the dermal papilla.

DERMAL PAPILLA

At the base of the hair follicle is a mass of loose connective tissue which contains tiny capillaries to nourish all the cells of the follicle. Just above the papilla is a group of cells which produce the hair.

GERMINAL MATRIX

This is an area of cells around the dermal papilla where the cells divide by mitosis to produce new hair. It is also where melanin is transferred to the hair to give it pigmentation. This area is very active during the **anagen** stage of hair growth.

Anagen
The growing phase of a hair follicle

SEBACEOUS GLAND

The sebaceous gland is usually located two-thirds of the way up the hair follicle. It produces sebum which is secreted into the follicle. In larger hair follicles there might be more than one sebaceous gland.

ARRECTOR PILI MUSCLE

This is a small muscle that is attached to the hair shaft. It supports the hair follicle and when we are cold, it pulls the hair upright so that the hair stands on end producing goose bumps.

STRUCTURE OF THE HAIR SHAFT

The hair shaft is the part of the hair that is visible above the skin. The part below the skin is called the root. The hair shaft is made up of three layers of keratinised cells:

- the medulla
- the cortex
- the cuticle.

MEDULLA

The medulla is the most central layer of the hair shaft. It is not always present in **vellus** hair (ie in fine body hair). It reflects the light making hair look shiny.

Vellus
Short, fine, light-coloured hair that develops in childhood

CORTEX

The cortex surrounds the medulla and creates the bulk of the hair. It contains melanin and gives the hair its colour. It is made up of elongated keratinised cells that are twisted together. These strands are able to stretch and flex and return back to their original shape.

CUTICLE

The cuticle is the outermost layer of the hair shaft. It is made up of overlapping scales of keratinised cells which provide a protective coat. If you take a strand of hair and run your fingers towards the root you will feel these scales. The cuticle has no colour and is quite a thin layer.

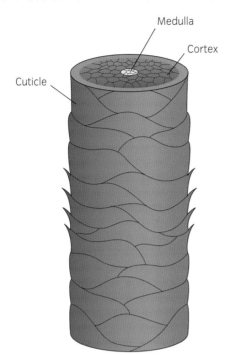

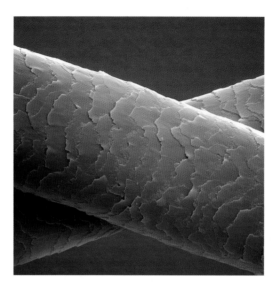

HAIR TEXTURE

The texture or thickness of a hair depends on:

- the diameter and shape of the hair follicle
- the proportion of the cuticle around the hair.

In coarse hair, the cuticle makes up around 10% of the volume of the hair and the cortex around 90%. In fine hair the cuticle makes up around 40% of the hair and the cortex around 60%.

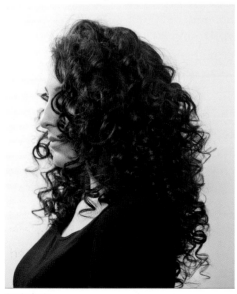

Curly hair

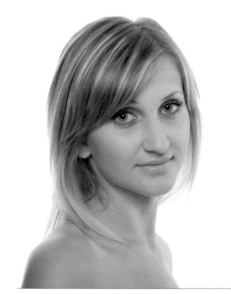

Straight hair

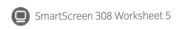
HAIR GROWTH CYCLE

The hair follicle has three stages of growth. These stages include periods of activity and rest and vary from person to person. The growth rate also varies in different parts of the body. The hair on the head has a growth cycle of between two to eight years while the growth rate of the eyelashes is about four months. The three stages of the hair growth cycle are:

- anagen
- catagen
- telogen.

> **INDUSTRY TIP**
>
> The word ACT will help you to remember the hair growth cycle and its sequence.

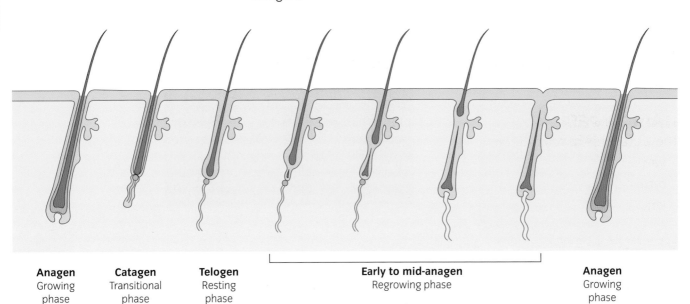

| **Anagen** Growing phase | **Catagen** Transitional phase | **Telogen** Resting phase | **Early to mid-anagen** Regrowing phase | **Anagen** Growing phase |

The hair growth cycle

ANAGEN

During anagen the hair is in the active growth stage. The cells in the root sheath divide and grow down deeper into the dermis. At the same time cells grow up the follicle to form the inner root sheath and the hair itself. The hair becomes injected with keratin and becomes keratinised. As the hair matures the growth slows down. Around 80 to 90% of the hair on our head is in the anagen phase of growth at any one time.

CATAGEN

When the hair growth is complete, the hair goes through a state of change which lasts about two weeks. During this time the cell activity slows down until no new cells are produced. There is no melanin pigmentation so the hair produced in these final stages of growth has no colour. The hair bulb begins to wither and die and forms a club shape at its end. The follicle begins to shorten, shrink and becomes detached from the dermal papilla. A small cord forms between the dermal papilla and the club end of the hair. Around 1% of the hair on the scalp is in the catagen phase of growth.

> **WHY DON'T YOU...**
>
> run your fingers through your hair and pull at the ends gently. Look at the hair that comes away. The telogen hair will have a distinct white ball at the end and you will see the loss of hair colour towards the final hair growth. Compare this to a hair that has been removed from an eyebrow using tweezers.

TELOGEN

In this final stage, the hair is dead and is shed from the hair follicle. The follicle rests until it is stimulated to begin the cycle again. This stage lasts around three to four months. Sometimes a new hair begins to grow, pushing the old hair out of the skin straight away. Around 13% of hair on the head is resting in the telogen phase of growth.

ACTIVITY

Wax an underarm with hot wax. Turn the wax over and look at the hairs. Can you clearly see the different hair growth stages?

ACTIVITY

Discuss with your colleagues what impact waxing has on the hair growth cycle.

HAIR TYPES

There are three hair types:

- vellus
- terminal
- lanugo.

VELLUS HAIR

This is the soft fine downy hair which is found all over the body with the exception of the soles of the feet and palms of the hands. It usually lacks any pigmentation. This hair has shallow roots.

TERMINAL HAIR

At birth, this type of hair is found on the scalp, eyelashes and eyebrows. During puberty it grows under the arms and in the groin areas. During male puberty it grows on the lower legs and chest and as a beard. This type of hair has a well-developed root and bulb with a strong blood supply. The follicle extends deep into the dermis during anagen growth.

LANUGO HAIR

Lanugo hair is very soft fine hair that covers a baby in the womb and disappears a few months after birth.

ACTIVITY

Ask some of your colleagues with different hair colour, shape and thickness to brush their hair and collect any loose hairs. Compare the hairs. Discuss your findings.

CHANGES IN HAIR GROWTH

Hair growth and changes in hair growth can be caused by a number of different factors such as:

- hereditary/congenital factors (eg genetics will determine hair colour, type, amount and hair growth cycles)
- topical stimulation (eg from sunburn, waxing, scars)

WHY DON'T YOU...
draw a table with two columns. Head one 'Vellus' and the other 'Terminal'. In the relevant column, write down the differences between vellus and terminal hair.

- normal systemic changes (eg changes in hormones during puberty, pregnancy and menopause can cause excessive hair growth)
- abnormal systemic changes (eg diseases or disorders of the endocrine system)
- severe emotional trauma (eg stress can stimulate the adrenal glands which can cause the hair to become more coarse)
- surgical changes and medication (eg some surgical procedures, such as removal of an ovary, and some medication, such as birth control pills or some steroids, can cause excessive hair growth).

HIRSUTISM AND HYPERTRICHOSIS

Hirsutism is excessive hair growth, usually in females. It is caused by an excess of the male sex hormone, androgen. The hair is usually dark and thick and grows on the face (upper lip and chin), chest, lower back and buttocks.

Hypertrichosis also describes excessive hair growth and affects both men and women. It can be hereditary or it can develop later in life.

HAIR DISEASES AND DISORDERS

PARASITIC INFECTIONS OF THE SCALP

Parasitic infections of the scalp are very common. We tend to think of them affecting children but adults can get them just as easily.

Disorder	Description and cause	Contra-indications and general precautions	Advice for client
Pediculosis capitis (head lice)	Caused by a small wingless flat insect which feeds on blood. The eggs (nits) take 7–10 days to hatch. It takes 7–14 days for the lice to mature and mate. They survive for several weeks. Symptoms include intense itching at the site of infection. Nits look like grey-coloured beads attached to the hair shaft close to the scalp.	Contra-indicated. Contagious. Direct contact is required for the lice to jump from head to head.	Seek medical advice. Treatment must be ongoing for a minimum of 14 days. Use a special comb to loosen and remove nits and lice.
Pediculosis pubis (pubic lice)	These tiny insects look like crabs or scabs. The females lay eggs that hatch after eight days. Pubic lice can be found under the arms, in beards and in eyebrows. Symptoms include Intense itching at the site of the infestation.	Contra-indicated. Contagious. Transmitted by direct contact.	Seek medical advice

BACTERIAL INFECTIONS AFFECTING THE HAIR FOLLICLE

Disorder	Description and cause	Contra-indications and general precautions	Advice for client
Folliculitis	A common result of poor hygiene. Can occur following waxing and shaving. Inflammation of one or more hair follicles. Commonly found around the neck, bikini line, beard and armpits. The hair may grow inwards causing further inflammation and a condition called pseudo-folliculitis.	Contra-indicated. There is a risk of cross-infection. Give very thorough aftercare advice.	Seek medical advice. Follow very thorough aftercare advice.

COMMON SCALP AND HAIR CONDITIONS

While you do not generally deal with the head during treatments, it is useful to understand common conditions that affect the hair and scalp.

Disorder	Description and cause	Contra-indications and general precautions	Advice for client
Alopecia	Can be patches of hair loss (alopecia areata) or total hair loss (alopecia universalis). Can be caused by stress, shock, illness or medication (chemotherapy).	Not contra-indicated.	Stimulate the blood supply to the area to encourage healthy circulation. Recommend they see a **trichologist** for additional advice and treatment.

INDUSTRY TIP

Androgenic alopecia is male pattern baldness in women. The hair growth begins to thin often starting at the crown and the hair line recedes. It can be hereditary, or caused by hormonal changes. Androgens cause the hair growth to alter and the hair becomes shorter and finer until it stops growing leaving the scalp hairless or with a fine covering of vellus hair.

Trichologist

A person who specialises in hair and scalp problems

NAILS

A perfect healthy nail is smooth, unmarked and can be flexed without breaking or splitting. It is usually a delicate pink colour which shows that there is a healthy circulation to the nail bed. The nail is an extension of the stratum lucidum (clear layer). It is made up of dense keratinised cells, water, minerals (including calcium and zinc) and a small quantity of lipids.

In this part of the chapter you will learn about:

- the functions of the nails
- the structure of the nail
- the growth cycle of the nail

- nail shapes
- diseases and disorders of the nail and their appearance and causes.

FUNCTIONS OF THE NAILS
Nails have three functions:
- to protect the nail bed, and through the nail plate, to protect the soft sensitive fingers and toes
- to enhance the fingertips' sensitivity
- to assist the fingers when picking up objects or scratching.

STRUCTURE OF THE NAIL
The structure of the nail can be divided into three main sections:
- the matrix
- the nail plate
- the free edge.

MATRIX
The matrix is the living part of the nail structure and is an extension of the stratum germinativum. The matrix is sometimes referred to as the root of the nail and lies underneath the nail fold or mantle. It is nourished by an abundant supply of blood vessels. It is here that new cells divide by mitosis to produce the nail. Any injury to the area can cause damage to the nail's structure. The shape of the matrix determines the size and shape of the nail.

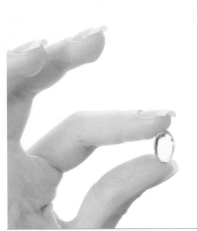
Nails assist the fingers in picking up objects

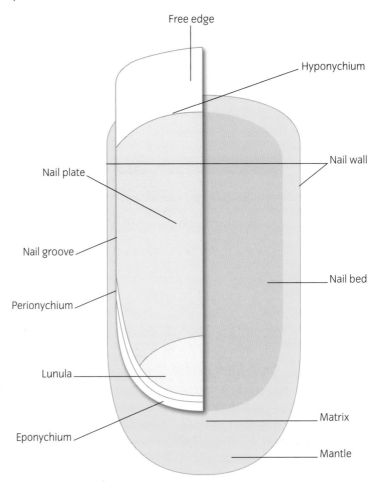

THE CITY & GUILDS TEXTBOOK

NAIL PLATE

The nail plate is the visible part of the nail and is made up of hundreds of layers. These are found in three sections of keratinised cells bound together by sulphur bonds, moisture and fat. The middle section makes up 75% of the nail plate. Unlike the skin, the nails cells cannot be easily exfoliated. The nail plate is attached to the finger by the nail bed. It is dead and has no nerves or blood supply. The cells of the nail plate are able to absorb moisture but too much moisture can cause the nail to split or peel.

FREE EDGE

This is the part of the nail plate that extends beyond the fingertip. It protects the hyponychium at the edge of the nail bed. This is the part of the nail that can be filed into shape.

THE HYPONYCHIUM

The hyponychium is the part of the epidermis that is visible under the free edge of the nail. The hyponychium lies at the edge of the nail bed just beneath the free edge. It has a seal that protects it from infection.

THE MANTLE OR PROXIMAL NAIL FOLD

This is a fold of skin that protects the base of the nail and the matrix.

NAIL BED

The nail bed lies under the nail plate. The nail plate is held in place by a series of ridges and grooves.

ACTIVITY

Look carefully under the free edge of one of your nails. Can you see the thickened area and some ripples in the skin's structure? This is the nail bed.

NAIL GROOVES

These are tiny depressions at the side of the nail beneath the nail wall. They guide the nail as it grows up the nail bed.

LATERAL NAIL FOLD OR SIDE WALL

The skin along the sides of the nail folds back to form a protective wall and seal around the sides of the nail.

LUNULA

This is the visible part of the matrix. It is the very pale pink area at the base of the nail plate. It is a different colour because the circulation is less efficient and also because the cells are not fully keratinised. Most people only have lunulae visible on their thumbs.

CUTICLE

The cuticle is formed from thickened stratum corneum (the horny layer) and is constantly being shed. It is found at the base of the nail and grows up with the nail. The cuticle has two parts: the eponychium and the perionychium.

Eponychium

The eponychium is the fold of skin which overlaps the lunula at the base of the nail plate. It forms a seal to prevent micro-organisms entering into the surrounding tissues. A healthy eponychium should be soft, supple and secure. This is the part of the nail that is freed from the nail plate during a manicure.

SmartScreen 312 Worksheet 4

Perionychium

This covers the outer portion and sides of the nail.

NAIL GROWTH

The nail grows at a rate of about 3–5mm a month. It will take about three to five months to grow from the matrix to the free edge. Toenails grow at about half this speed. It will take about eight to nine months to grow a full new toenail.

HANDY HINT

Nail disorders are covered briefly as it is important to be aware of them. However, it is not necessary to cover them in depth as you will not come across them in the units covered within this book.

NAIL DISEASES AND DISORDERS

Disorder	Description and cause	Contra-indications and general precautions	Advice for client
Onychia (oh-nik-ee-uh)	Bacterial infection of the nail fold causing the skin around the base of the nail to become red and inflamed. Pus might be visible.	Contra-indicated. Contagious.	Seek medical advice.
Paronychia (parr-uh-NIK-ee-uh)	A bacterial infection of the cuticle. Symptoms include tenderness, redness and swelling in the infected area. A small pus-filled spot will appear if the condition is not treated.	Contra-indicated. Avoid the skin around the infected toenail.	Consult a podiatrist who will remove the part of the nail with the disorder. If very infected, the client might need to seek medical advice.
Onychocryptosis (ingrown nail) (on-i-koh-krip-toe-sis)	Symptoms include discomfort or pain around the side of the nail as well as redness and swelling. It is caused by poorly fitting shoes and incorrect nail care, in particular incorrect filing or cutting of the nail. It is often seen on the big toe.	Contra-indicated.	Seek medical advice if infected or see a chiropodist for treatment.

SKELETAL SYSTEM

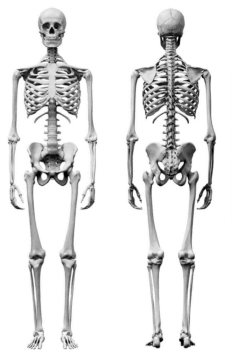

In this part of the chapter you will learn about:

- the functions of the skeleton
- the types of bone
- the structure of bone
- bone formation
- the effects of ageing on the skeletal system
- the structure of the skeleton
- joints
- skeletal conditions that restrict or prevent treatment.

Bone is the hardest tissue in the human body. Bone is made from specialised cells called osteocytes which create a rigid non-elastic tissue. These cells are surrounded by a matrix of collagen fibres strengthened by **calcium** and **phosphate**. Bones have lots of hollow spaces within their structure which make them light and provide tiny spaces for blood vessels and nerves to supply the bone tissue.

Bone tissue is not completely **rigid**. If it is injured, it breaks down and rebuilds, renewing its shape and structure during growth and repair.

Calcium
A mineral necessary for the healthy function of the heart, muscles and nerves and an essential part of the structure of bones and teeth

phosphate
A chemical compound containing phosphorous

Rigid
Unable to bend; not flexible

FUNCTIONS OF THE SKELETON

There are six main functions of the skeleton:

- Protection – the skull protects the brain; the spine protects the spinal cord; the rib cage protects the heart and lungs.
- Support/shape – bones give support for the muscles of the body and give shape to the body contours and the characteristics of our face shape.
- Movement – bones have ridges where muscles attach to allow bones and joints to provide flexible movement.
- Formation of blood cells – all red blood cells and some of the white blood cells are made in specialised tissue called bone marrow.
- Storage and release of certain vitamins and minerals, including calcium and phosphorous.

TYPES OF BONE

There are 206 bones in the human body and these are shaped according to the function they need to perform. There are five different shapes or types of bone:

- Long bones act as levers to raise and lower limbs. They have a shaft, made of compact bone with a central canal which contains bone marrow, and two ends, which have an outer covering of compact bone. Long bones contain bone marrow.

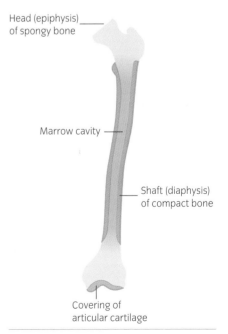

Head (epiphysis) of spongy bone

Marrow cavity

Shaft (diaphysis) of compact bone

Covering of articular cartilage

Long bone

- Short bones often form bridges and are subject to pressure type forces (eg the wrist and ankle).

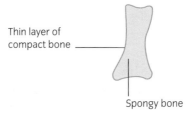

Thin layer of compact bone

Spongy bone

- Irregular bones often have complex shapes (eg the vertebrae).

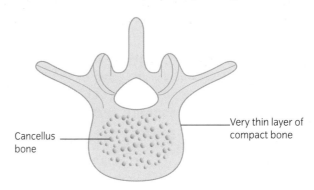

Cancellus bone

Very thin layer of compact bone

- Flat bones are good for creating protective shells (eg the bones of the cranium and sternum and scapula in the torso).

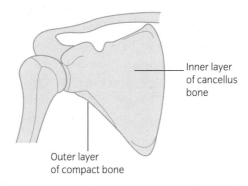

Inner layer of cancellus bone

Outer layer of compact bone

- Sesamoid bones are often rounded bones and sit inside tendons or synovial joints (eg the patella/knee cap).

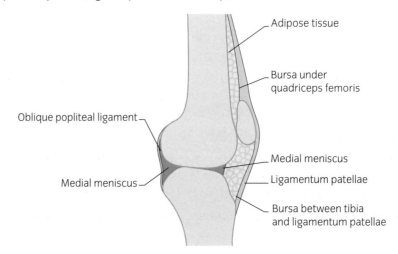

Adipose tissue

Bursa under quadriceps femoris

Oblique popliteal ligament

Medial meniscus

Ligamentum patellae

Medial meniscus

Bursa between tibia and ligamentum patellae

STRUCTURE OF BONE

There are two types of bone tissue:

- compact hard bone
- cancellous (spongy) bone.

COMPACT (HARD) BONE

This forms the surface layer of all bones and the tubular shafts inside long bones. It makes up around 80% of the bone in the body. Compact bone is made up of osteons. Osteons consist of **concentric** layers of bone called **lamellae** which surround a long hollow central passage (the **Haversian canal**). The central canal contains blood vessels, lymph vessels and nerves which supply the individual bone cells (**osteocytes**).

CANCELLOUS (SPONGY) BONE

This type of bone is sponge-like and is lighter than compact bone.

BONE MARROW

Bone marrow is found inside long bones, flat bones and vertebra. Most of the cells in the blood are made in the bone marrow.

Erythrocytes

Erythrocytes are red blood cells. Red blood cells start as immature cells in the bone marrow. Once they have matured (after about seven days), they are released into the bloodstream. Red blood cells contain a special protein called haemoglobin. Haemoglobin is essential for transporting oxygen from the lungs around the body and for carrying carbon dioxide back to the lungs so that it can be exhaled.

Lymphocytes

Lymphocytes are a type of white blood cell that help protect the body against diseases and fight infections. Lymphocytes are formed in lymphoid tissue throughout the body.

Thrombocytes

Also known as platelets, thrombocytes are tiny pieces of large bone marrow cells that are essential in the blood clotting process.

STRUCTURE OF A LONG BONE

A long bone has:

- two **epiphyses** which form the rounded ends of the bone. They are made up of compact bone inside
- a **diaphysis** – the main shaft which is made up from compact bone and forms the length of the bone structure
- a central space (cavity) called the **medullary canal** which contains special fatty yellow bone marrow
- a **periosteum** – a membrane that protects the bone. The periosteum contains **osteoblasts** and **osteoclasts** that are responsible for producing new bone and breaking down old bone respectively
- **hyaline cartilage** – a bluish-white type of cartilage found at the joints.

Concentric
Circular shapes sharing the same centre

Lamellae
Concentric layers of bone

Haversian canal
The central passage of compact bone containing small blood vessels, lymph vessels and nerves

Osteocytes
Individual blood cells

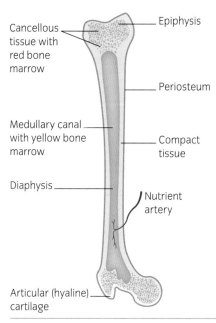

Cancellous tissue with red bone marrow

Epiphysis

Periosteum

Medullary canal with yellow bone marrow

Compact tissue

Diaphysis

Nutrient artery

Articular (hyaline) cartilage

Structure of a bone

Epiphysis
The rounded end of a long bone

Diaphysis
The main shaft of a long bone

Medullary canal
The central cavity containing fatty yellow bone marrow

Periosteum
A membrane that protects the bone

Osteoblasts
Cells responsible for bone formation

Osteoclasts
Cells that break down bone

hyaline cartilage
A type of cartilage found at the joints

Ossification
The process of bone formation

Chondrocytes
Cartilage-forming cells

Osteocytes
Mature osteoblasts that no longer form bones but assist with blood flow through the bones

Dense
Closely packed together

BONE FORMATION

Ossification is the formation of bone by the activity of osteoblasts, **chondrocytes** and osteoclasts.

Chondrocytes can be found close to the end of the long bones. Chondrocytes multiply and become enlarged.

Osteoblasts can be found:
- in the periosteum
- in new bone
- at the ends of the diaphysis
- at the site of a bone fracture.

Osteoblasts begin laying down spongy bone. Calcium is deposited to form new hardened bone cells. Once osteoblasts stop forming new bone they become **osteocytes** which assist with blood flow through the bones**.**

Osteoclasts are cells that break down bone tissue and absorb it back into the body to maintain the skeleton. The maintenance of bone is therefore a balance between osteoblast and osteoclast activity (ie osteoblasts create new bone and osteoclasts break down old bone tissue).

EFFECTS OF AGEING ON THE SKELETAL SYSTEM

As we age, our bones become more fragile. The calcium content of the bones decreases and as a result the bones become less **dense**, lighter and weaker. This means that bones break more easily. Any damage will take much longer to repair because bone growth and repair slow down with age.

STRUCTURE OF THE SKELETON

The skeleton can be divided into two parts:
- the axial skeleton, which includes the skull, the spine and the thorax
- the appendicular skeleton, which includes the shoulder girdle, the arms and hands, the pelvic girdle and the legs and feet.

BONES OF THE SKULL AND FACE

The skull consists of:
- the cranium, which encloses and protects the brain
- the mandible – the jawbone.

The cranium consists of eight bones, which are fused together:

Bones of the cranium	Position
Frontal	Front of the cranium. Forms the forehead.
Occipital	At the back of the head. Forms the back of the skull.
Parietal	Two bones forming the sides and roof of the cranium.
Sphenoid	One bone forming the back of the eye sockets and the middle of the cranium.
Temporal	Two bones on either side of the cranium. They sit under the ears.
Ethmoid	One bone between the nasal cavity and brain. Forms part of the eye socket cavity.

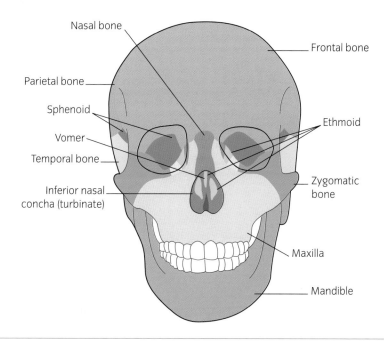

Front view of the skull

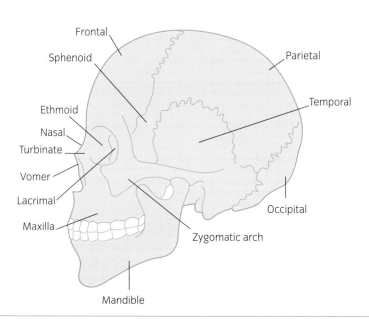

Profile view of the skull

HANDY HINT

The shape of the facial bones gives rise to our facial characteristics and individual features.

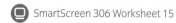

SmartScreen 306 Worksheet 15

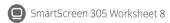

SmartScreen 305 Worksheet 8

There are also 14 facial bones:

Facial bones	Position
Maxillae	Two bones forming the upper jaw.
Zygomatic arch	Two bones forming the cheekbones.
Nasal	Two bones forming the bridge of the nose
Mandible	Lower jaw bone.
Palatine	Two bones forming the floor of the nose and the roof of the mouth.
Inferior conchae	Two bones forming the sides of the nasal cavity.
Vomer	One thin bone forming the nasal septum.
Lacrimal	Two bones forming the inner wall of the eye sockets.

Sinus

A hollow cavity

The facial sinuses

There are four air-filled spaces within the skull which form the facial **sinuses**. The sinuses:

- lighten the weight of the head
- protect the skull from impacts to the face
- give tone and quality to the sound of our voices
- secrete mucus to trap dust and germs that enter through the nose.

The sinuses form one of the body's first lines of defence against infection.

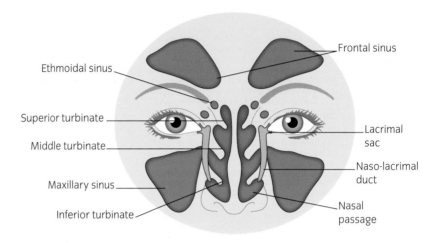

VERTEBRAL COLUMN

The vertebral column is made up of 33 vertebrae bones. Of these, 24 bones are moveable.

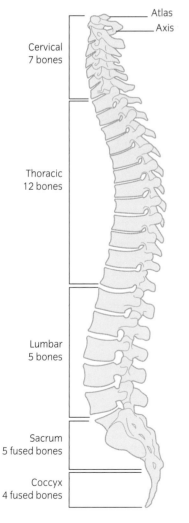

Bones of the spine	Position
Cervical	Seven bones. The first cervical bone is called the atlas. This sits on the second cervical vertebra known as the axis. The axis allows the head to rotate and the atlas supports the position of the skull.
Thoracic	Twelve bones. The ribs are attached to the thoracic vertebrae.
Lumbar	Five bones between the ribs and pelvis.
Sacral	Five fused bones between the pelvis.
Coccyx	Four fused bones that form a small tail at the base of the spine.

ACTIVITY

Working with a partner, ask them if they would be willing to remove their top and lean forward so that their vertebrae stand out. Try to locate each of the different types of vertebra.

Functions of the vertebral column

The functions of the vertebral column are to:

- protect the spinal cord
- provide a pathway for delicate spinal nerves to sit in while being protected
- allow flexion, extension and rotation
- support the skull
- absorb shock during movement to prevent tissue damage – there are soft intervertebral discs which sit in between the vertebrae to absorb shock during movement and prevent tissue damage
- provide attachment for other bones including the ribs, shoulder girdle, arms and pelvis
- provide attachment for muscles.

BONE STRUCTURE OF THE TORSO

Thorax

The thorax is the protective cavity for the chest and includes the ribs and sternum. The sternum runs down the centre of the chest and is commonly known as the breastbone. The ribs are long flat bones that run across the sides of the chest and there are 12 pairs in total. At the front of the body they are attached to the sternum and at the back of the body they are attached to the vertebrae.

Shoulder girdle

The shoulder girdle includes:

- two scapulae – the large bones at the top of the back that look like wings
- two clavicles – the bones at the front that sit across the shoulders
- the upper ends of the two humerus bones – the bones of the upper arm.

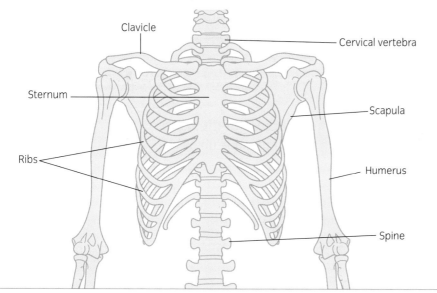

Front view of the chest, neck and shoulders

INDUSTRY TIP

The female pelvic girdle is wider and lighter than the male pelvic girdle to make childbirth easier.

Pelvic girdle

The pelvic girdle is made up of:

- the sacrum – the large, triangular bone at the base of the spine
- the pelvis which consists of two hip bones.

Each hip bone is made up of three fused bones:

- the ilium, which is the largest bone of the pelvis, forms the synovial joint (sacroiliac joint) with the sacrum
- the ischium which takes the weight of the body when sitting down
- the pubis – the pubic bones are found between the legs.

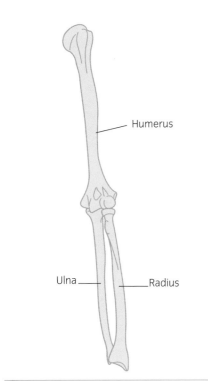

Bones of the arm

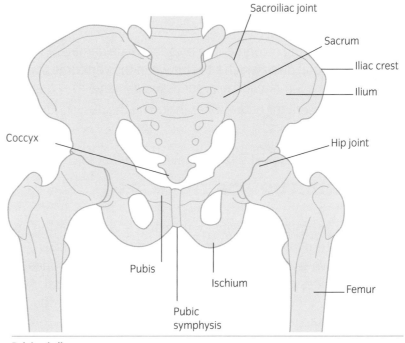

Pelvic girdle

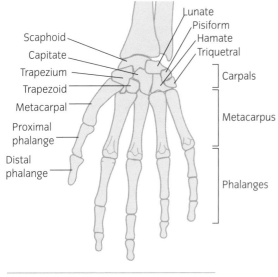

Bones of the hand

Metacarpals

Bones of the hand

BONE STRUCTURE OF THE UPPER LIMBS

Bone structure of the arms

The arms are made up of the:

- humerus – upper arm
- ulna (forearm) – runs along the little finger side of the forearm
- radius (forearm) – runs along the side of the thumb in the forearm.

Bone structure of the hands

The hands are made up of:

- eight carpals (wrist): triquetral, lunate, scaphoid, trapezium, trapezoid, pisiform, hamate and capitate (these form the wrist)
- five **metacarpals** (these form the palm of the hand)
- 14 phalanges (these form the fingers).

BONE STRUCTURE OF THE LOWER LIMBS

Bone structure of the legs

The legs are made up of the:

- femur – forms the thigh and is the longest bone in the body
- patella – the knee cap
- tibia – on the big toe side of the lower leg and commonly called the shin bone
- fibula – on the little toe side of the lower leg.

Bone structure of the feet

The feet are made up of:

- seven tarsals (the ankle): talus, calcaneus (or heel bone), cuboid, central cuneiform, medial cuneiform, lateral cuneiform, navicular
- five **metatarsals** (the main part of the foot)
- 14 phalanges (form the toes).

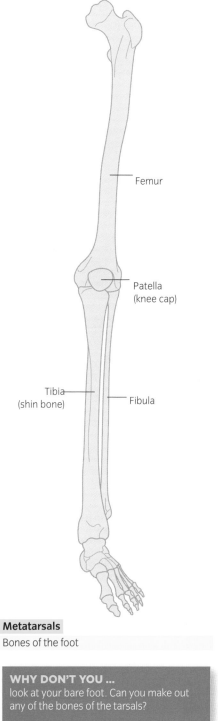

Femur

Patella (knee cap)

Tibia (shin bone)

Fibula

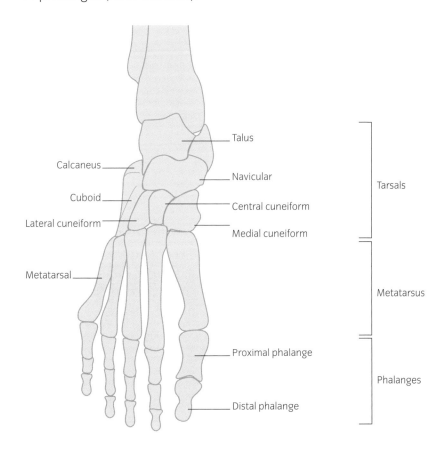

Talus

Calcaneus

Navicular

Cuboid

Central cuneiform

Lateral cuneiform

Medial cuneiform

Metatarsal

Proximal phalange

Distal phalange

Tarsals

Metatarsus

Phalanges

Metatarsals
Bones of the foot

WHY DON'T YOU ...
look at your bare foot. Can you make out any of the bones of the tarsals?

JOINTS

A joint is where two bones meet. Muscles and tendons stretch across joints when they move. Joints are **classified** by their structure or by the way they move. There are three main types of joints:

- fibrous or fixed joints
- cartilaginous/slightly moveable joints
- synovial/freely moveable joints.

FIBROUS/FIXED JOINTS

These joints are tightly linked with a tough fibrous material and have virtually no movement (eg the skull).

Classified
Grouped or arranged by a particular category or type

CARTILAGINOUS/SLIGHTLY MOVEABLE JOINTS

These joints are formed by a pad of tough fibrous cartilage and have no movement or only a limited range of movement. The pad acts as a shock absorber (eg joints between the vertebrae).

SYNOVIAL JOINTS/FREELY MOVEABLE JOINTS

These joints have a range of movement. The majority of joints in the body are synovial. Each bone end is covered with a smooth coating of cartilage. In the small space between the bones is a liquid called synovial fluid which is a **lubricant**. Around the synovial fluid is a capsule to hold the joint in place. Ligaments provide stability to the joint.

Lubricant

A substance that reduces friction and allows smooth movement

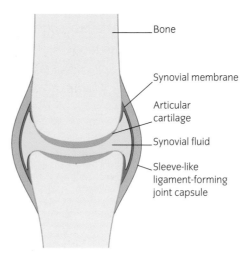

- Bone
- Synovial membrane
- Articular cartilage
- Synovial fluid
- Sleeve-like ligament-forming joint capsule

Types of synovial joints

Type of synovial joint	Description	Movement range
Ball and socket	The rounded end of one bone fits into a neat cup-shaped cavity in another bone (eg the shoulder and hip).	Flexion, extension, adduction, abduction, rotation and circumduction. See page 68 for more details.
Hinge	The convex (rounded outward) surface of the end of one bone fits into the concave surface of a second bone (or bones), eg elbow and knee. (Think of the hinge of a door.)	Flexion and extension.

Type of synovial joint	Description	Movement range
Pivot	A bony projection from one joint turns within the ring-shaped socket of another. The top two cervical vertebrae allow the head to turn from side to side.	Rotation.
Gliding/plane	The surfaces of the bone are almost flat and glide over each other (eg **tarsals** and **metatarsals**).	Range is limited.
Condyloid	This is a smooth rounded **projection** on a bone which sits into a cup-shaped depression on another bone (eg mandible and temporal bone, metacarpal and phalange).	Flexion, extension, abduction, adduction and circumduction.
Saddle	The surfaces of the two bones that meet have both concave and convex surfaces. There is only one saddle joint in the body at the base of the thumb.	Movement range is similar to condyloid.

Tarsals
Bones of the ankle and heel

Metatarsals
Bones of the foot

Projection
A part that sticks out

TYPES OF JOINT MOVEMENT

Type of movement	Description
Abduction	A movement away from the body.
Adduction	A movement towards the body.
Flexion	A bending movement bringing two level joints together.
Extension	Straightening a joint (ie taking two levers away from each other).
Rotation	The movement of a bone in a circle around fixed points.
Circumduction	The movement of a limb or finger with little movement where it is attached and greater movement at the end. For example, where the little finger is attached to the hand its movement is small but the finer tip can draw a large circle.

ACTIVITY

Stand up and go through each of the types of movement so that you are familiar with them.

SKELETAL CONDITIONS THAT RESTRICT OR PREVENT TREATMENT

Skeletal conditions can be easily overlooked as they are hidden away from view inside the body. It is important to remember that whether something is inside or not the body needs time to repair itself. Damage can be done if the body is not allowed time to heal properly. The conditions below will require you to **modify** your treatment. You should not work over the area directly around a sprain or broken bone.

Modify

adapt or make changes to your treatment

Skeletal condition/disorder	Description and cause	Contra-indications and general precautions	Advice for client
Bunion	A displacement and inflammation of the big toe joint. Fluid collects around the joint. Caused by repeated pressure on the side of the first metatarsal, commonly from wearing tight, poorly fitting shoes.	Not contra-indicated. Take extra care as the joint might be very tender. Massage should be very gentle.	Seek advice from a medical practitioner or chiropodist if bunion is painful.
Broken and fractured bones	A fracture is a crack or break in the bone either across its width or diagonally across the bone shaft.\n\nA **compound break** or open fracture occurs when the bone breaks through the skin's surface. Closed fractures happen when the bone is still within the body. These can cause a lot of tissue damage in the area of the break. A greenstick fracture is where a long bone is fractured along the bone but not all the way through.	Contra-indicated. Do not treat the area until fully healed to prevent further damage.	Rebook the treatment once area has healed.
Sprains	Occurs when a ligament is over-stretched or torn. A common area for sprains is around the ankle joint. A sprain can occur as the result of a fall when the full force of the body's weight is placed onto a joint.	Contra-indicated. Do not treat until it is fully healed to prevent any further tissue damage or discomfort to the client.	Rebook the treatment once area has healed.

Compound break

An injury where there is a break in the skin around a broken bone

Skeletal condition/disorder	Description and cause	Contra-indications and general precautions	Advice for client
Rheumatoid arthritis	A **chronic**, **progressive** disorder of the immune system. The synovial joints and surrounding tissues become damaged and inflamed. Symptoms include inflammation of the synovial joints. The joints become deformed and painful and there is loss of movement.	Contra-indicated. Avoid the affected area.	Seek medical advice.
Osteoarthritis	Causes restricted movement and pain in the affected joints. The **articular cartilage** thins and eventually the surfaces rub against each other. Symptoms include pain, swelling, stiffness and enlarged joints with some loss of joint movement.	Contra-indicated. Treat joints gently and with extra care.	Seek medical advice.
Gout	A disorder related to the metabolism. Uric acid crystals are deposited in the joints and tendons. It can be related to kidney problems. The joint becomes red, swollen and very tender. It usually affects a single joint.	Contra-indicated. Avoid the affected area.	Seek medical advice.
Bursitis	Inflammation of the **bursa**. Usually the result of friction or slight injury to the membrane surrounding the joint.	Contra-indicated. Avoid the affected area. Advise client to seek medical advice.	Seek medical advice and treatment.
Torn cartilage	Cartilage can tear when a sudden load is applied to a joint. It might cause the cartilage to fail completely. Symptoms include pain, swelling and restricted joint movement.	Contra-indicated. Avoid the affected area.	Seek specialist advice and treatment.

Skeletal condition/disorder	Description and cause	Contra-indications and general precautions	Advice for client
Tendonitis	Inflammation of the tendon causing pain and possibly restricted movement.	Contra-indicated. Avoid the affected area.	Seek specialist advice and treatment.
Dislocation	Damage to the soft tissue, tendons and ligaments around the bones causing the two joints to become **displaced**.	Contra-indicated. Avoid the affected limb and area. The joint will be painful with restricted movement.	Seek specialist advice and treatment.
Osteoporosis	Bone **density** is reduced making the bone weak and brittle. Bone is broken down at a greater rate than new bone is produced. The disease is associated with ageing, certain medication (eg steroids) and the menopause. There are no obvious symptoms.	Contra-indicated to mechanical massage. Treat gently and lightly to avoid any damage.	Refer client to a medical practitioner. A bone scan will confirm diagnosis. Regular **weight-bearing exercise** will be beneficial as it helps to build and support the bones.
Rickets	Caused by a deficiency of calcium, phosphate and vitamin D in the diet. Causes a condition called **osteomalacia** in adults.	Treat with caution.	Seek specialist advice and treatment.

Chronic
Long term

Progressive
Increasing in severity

Articular cartilage
Smooth white tissue that covers the ends of bones where they form joints

Bursa
A fluid-filled sac between the bone and tendon that prevents friction

Displaced
Moved from its original position

Density
Compactness

Weight-bearing exercise
Exercise that places weight on bones (eg walking)

Osteomalacia
A softening of the bones

Skeletal condition/disorder	Description and cause	Contra-indications and general precautions	Advice for client
Hammer toes	A **deformity** of the tendons in the toe joints. Causes the toes to become bent.	Treat with caution.	Seek specialist advice and treatment.

Deformity

Distortion or imperfection

DISORDERS OF THE SPINE

Disorder	Description and cause	Contra-indications and general precautions	Advice for client
Scoliosis	A **lateral** curvature of the spine in the thoracic region of the spine. May be caused by deformities of the bones and spine and poor posture. Signs of scoliosis include: ■ a difference in height between both ears and both shoulders. ■ twisted scapula and torso ■ curved spine ■ twisted pelvis with one leg shorter than the other.	Treat with caution. Might be visible when carrying out a full body consultation.	Seek professional advice from a medical practitioner or an alternative practitioner, such as an osteopath. Balancing and strengthening exercises and yoga and Pilates are beneficial.
Kyphosis	Rounding of the shoulders and back in the thoracic region. The pectoral muscles become tight and the back muscles are over-stretched. Might cause back pain in the thoracic region. Causes include poor posture (eg as a result of leaning over a keyboard) and disease of the joints.	Not contra-indicated.	Seek professional advice from a medical practitioner or an alternative practitioner, such as an osteopath. Balancing and strengthening exercises and yoga and Pilates are beneficial.

Disorder	Description and cause	Contra-indications and general precautions	Advice for client
Lordosis	Curvature of the lumbar spine. Can be seen as a hollow in the lower back. The pelvis tilts forward and the **gluteal muscles** stick out.	Not contra-indicated.	Seek professional advice from a medical practitioner or an alternative practitioner, such as an osteopath. Balancing and strengthening exercises and yoga and Pilates are beneficial for correction of the pelvic tilt and to strengthen the abdominal, core and back muscles.
Herniated or prolapsed disc (slipped disc)	An intervertebral disc ruptures and part of the disc **protrudes** placing pressure on the nerve. Often caused by sudden strenuous activity. Can be part of the ageing process as the result of the wearing out of the discs.	Contra-indicated. Avoid back area and mechanical G5 massage. Provide additional support for the client.	Seek medical advice.

Lateral
From side to side

Gluteal muscles
Buttock muscles

Protrudes
Sticks out

ACTIVITY

Working with a partner, try to identify the curves of the spine. Make a note of whether the curve is a natural curve, flattened or exaggerated.

MUSCULAR SYSTEM

Our muscular system includes all the muscle tissue in the body. Muscle tissue enables movement, maintains posture and is vital for the function of the organs of the body. All muscle tissue has four common properties. It can:

- respond to stimuli from the nervous system
- contract in response to a stimulus
- be stretched without damaging its structure
- return to its original shape after contraction (ie it is elastic).

In this part of the chapter you will learn about:

- the types of muscle tissue
- the functions of the muscular system
- muscles of the body
- disorders of the muscular system.

Conscious

When you are aware of what you are doing; deliberate

Respiratory

Relating to the system for taking in oxygen and giving out carbon dioxide (ie breathing)

TYPES OF MUSCLE TISSUE

There are three types of muscle tissue:

- cardiac muscle
- smooth, involuntary muscle
- skeletal, striated or voluntary muscle.

CARDIAC MUSCLE

This is a specialised type of muscle tissue found only in the heart.

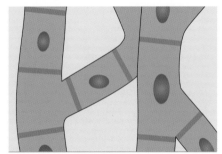

Cardiac muscle tissue

SMOOTH, INVOLUNTARY MUSCLE

This is not under **conscious** control and is found in the walls of hollow organs (ie blood and lymph vessels, the alimentary canal (digestive system), the **respiratory** tract, bladder, uterus and ducts of glands).

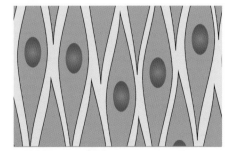

Involuntary muscle tissue

SKELETAL, STRIATED OR VOLUNTARY MUSCLE

These muscles are under conscious control. A tiny motor nerve carries messages from the central nervous system to the muscles to stimulate them into action. There are 650 named muscles in our body; 150 of these muscles are in the head and neck. Skeletal muscles make up about 40 to 50% of our body weight. Each muscle is made up of thousands of long narrow cells which look like fibres. These cells are surrounded by a tough sheath.

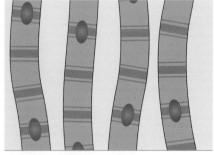

Skeletal muscle tissue

The structure of the cells in skeletal muscles

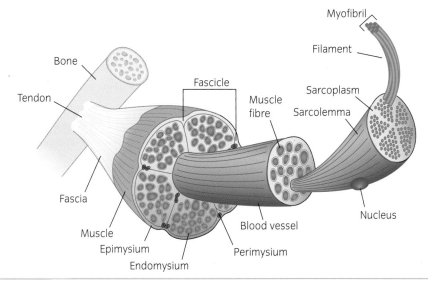

A cross-section of a skeletal muscle

Muscles are covered in a layer called the epimysium or muscle fascia. The epimysium has a smooth surface which protects the muscle from friction against other muscles and bones and allows it to move easily against other structures.

Each muscle is made up of hundreds of small fibres called myofibrils. Myofibrils are made up of even smaller protein filaments called actin and myosin. Myosin forms thick filaments and actin forms thin filaments. It is bundles of the thick filaments and thin filaments that give muscle tissue its striped appearance. A sarcomere is the smallest unit of skeletal muscle that can contract. Myofibrils are made up of rows of sarcomeres.

Myofibrils are bundled together (in bundles of between 10 and 100 muscle fibres) to form a fascicle. Each individual muscle fibre within the fascicle is covered by a fibrous connective tissue called endomysium which insulates the fibres and helps to keep the muscle in an organised structure.

The whole fascicle is also surrounded by a layer of protective tissue called the perimysium.

Nerves and blood vessels run along and through the layers of connective tissue to supply the muscle fibres. Each fibre is linked to the central nervous system by a tiny nerve. **Motor nerves** carry messages from the central nervous system to the muscles to stimulate them to contract.

Motor nerve
A nerve carrying impulses from the brain or spinal cord to a muscle

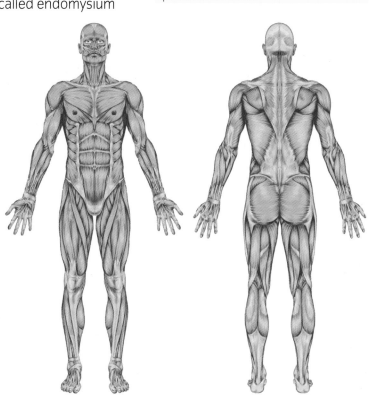

THE FUNCTIONS OF THE MUSCULAR SYSTEM

The muscular system has several functions:

- Movement – movement happens as a result of the shortening (contracting) and the lengthening (relaxing) of muscle tissue.

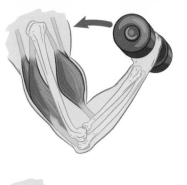

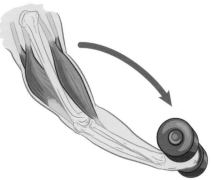

A muscle contracting and relaxing during exercise

Glycogen
A polysaccharide stored in the liver and muscles. It is converted to glucose to provide skeletal muscles with energy

SmartScreen 307 Worksheet 3

SmartScreen 305 Worksheets 7 and 8

- Posture – some of the muscle's fibres are always contracted even when the muscle is at rest. Otherwise the body would not be able to function. This is essential for maintaining posture. This muscle tone is weakest when we are sleeping and in a relaxed state. Muscle tone makes sure enough blood supply reaches the muscles.
- Creation of heat – muscular activity creates heat in the cellular tissues.
- Assists with blood flow and lymphatic movement – muscular movement squeezes the blood and lymph vessels, which helps both blood flow and lymphatic movement.
- Protection – some muscles also help to provide protection for some of the abdominal organs.

MUSCLE CONTRACTION

Muscle contractions occur every time we move. Muscles contract (shorten) when they are stimulated by a nerve. A stronger muscle contraction will take place when more muscle fibres are stimulated. Contraction needs energy in the form of adenosine triphosphate (ATP) which is made from glucose.

Glucose from our food is taken to the muscles by the blood and stored as glycogen until it is needed. When muscles require energy, a metabolic process breaks down the **glycogen** to release energy. The glycogen is combined with oxygen from the blood and forms ATP to provide energy for the contraction. If there is not enough oxygen to keep this process going lactic acid is formed which causes tiredness (fatigue) in the muscles. Lactic acid can cause the muscles to ache and feel weak.

MUSCLES OF THE BODY

MUSCLES OF THE HEAD AND FACE

The muscles of our face define our features. They give us expression and show our age. You will find it particularly helpful to know the location and action of each muscle during massage treatments.

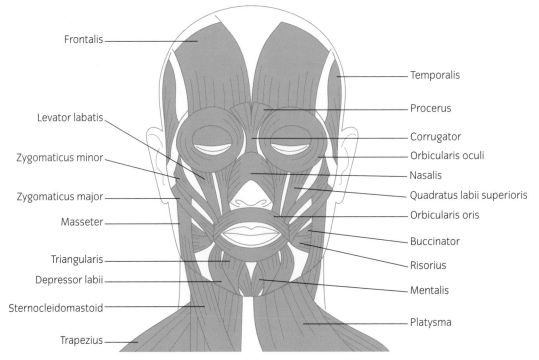

Frontalis
Temporalis
Procerus
Levator labatis
Corrugator
Zygomaticus minor
Orbicularis oculi
Nasalis
Zygomaticus major
Quadratus labii superioris
Masseter
Orbicularis oris
Buccinator
Triangularis
Risorius
Depressor labii
Mentalis
Sternocleidomastoid
Platysma
Trapezius

Facial muscle	Position	Action
Occipitalis	At the back of the cranium at the base.	Moves the scalp.
Frontalis	Runs along the forehead.	Raises the eyebrows and helps you frown by wrinkling forehead.
Temporalis	Side of the head stretching to the mandible (jaw).	Raises the mandible during chewing.
Orbicularis oculi	Surrounds the eye socket.	Closes the eyelids.
Corrugator	Between the eyebrows.	**Depresses** the forehead to frown.
Buccinator	At the sides of the cheek.	Squeezes the cheeks together during chewing.
Risorius	Found at the corners of the mouth.	Lifts the corner of the mouth into a smile.
Quadratus labii superioris	At the sides of the upper lip across the top of the maxilla and zygomatic bone.	Lifts the upper lip.
Depressor labii	Runs down the chin from the lower lip.	Pulls the lower lip down.
Procerus	Between the brows, extending down to the nasal bone.	Draws the eyebrows down in a frown and wrinkles nose.
Nasalis	Crosses of the bridge of the nose.	There are two parts to this muscle – one part dilates the nostrils and one part constricts the nostrils.
Triangularis	Outer part of the mandible.	Draws the sides of mouth down.
Orbicularis oris	Around the mouth.	Closes the mouth and pouts the lips.
Masseter	Sides of face.	Raises the lower jaw and helps us to chew food.
Zygomaticus major/minor	Along the cheek.	Raises the corner of the mouth into a smile.
Mentalis	Over the chin.	Allows the lower lip to pout.
Sternocleidomastoid	Sides of neck.	When the muscles work singularly they help to rotate the head. Together they pull the head forward (chin down).
Platysma	From the chin down the front of neck.	Draws the corners of mouth down, lowers the mandible and maintains skin texture.

INDUSTRY TIP

If you confuse orbicularis oris and oculi remember the i at the end of oculi for eye.

Depresses

Pushes down into a lower position

 SmartScreen 306 Worksheet 5

MUSCLES OF THE SHOULDER, ARM AND HAND

It is important to be aware of these muscles during body treatments that include the shoulders, arms and hands.

SmartScreen 207 Worksheet 3

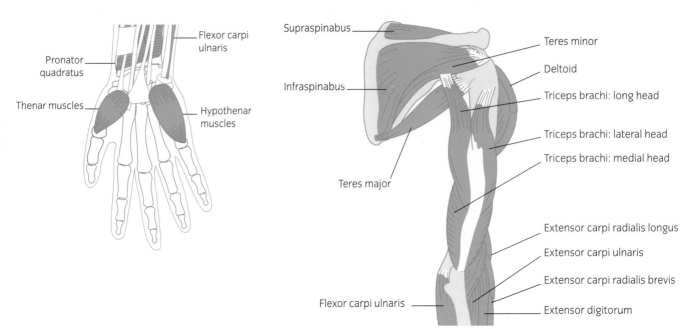

Muscles in the shoulder, arm and hand	Position	Action
Deltoid	Lies over the shoulder (like a shoulder pad).	Draws the arm backwards and forwards. **Abducts** the arm.
Levator scapula	At the back of the neck between the cervical vertebrae and the scapula.	Lifts the shoulder and rotates the scapula.
Biceps	Front of the upper arm.	Turns and flexes the forearm. Flexion of the forearm at the elbow.
Triceps	Back of the upper arm.	Extension of the arm at the elbow.
Extensor carpi radialis longus	Covering the back of the forearm.	Extends and abducts the wrist.
Extensor carpi ulnaris	Covering the back of the forearm.	Extends the wrist and **adducts** the hand.
Extensor carpi radialis brevis	Inner side of the forearm.	Extends and abducts the wrist and flexes the forearm.
Flexor carpi radialis	Front of the forearm.	Flexes and abducts the hands.
Flexor carpi ulnaris	Front of the forearm.	Flexes and adducts the ulna.
Extensor digitorum	Back of the forearm.	Extends the fingers and the wrist.
Thenar eminence	This is a group of small muscles located in the thumb and palm of the hand.	Movement of the thumb.

Abduct

To move a muscle or limb away from the midline of the body or from another part of the body

Adduct

To move a muscle or limb towards the midline of the body or towards another part of the body

MUSCLES OF THE THORAX AND ABDOMEN

The muscles of the thorax and abdomen are involved in movement of the torso. It is important to be aware of these muscles during body treatments that include the back, chest and abdomen.

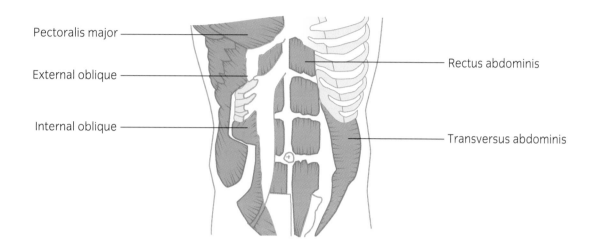

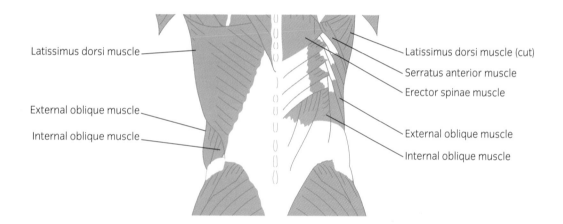

Muscles of the thorax and abdomen	Position	Action
Trapezius	A large diamond-shaped muscle that extends from the occipital bone to the vertebrae in the thoracic region.	Lifts and braces the shoulders and rotates the scapula.
Pectoralis major	Front of the chest.	Flexion, adduction and rotation of the upper arm. Draws the arm across chest.
Sacrospinalis (erector spinae)	Group of muscles either side of the spinal column.	Rotates the body and extends the spine. Maintains posture of the trunk.
Latissimus dorsi	Large, flat triangular muscle covering the lower back. Stretches from the lower part of the spine to the upper part of the humerus.	Draws upper arm downwards and backwards. Rotates the upper arm.
Serratus anterior	Starts on the upper ribs at the side of the chest along the side of the scapula.	Holds the scapula in position during movement. Pulls the shoulder forward. Rotates the shoulder.

Muscles of the thorax and abdomen	Position	Action
Quadratus lumborum	Forms part of the **posterior** abdominal wall.	Helps extend and stabilise the lower back. Allows straightening of the spine (ie standing straight). Adducts trunk.
External obliques	Either side of the rectus abdominis. Forms the sides of the abdomen.	Help maintain posture and **compresses** the abdomen. Allows rotation, flexion and sideways bending of the trunk.
Rectus abdominis	Forms the **anterior** wall of the abdomen. Runs from the pubis to the ribs.	Flexion of the spinal column and the trunk.
Internal obliques	A pair of muscles just below the external oblique muscles. Found at the sides of the abdomen.	Along with external obliques, help maintain posture and compress the abdomen. Allow rotation, flexion and sideways bending of the trunk.
Transversus abdominis	Wraps around the trunk from the front to the back. Extends from the ribs to the pubis.	Helps compress abdomen and internal organs. Stabilises the spine and helps with breathing.

Posterior
At the back of the body

Compress
To squeeze or press

Anterior
In the front of the body

MUSCLES OF THE HIP, LEG AND FOOT

There are some large muscles that give the leg its shape and definition. There are lots of smaller muscles that attach to different bones to flex and extend the leg, foot and toes.

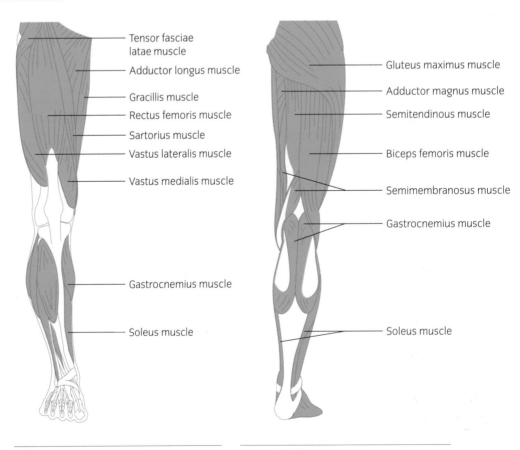

Tensor fasciae latae muscle
Adductor longus muscle
Gracillis muscle
Rectus femoris muscle
Sartorius muscle
Vastus lateralis muscle
Vastus medialis muscle
Gastrocnemius muscle
Soleus muscle

Gluteus maximus muscle
Adductor magnus muscle
Semitendinous muscle
Biceps femoris muscle
Semimembranosus muscle
Gastrocnemius muscle
Soleus muscle

Anterior of the leg

Posterior of the leg

Anterior muscles of the leg and hip

Anterior muscles of the leg and hip	Position	Action
Tensor fasciae latae	**Lateral** side of the outer thigh. Runs from the ilium down into a tendon that attaches to the tibia.	Flexes and abducts the hip. Rotates the lower leg.
Sartorius	Runs diagonally across the front of the thigh.	Abducts thigh and hip, flexes hip and knee and external rotation of the thigh.
Hip adductors: • Adductor longus • Adductor brevis • Adductor magnus • Pectineus	Upper inner thigh.	Adducts hip, rotates thigh and extends hip.
Gracilis	Runs down the inner thigh from the pelvis to the top of the tibia.	Adducts leg and flexes hip and knee joints.
Quadriceps: • Vastus lateralis • Vastus intermedius • Vastus medialis • Rectus femoris	Front of the thigh.	Extend the knee and flex the hip.
Tibialis anterior	Runs along the outside of the tibia.	Inverts the foot, flexes the foot.

Posterior muscles of the leg and hip

Posterior muscles of the leg and hip	Position	Action
Gluteus maximus	Forms the buttocks.	Extends, flexes, rotates and adducts hip joints and the legs.
Hamstrings: • Biceps femoris • Semimembranosus • Semitendinosus	Back of the thigh. Semimembranosus and semitendinosus are on inner thigh and biceps femoris is on outside of thigh.	Extend thigh and hip and flex the knee.
Gastrocnemius	Forms the bulk of the calf at the back of the lower leg.	**Plantar** flexion of the ankle. Flexes the leg at the knee joint.
Soleus	Lies under the gastrocnemius.	Plantar flexion of the foot.

Muscles of the foot

Muscles of the foot	Position	Action
Flexors of the toes – flexor digitorium brevis, flexor digitorium accessories, flexor hallucis brevis	The lower leg and to the heel of the foot.	Flexes the toes.
Extensors of the toes – extensor digitorium brevis, extensor digitorum, longus, entensor hallucis longus	The lower leg and the foot.	Extends the toes and flexes the ankle.

Plantar Sole of the foot		**Lateral** On one side of the body or other

DISORDERS OF THE MUSCULAR SYSTEM

Disorder	Description and cause	Contra-indications and general precautions	Advice for client
Fibrositis	Pain and stiffness in the muscles. Movement is not restricted.	Not contra-indicated. Treat with caution if painful.	Seek professional advice from a medical practitioner or an alternative practitioner, such as an osteopath.
Lumbago	Lower back pain.	Contra-indicated depending on cause. Treat with caution.	Seek professional advice from a medical practitioner or an alternative practitioner, such as an osteopath, if the cause is unknown.
Muscular dystrophy	Progressive muscle wasting and weakness. Can affect the muscles and nerves of the limbs or the heart and lungs. Symptoms vary depending on the type of muscular dystrophy.	Contra-indicated without medical advice.	Seek medical advice before treatment.
Repetitive strain injuries (RSIs)	Soft tissue injury (eg tennis/golfer's elbow, tendonitis, carpal tunnel syndrome) caused by over-use. Symptoms include pain, tenderness and weakness in the joint.	Not contra-indicated. Treat with caution. Massage is very beneficial.	Rest the affected area. Seek professional advice from a medical practitioner or an alternative practitioner, such as an osteopath.

CARDIOVASCULAR SYSTEM

Nutrients
Substances that help us live and grow

Immunity
Protection from a disease

The cardiovascular system includes the heart, blood vessels and blood cells. The blood is the transport system of the body making sure that the body is provided with the essential **nutrients** it needs to function. The blood cells play a crucial role in fighting infection and proving **immunity**.

In this part of the chapter you will learn about:
- the heart
- the functions of blood
- the composition of blood
- blood vessels
- blood pressure
- disorders of the cardiovascular system.

HEART

The heart is a powerful pear-shaped muscular organ that sits in the centre of the chest, tilted at its base slightly to the left side. It sits behind the sternum between the lungs. It is surrounded by a protective membrane called the pericardium. The pericardium is a fluid-filled cavity which prevents any friction between the heart and the surrounding tissues. The four chambers of the heart vary in size according to the work being done. The atrium walls are very thin, as they only have to push blood into the ventricles. The ventricles are very thick as they have to push blood around the body.

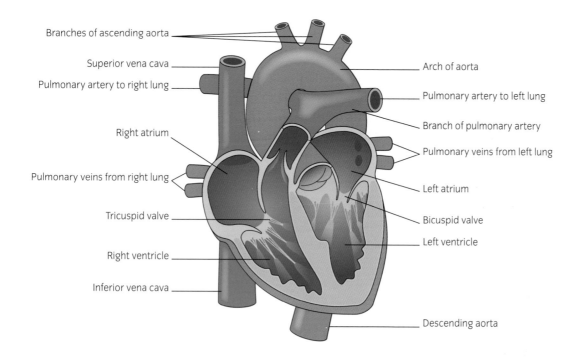

Branches of ascending aorta
Superior vena cava
Pulmonary artery to right lung
Right atrium
Pulmonary veins from right lung
Tricuspid valve
Right ventricle
Inferior vena cava

Arch of aorta
Pulmonary artery to left lung
Branch of pulmonary artery
Pulmonary veins from left lung
Left atrium
Bicuspid valve
Left ventricle
Descending aorta

BLOOD VESSELS OF THE HEART

The most important blood vessels in the **coronary circulatory system** are:

- the vena cava which carries blood from the body into the right atrium
- the pulmonary vein which carries blood from the lungs into the left atrium
- the aorta which carries blood from the left ventricle to the tissues on the left side of the body
- the pulmonary artery which carries blood from the right ventricle to the lungs.

Coronary circulatory system
The system that provides blood to the heart

FUNCTIONS OF BLOOD

Our blood can be described as our life force, making sure our cells have all the essential supplies they need and keeping **micro-organisms** at bay.

The blood has several essential functions which are important for the body to survive. These functions can be divided into two main areas:

- transportation
- protection.

Micro-organism
A very small living thing that can only be seen through a microscope

Haemoglobin
A protein that gives red blood cells their colour. Their main function is to transport oxygen from the lungs to the body's tissues

Elimination
Getting rid of something

Excretion
The process of getting rid of waste

Invasion
Entering uninvited

Phagocytic
Describing the process in which a **phagocyte** absorbs bacteria

Phagocyte
A type of cell within the body capable of absorbing bacteria

Neutrophil
A type of white blood cell

Monocyte
A type of white blood cell

Antibody
Proteins produced in response to an **antigen** to neutralise it

Antigen
A foreign body or toxin which stimulates an immune response in the body

Antitoxin
A protein produced in response to a toxin to neutralise it

Conduction
The passing of heat or electricity from one object to another

Convection
The movement of heat through a liquid or gas

Superficial
On the surface; not deep penetrating

Concentration
The amount of something within a liquid

Homeostasis
The body needs to maintain a constant state of internal balance. If one or more of the systems of the body gets out of balance, ill health and disease can occur

Anticoagulant
A substance that prevents clotting

TRANSPORTATION

The erythrocytes transport oxygen attached to **haemoglobin** from the lungs to the body's cells and return carbon dioxide from the cells to the lungs for **elimination**. Hormones and enzymes are transported from their cells of production to their target organs and tissues.

The blood supplies nourishment to the cells. Nutrients are absorbed from the small intestine into the bloodstream and are transported to where they are needed.

The circulation removes waste products from the cells and surrounding tissues. These waste materials are transported to liver to be prepared for removal and to the kidneys for **excretion**.

PROTECTION

White blood cells defend the body against the **invasion** of micro-organisms and their toxins. They achieve this through:

- the **phagocytic** action of **neutrophils** and **monocytes**
- the presence of **antibodies** and **antitoxins**.

Blood clotting prevents the loss of any body fluid and blood cells when the tissues are injured.

The blood helps to maintain the body's temperature. Chemical activity in the cells and tissues produces heat. This heat makes the blood warm as it circulates. If the body produces too much heat the blood vessels near the surface of the body dilate and heat is lost by radiation, **conduction, convection** and the evaporation of sweat. If the external temperature is cold, the **superficial** blood vessels constrict to prevent heat loss.

COMPOSITION OF BLOOD

Blood accounts for 7–9% of our total body weight and we have approximately 5.6 litres of this red viscous liquid flowing around our bodies. Around 55% of blood is plasma and the other 45% is made up from the different blood cells. The volume and **concentration** of our blood must be kept within narrow limits to maintain **homeostasis**.

RED BLOOD CELLS (ERYTHROCYTES)

Red blood cells account for 45% of all the blood cells. They contain the molecule haemoglobin which combines with oxygen to allow it to be transported around the body. Red blood cells are manufactured in the bone marrow of the short bones (ribs) and the ends of the long bones.

WHITE BLOOD CELLS (LEUKOCYTES)

White blood cells, also called leukocytes or white corpuscles, account for 1% of the blood. They vary in size, shape and function.

Granulocytes are the most numerous type of white blood cells. They are formed in the bone marrow. There are three different types of granulocytes. Each type has a specific function in response to injury and inflammation:

- eosinophils protect the body from foreign pathogens
- basophils contain an **anticoagulant** and histamine and are important in allergic reactions

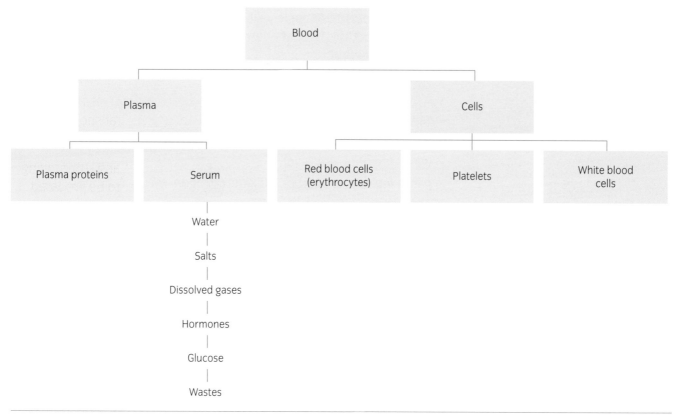

Components of blood

- neutrophils are attracted to the site being invaded by micro-organisms and ingest foreign particles and damaged tissue through the process of **phagocytosis.**

Agranulocytes
These account for 25–50% of all leukocytes. There are two types of agranulocytes.

Monocytes
These cells are formed in the red bone marrow. There are two different types of monocytes:

- a phagocytic monocyte that engulfs germs
- a macrophage which has an important function in inflammation and immunity.

Lymphocytes
Lymphocytes circulate within the blood and are also found in lymphoid tissue. Unlike other blood cells they are also developed in the lymphoid tissue as well in the red bone marrow. Larger lymphocytes play an essential role in immunity and help the body to recover. Lymphocytes respond to specific antigens and produce antibodies. Antigens and antibodies work together. There are two different types of lymphocytes:

- **T-lymphocytes** combat and destroy cells containing antigens.
- **B-lymphocytes** are involved in the production of the antibodies that neutralise antigens.

> **Phagocytosis**
> Phagocytes absorb bacteria and digest them to help the body to dispose of unwanted matter such as dirt and dead body cells

PLASMA

Plasma is a transparent pale yellow fluid. If you remove all the blood cells from the blood, this is what is left. Plasma is made up of many important elements including:

- water
- blood proteins
- salts and minerals (eg sodium chloride)
- food substances (eg amino acids, glucose, fats)
- waste (eg urea, uric acid)
- gases (eg oxygen, carbon dioxide, nitrogen)
- enzymes
- antibodies
- hormones
- antitoxins.

THROMBOCYTES (PLATELETS)

These are small fragments in the blood and play an essential role in blood clotting. When a blood vessel is damaged the blood vessels constrict and the thrombocytes stick to the damaged wall. They form a thread-like mesh to prevent any further blood escaping.

ACTIVITY

Discuss with your tutor or manager what effect you think a poor circulation will have on a client and how this may be noticed during our treatment. Which treatments do you think will be beneficial and why?

BLOOD VESSELS

The blood vessels are our transport system and are responsible for transporting blood around the body. They carry blood from the heart to the tissues and back to the heart again.

ARTERIES

Arteries are blood vessels that carry oxygenated blood *away* from the heart (with the exception of the pulmonary artery). The oxygen the blood is transporting is what gives it a bright red colour. Arteries are designed to withstand the high pressure **exerted** from the blood as it is pumped from the heart. Arteries vary in size but all have thick walls consisting of three layers of tissue. The middle layer is a thick layer of muscle. Arterioles are smaller blood vessels that branch out from an artery that lead to capillaries.

VEINS

Veins are the blood vessels that transport blood to the heart and carry deoxygenated blood (with the exception of the pulmonary vein). The blood is a dark purplish red as it is no longer carrying oxygen. The walls of the veins are much thinner than those of arteries and they have less muscle and elastic tissue. Muscular movement and breathing help to move blood along the veins in the body. The blood within veins is not under pressure unlike the blood flow in the arteries. Most veins contain

Exert

To apply pressure

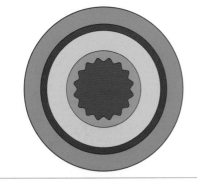

Artery

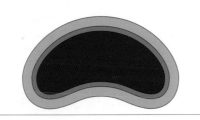

Vein

special valves which prevent blood from flowing back along the vein. The smallest veins are called venules.

CAPILLARIES

Capillaries are the smallest blood vessels. They link the arteries (carrying blood away from the heart) back to the veins (to return blood back to the heart). Capillary walls are only a single cell layer thick, and are **semipermeable**. Substances such as oxygen, vitamins, minerals, water and amino acids are able to move easily from the capillaries into the surrounding tissues to nourish and feed the cells. Substances such as carbon dioxide, cellular waste and water pass back into the capillaries to be removed. This simple process is known as capillary exchange. Due to their size, blood cells and large substances, such as plasma proteins, remain in the capillaries and cannot move out into the surrounding tissue unless the blood vessel is damaged.

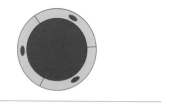

Capillary

Semipermeable
Allowing certain substances to pass through but not others

PRIMARY BLOOD VESSELS

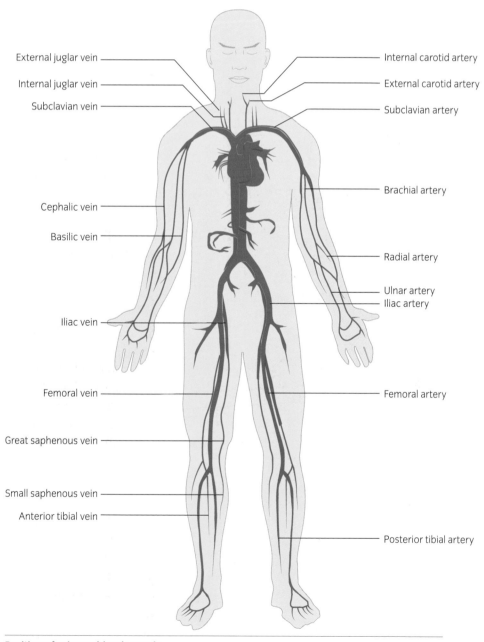

External juglar vein
Internal juglar vein
Subclavian vein
Cephalic vein
Basilic vein
Iliac vein
Femoral vein
Great saphenous vein
Small saphenous vein
Anterior tibial vein

Internal carotid artery
External carotid artery
Subclavian artery
Brachial artery
Radial artery
Ulnar artery
Iliac artery
Femoral artery
Posterior tibial artery

Position of primary blood vessels

You need to be familiar with the location of each of the blood vessels in the following tables.

BLOOD VESSELS OF THE HEAD, FACE AND NECK

The following blood vessels supply and remove blood from the tissues in head, face and neck.

Primary blood vessels in the head, face and neck	Position
Common carotid artery	Starts at the aorta and travels up either side of the neck. The vessels divide to become the internal and external carotid arteries.
External carotid artery	Travels up the side of the neck to the base of the skull where it divides into smaller vessels which branch off to supply the brain, eyes, forehead and nose.
Internal carotid artery	Travels up the inner side of the neck where it divides into smaller vessels which branch off to supply the superficial tissues of the head and neck.
External jugular vein	Starts at the jawline and travels down in front of the sternocleidomastoid muscle and behind the clavicle where it joins the subclavian vein.
Internal jugular vein	Begins in the middle of the cranium and travels down the neck behind the sternocleidomastoid muscle and the clavicle where it joins the subclavian vein.

ACTIVITY

If you feel the inside of your neck and press gently along the line of the sternocleidomastoid muscle with two fingers, you will feel the pulse of the carotid artery.

Primary blood vessels in the forearm, wrist and hand	Position
Brachial artery	Runs down the inner (medial) side of the upper arm, past the elbow where it divides into the radial and ulna arteries.
Radial artery	Travels down the ulnar side of the forearm to cross the wrist and into the hand.
Ulnar artery	Travels down the radial side of the forearm over the wrist and into the palm of the hand.

BLOOD VESSELS OF THE LOWER LEG, ANKLE AND FOOT

Primary blood vessels in the lower leg, ankle and foot	Position
Femoral artery	Begins at the ligament in the groin and travels down the front of the leg, it then runs **medially** across the thigh where it finishes in the popliteal space and becomes the popliteal artery
Anterior tibial artery	Travels from the tibia and fibula; it lies on the tibia and runs across the ankle joint.
Posterior tibial artery	Runs down the back of the leg and turns medially to the sole of the foot where it becomes the plantar artery.
Saphenous vein	The great saphenous vein is the longest vein in the body. It begins halfway up the top of the foot, travels up the medial side of the tibia and inner side of the thigh. It joins the femoral vein in the groin. The small saphenous vein starts behind the ankle joint. It travels up the back of the leg and joins the deep popliteal vein at the back of the knee.
Femoral vein	In the groin.

Medially
In the middle

ACTIVITY

If you feel the inside of your wrist and press gently with two fingers, you will feel the pulse of the radial artery.

WHY DON'T YOU ...
find the pulse in your wrist or neck. Compare your pulse with those of other colleagues and discuss your findings.

BLOOD PRESSURE

Blood pressure is the force or pressure the blood exerts on the walls of the blood vessels in which it is contained. Normal blood pressure is dependent on several factors:

- the function of the heart
- the blood volume
- the elasticity of the artery walls
- the **venous return**.

Simple changes can make the blood pressure go up or down.

Blood pressure will drop:

- if there is a loss in the volume of blood (eg from severe dehydration or blood loss)
- if you go into **shock**
- during deep relaxation.

It will increase:

- if there is fluid retention
- if there is excessive heat
- as a result of increased physical activity/exercise
- during vigorous massage.

Venous return
The blood flow back to the heart via the veins

Shock
A condition that occurs when the body isn't getting enough blood flow

 SmartScreen 306 Worksheet 12

 SmartScreen 307 Worksheet 7

DISORDERS OF THE CARDIOVASCULAR SYSTEM

The following medical conditions might require you to adapt or modify your treatment so it is important you are familiar with each of the following conditions.

Disorder	Description and cause	Contra-indications and general precautions	Advice for client
Low blood pressure (hypotension)	If blood pressure is too low, the vital organs will be unable to function properly. Can be caused by relaxation, heat, eating. Postural hypotension can be caused by getting up too quickly. There is a sudden drop in blood pressure as the body adjusts.	Not contra-indicated.	Take their time getting up or sitting up.
High blood pressure (hypertension)	Blood is pushing against the walls of the arteries too strongly. There is an increased risk of damage to the blood vessels and a risk of internal bleeding. Often caused by a hardening of the artery walls due to ageing. Other causes include being overweight, a lack of exercise, eating too much salt and stress.	Contra-indicated. There is a slightly higher risk of the client bruising more easily when they have high blood pressure. Make sure that their high blood pressure is being stabilised with medication before carrying out any treatments.	Seek medical advice if necessary.
Bruising	Caused by damage to the blood vessels allowing the blood to flow freely into the surrounding tissues. The skin tissue appears blue, black or yellow coloured. Caused by a sharp blow or by too much pressure being exerted on the body. Some medical conditions cause people to bruise more easily.	Contra-indicated. Modify treatment. Avoid bruised area to allow the body to repair and to prevent any further blood vessel damage.	None.

Disorder	Description and cause	Contra-indications and general precautions	Advice for client
Varicose veins	If one of the valves in the legs stops functioning properly the blood will collect in the vein and become swollen. During muscle movement the blood seeps into the surrounding tissues.	Contra-indicated. Avoid areas where there are visible varicose veins. Do not apply pressure to the area.	If client is concerned, seek medical advice before treatment. Raise the legs to help the blood flow return.
Deep vein thrombosis	A blood clot that partially or fully blocks a blood vessel. Caused by changes in the blood chemistry and long periods of inactivity.	Contra-indicated. If the client is not on medication and the thrombosis occurred over a year ago, treatment may be given with caution.	Seek medical advice.
Stroke	Damage to the brain caused by the blood supply to the brain being disrupted by a **thrombosis, embolism** or **haemorrhage**. May cause some damage to certain body functions and weakness or paralysis on one side of the body.	Contra-indicated until medical advice has been given.	Seek medical advice before treatment.

Thrombosis

Clotting of the blood in the circulatory system

Embolism

Blockage of an artery by a fragment of material travelling in the blood. This could be a thrombus (blood clot), air bubble or other fragment, such as bone

Haemorrhage

An escape of blood from a ruptured blood vessel

INDUSTRY TIP

If you suspect someone has had a stroke think FAST:

- **F**ace – Is it dropped on one side? Can they smile or stick their tongue out straight?
- **A**rms – Can they raise their arms above their head?
- **S**peech – Can they speak clearly without slurring?
- **T**rouble – If they have trouble with any of these tasks, call 999.

Disorder	Description and cause	Contra-indications and general precautions	Advice for client
Angina	Heaviness and pain in the chest. Caused by insufficient blood supply to the heart due to heart disease or **arteriosclerosis**.	Contra-indicated until medical advice has been given.	Seek medical advice before treatment.
Erythema	Increased circulation in the tiny capillaries near the skin's surface due to massage or trauma following waxing or eyebrow shaping. Appears as a reddening of the skin. In combination with irritation and tingling, it can be a sign of an adverse reaction.	Contra-indicated. Treatment might need to be adapted or rebooked. If erythema is present before treatment it may be a sign of skin damage (eg sunburn). Tactfully question the client and avoid the area during treatment. If erythema is severe avoid treatment.	Suggest the client rebooks once their skin has returned to normal.

Arteriosclerosis
Thickening and hardening of the walls of the arteries in old age

LYMPHATIC SYSTEM

The lymphatic system is a network of lymphatic vessels and lymphatic organs that stretches throughout the entire body. It provides transportation of nutrients to the tissues and drains excess fluid from the spaces between cells. The lymphatic system is one-way; it returns fluid to the bloodstream but cannot collect lymph from the bloodstream.

In this section you will learn about:
- the functions of the lymphatic system
- the structure of the lymphatic system
- the location and function of the major lymphatic nodes in the body
- disorders of the lymphatic system.

FUNCTIONS OF THE LYMPHATIC SYSTEM

The main function of the lymph nodes is to filter lymph and prevent infection. The lymphatic system has a crucial role in immunity, producing T- and B-lymphocytes and antibodies in the lymph nodes.

The system also helps to remove fluids from tissue in the body and remove fat into the bloodstream. Special lymphatic capillaries, called lacteals, collect microscopic molecules of fat from the small intestine. The fat then travels through the lymphatic system and is slowly emptied into the bloodstream.

IMMUNITY

One of the main functions of the lymphatic system is to create cells to help remove and destroy waste, toxins and debris. Immunity involves the interaction of antigens and antibodies.

Antigens

An antigen is a specialised protein that stimulates an immune response. Bacteria or viruses give off antigens which are recognised by the immune system as being harmful. The immune system then stimulates the production of antibodies.

Antibodies

Antibodies (immunoglobulins) are specialised **glycoproteins** that are secreted by white blood cells (lymphocytes) in the lymph nodes. They bind to receptors that **protrude** from the surface of the antigens and neutralise them.

Glycoprotein

A protein molecule that contains a carbohydrate

Protrude

Stick out from

Types of immunity

There are two types of immunity:

- Innate immunity – this type of immunity is present in humans at birth before they are exposed to pathogens or antigens.
- Adaptive immunity – this type of immunity develops when we have had contact with a pathogen. The body develops a defensive response and an army of immune cells attack the antigens given off by the pathogen. Our immune system remembers the pathogen for future responses.

Immunity to a specific pathogen can also be developed through immunisation. When we are immunised against a disease, the pathogen is deliberately introduced into the body. This causes an immune response in the body and antibodies are produced as a result of being immunised. For example, if you have the MMR immunisation, a very small amount of the measles, mumps and rubella viruses are introduced into the body and the body fights the viruses. This should mean that you are protected against measles, mumps and rubella in the future.

Autoimmune diseases

Antibodies are not always beneficial. The body can sometimes attack and destroy healthy body tissue by mistake. Rheumatoid arthritis is an example of an autoimmune disorder.

Allergies

Sometimes the immune system causes reactions that make the body very sensitive to a particular allergen that would not normally be dangerous (eg pollen). When this happens, we have an allergic reaction. Reactions can be so mild that they aren't noticeable or they can be life-threatening. An extremely severe allergic reaction is called an anaphylactic shock. Anaphylactic shock can be caused by insect stings and nut allergies.

INDUSTRY TIP

Remember the difference between the movement of blood (faster moving) and lymph (slower moving) as it might affect the technique you are using during your treatments. You might also be trying to target either the lymphatic system or the cardiovascular system during the treatment. You cannot make lymph flow faster but you can assist its flow to make it more responsive.

STRUCTURE OF THE LYMPHATIC SYSTEM

Lymph is a pale milky-coloured fluid that is made up of approximately 95% water and 5% lymphocyte cells. Lymph is also known as tissue fluid and it bathes the tissues of the body. It is formed from plasma seeping out of our blood capillaries. Lymph also contains additional substances that are too large to pass through blood capillary walls (eg debris from areas of infection and cells damaged by disease).

Lymph is a means of transferring nutrients such as food, oxygen and water and a means of collecting up waste, such as urea and carbon dioxide. It creates the essential environment that cells need to survive. Most lymph returns to the bloodstream via the capillary walls, but the rest becomes lymph and enters the lymphatic system. Lymph moves very slowly as a result of contraction of the skeletal muscles and movement of the thorax during breathing.

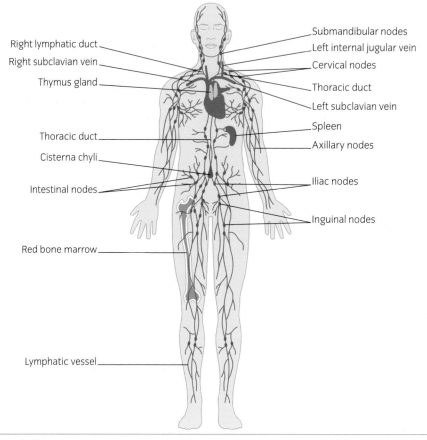

Lymphatic system

ACTIVITY

What signs are you likely to see if a client has a problem with their lymphatic system? Discuss your answer with your tutor or manager. What benefits will certain beauty treatments have for the lymphatic system?

The lymphatic system is made up of the following:

- lymphatic capillaries
- lymphatic vessels and lymphatic fluid (lymph)
- lymph ducts
- lymph nodes or glands
- lymphoid tissue:
    - the tonsils
    - the thymus
    - the spleen
    - the vermiform appendix
    - Peyer's patches.

LYMPHATIC CAPILLARIES

Lymphatic capillaries are located throughout the body. They start as tubes with a dead end **projecting** into the tissues. Their structure is similar to that of blood capillaries, in that they are composed of a single layer of cells. Their walls are more **permeable** and allow larger particles, such as cell debris and proteins, to be absorbed. They differ from blood capillaries in that blood capillaries have a venous end (an end connected to a vein) and an arterial end (an end connected to an artery), whereas lymph capillaries do not.

LYMPHATIC VESSELS

These vessels have thin **collapsible** walls and are similar to veins in structure. The lymphatic system, unlike the circulatory system, does not rely on the heart to pump the fluid along. Lymph is pushed towards the heart by the contraction of nearby muscles. Lymph vessels have many valves that prevent the backflow of lymph and make sure that the lymph moves in the right direction.

LYMPHATIC DUCTS

The lymphatic vessels gradually get larger and eventually form two large ducts called:

- the thoracic duct
- the right lymphatic duct.

The thoracic duct drains lymph from both legs, the pelvic and abdominal cavities, the left half of the head, the neck, the thorax and the left arm. The right lymphatic duct drains lymph from the right half of the head, the neck, the right arm and thorax.

Lymph is then returned to the bloodstream via the subclavian veins.

LYMPH NODES

Lymph nodes are often referred to as lymph glands, even though glands usually secrete substances and lymph glands do not. Lymph nodes vary in size with some as small as a pinhead and larger nodes the size of an almond. These nodes are situated in specific locations throughout the body. Some are nearer to the surface and are called superficial; others are positioned deep in the tissues.

Lymph nodes are made up of reticular and lymphoid tissue that is enclosed inside a tough fibrous capsule. Each node contains a network of fibres and white blood cells called lymphocytes. Lymphocytes produce antibodies that destroy micro-organisms and fight infection. These cells work to filter and clean the lymph fluid before it is returned to the venous bloodstream.

Projecting
Extending or reaching into

Permeable
Porous, leaky

INDUSTRY TIP

Efferent lymph vessels carry lymph out of the lymph nodes and afferent lymph vessels carry lymph into the lymph nodes.

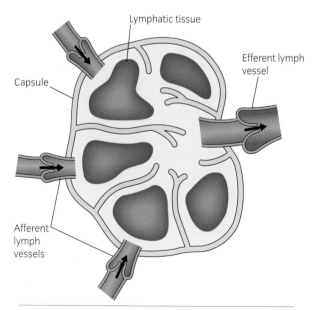

Lymph node

LYMPHATIC ORGANS

Thymus

The thymus is a gland that is located beneath the upper part of the sternum close to the heart. It is very large in young children and keeps growing until puberty. The thymus gland produces T-cells which fight infection. By adulthood the thymus is much smaller. Its exact function in adulthood is not clear.

Spleen

This is the largest of the lymph organs. It can be found below the diaphragm between the stomach and the duodenum. It contains lymph nodes that produce lymphocytes and **macrophages** which are **phagocytic** and fight infections. Blood passes through the spleen via a network of dilated blood vessels and is then taken to the liver.

Macrophage
A type of white blood cell

Phagocytic
Engulfing and absorbing bacteria

The spleen's main functions are to:

- break down and remove old red blood cells (erythrocytes) – the waste products, bilirubin and iron, are passed on to the liver
- filter and remove white blood cells (lymphocytes), platelets and tissue debris
- store mature lymphocytes mature which are released when needed to fight infection
- store blood which can be returned to the circulatory system at times of need.

The tonsils

The tonsils are a mass of lymphoid tissue. There are two tonsils at the back of the roof of the mouth and a small pair of tonsils at the base of the tongue. They help to protect the throat and airways from infection. Together with the adenoids they produce antibodies against **ingested** or inhaled organisms attempting to enter the body through the nose or mouth.

Ingested
Taken into the digestive system through the nose or mouth

Vermiform appendix

This is also known simply as the appendix. This is a worm-like fine tube connected to the caecum (a pouched area of the colon). It contains lymph nodes.

Peyer's patches

These are patches of lymphoid tissue located in the small intestine. They react to pathogens which have been ingested.

THE MAJOR LYMPH NODES OF THE BODY

There are many lymph nodes located throughout the body. The main lymph nodes are in the neck, armpit, breast, abdomen, groin, pelvis and behind the knee.

MAJOR LYMPH NODES OF THE HEAD, FACE AND NECK

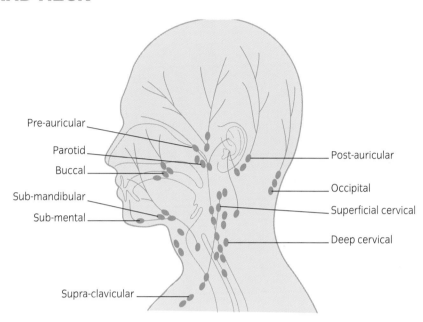

Pre-auricular
Parotid
Buccal
Sub-mandibular
Sub-mental
Supra-clavicular

Post-auricular
Occipital
Superficial cervical
Deep cervical

Lymphatic node	Position	Function
Buccal nodes	In the cheek area next to the buccinators.	Drains the cheeks.
Mandibular and submandibular nodes	Underneath the mandible.	Drain inner eye, nose, cheek and upper lip.
Post-auricular nodes (mastoid)	Behind the ear.	Drain the scalp.
Occipital nodes	At the base of the skull.	Drain back of scalp and neck.
Anterior/auricular nodes (parotid)	In front of the ears above the jaw.	Drain scalp, upper face, eyelids, nose and cheeks.
Superficial cervical nodes	At the side of the neck.	Drain the scalp, occipital nodes and mastoid nodes.
Deep cervical nodes	Deep within the neck. Form a chain along the neck.	All lymph passes directly or indirectly through these nodes. Drains the superficial nodes, tonsils and tongue.

SmartScreen 306 Worksheet 10

SmartScreen 307 Worksheet 2

OTHER MAJOR LYMPH NODES

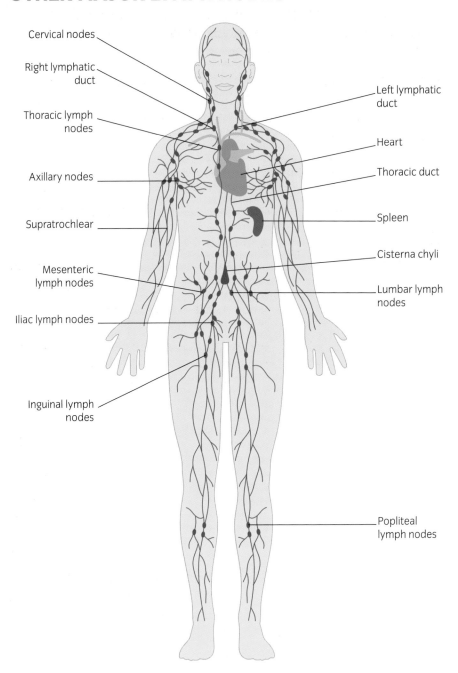

Cervical nodes

Right lymphatic duct

Thoracic lymph nodes

Axillary nodes

Supratrochlear

Mesenteric lymph nodes

Iliac lymph nodes

Inguinal lymph nodes

Left lymphatic duct

Heart

Thoracic duct

Spleen

Cisterna chyli

Lumbar lymph nodes

Popliteal lymph nodes

Lymph node	Position	Function
Cervical nodes	Deep within the neck.	Drain the head, tongue and mouth.
Axillary nodes	Under the arms.	Drain the upper limbs and breasts.
Mesenteric nodes	In the walls of the intestines.	Drain the colon and upper part of the rectum.
Iliac nodes	In the lateral parts of the pelvis.	Drain the leg and buttocks.
Inguinal nodes	In the groin.	Drain the lower limbs and abdominal walls.
Supratrochlear nodes	At the elbow joint.	Drain the lower arm.
Popliteal nodes	Behind the knee.	Drain the lower limbs.

DISORDERS OF THE LYMPHATIC SYSTEM

The lymphatic system's role in immunity and health means that any condition that a client has could have an impact on the lymph system and should be given time to recover.

There are many contra-indications that you will come across so it is important that you have a basic understanding of some of the common conditions. Insurance companies will expect you to carry out a full consultation before starting any treatment and the client should be referred to a medical practitioner before treatment if necessary. There are many conditions that can be treated with care and the treatment modified providing the client's medical practitioner has been consulted first. There are some conditions, however, that should not be treated.

Lymphatic disorder	Description and cause	Contra-indications and general precautions	Advice for client
Swollen glands	Inflamed, tender lymph nodes are usually an indication that the body is fighting an infection. The nodes might swell even before the effects of the infection are felt (eg glands in the neck might become tender and sore even before a sore throat is experienced).	Contra-indicated. The condition causing the swollen glands might be contagious. If the body is fighting an infection it should not be treated to allow the body to heal. Pressure over swollen nodes could affect the natural filtering of pathogens, forcing them through the nodes rather than being dealt with within the node itself by the lymphoid tissue.	Rest and recover.
Cancer	A broad term covering over 200 different types of the disease. Each cancer has different symptoms depending on the organ or part of the body affected. Caused by uncontrolled abnormal cell growth.	Contra-indicated. Do not carry out treatment.	Seek medical advice prior to treatment.
HIV (human immunodeficiency virus)/AIDS (acquired immunodeficiency syndrome)	The HIV virus is a retrovirus that infects the T-lymphocytes. Causes defects in immunity. Symptoms might include unexplained weight loss, fever, swollen lymph glands.	Contra-indicated for epilation and intimate waxing. As the treatments you are offering don't come into direct contact with blood (with the exception of epilation and intimate waxing), you should not be at any risk, unless you or the client has any open wounds.	Seek medical advice if needed.

Lymphatic disorder	Description and cause	Contra-indications and general precautions	Advice for client
Mastitis	Inflammation of the breast tissue. Causes swelling of the breast tissue, tenderness and discomfort. Can be caused by an infection, blocked milk glands while breastfeeding and hormonal changes.	Contra-indicated for all treatments.	Seek medical advice. Return when recovered.
Oedema	An abnormal accumulation of fluid in the body tissue. Associated with the lymphatic circulation but can also be due to problems with the blood circulation, heart or kidneys.	Contra-indicated if you are unsure of the cause. Avoid treatment until you are sure of the cause.	Seek medical advice before treatment.
Lymphoedema	Swelling caused by an accumulation of lymph in the tissues of a limb. Might be caused by blocked lymphatic vessels, damage to the lymph nodes or from removal of the lymph nodes.	Treating the affected limb is contra-indicated. There are specialised massage techniques but these should only be performed by a qualified practitioner.	Seek medical advice.

ACTIVITY

Discuss with your manager or tutor what might happen if you were to treat a client with swollen glands or undiagnosed lumps.

RESPIRATORY SYSTEM

HANDY HINT

During inspiration air is breathed in.

During expiration air is breathed out.

INDUSTRY TIP

When you are carrying out treatments make sure you breathe regularly and don't hold your breath. Often when we concentrate hard we hold our breath. You will suffer from fatigue if you don't breathe evenly.

Everything we do is made possible by the air that we breathe. We need to breathe effectively to provide our body with sufficient oxygen to enable basic cellular activity. Oxygen is needed for the brain to function.

In this part of the chapter you will learn about:

- the structure of the respiratory system
- the exchange of oxygen and carbon dioxide in the lungs
- how respiration works
- disorders of the respiratory system.

THE STRUCTURE OF THE RESPIRATORY SYSTEM

The following structures are needed to provide passageways for air to be transported to the lungs and then **exhaled**:

- nose
- naso-pharynx
- pharynx
- larynx
- trachea
- bronchi
- lungs.

Exhaled
Breathed out

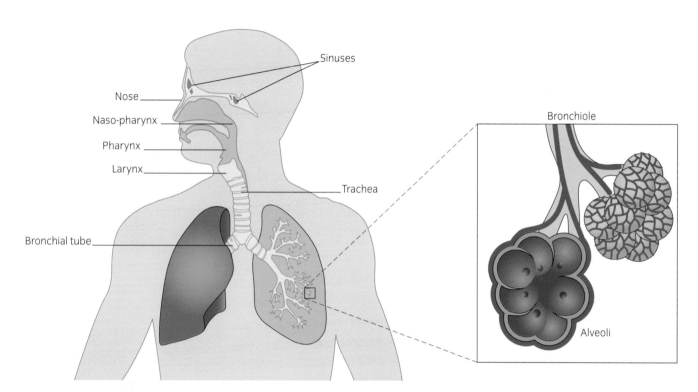

THE EXCHANGE OF OXYGEN AND CARBON DIOXIDE IN THE LUNGS

The main function of the respiratory system is the exchange of oxygen and carbon dioxide in the lungs. Oxygen, from the air that we breathe in, passes into the blood in the lungs. It is replaced by carbon dioxide which has been released by the body as a waste product of cell metabolism. The carbon dioxide is then exhaled.

HOW RESPIRATION WORKS

Air is breathed in through the nose and mouth and is transported into and out of the lungs by the combined action of the intercostal muscles and diaphragm.

Breathing is a passive process (ie we do it most of the time without even thinking about it). However, when we need more air our muscles can be stimulated to inhale or exhale more air. The rate at which we breathe is controlled by the respiratory centre in the brain and the levels of carbon dioxide circulating in the bloodstream.

DISORDERS OF THE RESPIRATORY SYSTEM

Disorder	Description and cause	Contra-indications and general precautions	Advice for client
Influenza (flu)	Flu is caused by a virus which is spread in the air. It can be caught by direct contact with an infected client or a colleague. Symptoms include feeling very unwell, aching, headache and a high temperature. Other symptoms may include a runny or blocked nose, watery eyes, sneezing, catarrh and a sore throat. Symptoms can also include a stomach upset and gastric flu.	Contra-indicated. Flu is a very contagious virus.	Advise client to go home and rest. Avoid contact to prevent further spread of the virus.
Sinusitis	Infection of the mucous membranes of the sinuses cavities. Symptoms include headache, facial pain and congestion of the nose and sinuses.	Advise client to go home and recover.	Suggest client seeks medical advice.
Bronchitis	Inflammation of the bronchi. Caused by a viral or bacterial infection or can be caused by air pollution and smoking. It can also be present alongside other lung diseases. Symptoms include wheeziness, shortness of breath and a persistent, possibly painful, chesty cough.	Might be contra-indicated depending on the cause. Keep the client's head raised where possible to avoid irritation in the lungs.	Seek medical advice if symptoms are persistent.
Asthma	Attacks of breathlessness and wheeziness caused by inflammation of the bronchi. The inflammation causes the lining of the bronchi to swell which reduces the amount of air flow in and out of the lungs. Symptoms include breathlessness, wheeziness, a dry cough and a tight feeling in the chest.	Products with strong smells, dust, cold air and stress can all trigger an asthma attack. Make sure clients keep their inhalers close by.	Seek medical advice if the client has a severe attack.

NERVOUS SYSTEM

The nervous system is responsible for receiving information from outside of the body and transmitting that information between different parts of the body. It is also responsible for transmitting information around the body. The nervous system works closely with the endocrine system to help maintain communication and **homeostasis** in the body.

Homeostasis
Control of internal conditions in the body

In this part of the chapter you will learn about:

- the organisation of the nervous system
- the structure and basic function of the nervous system
- diseases and disorders of the nervous system.

THE STRUCTURE OF THE NERVOUS SYSTEM

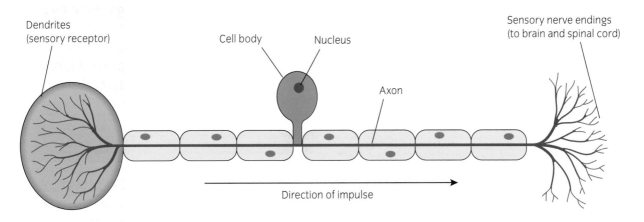

A nerve cell

NERVE CELL/NEURONE

A neurone is a specialised nerve cell designed to receive stimuli and transmit nerve impulses. Each neurone has a cell body, a central nucleus and special extensions called axons and dendrites.

DENDRITES

These are fine, branching extensions, which receive messages from other nerve cells.

AXON

This is a slender extension of the nerve cell which can be up to 100cm in length. The axon sends information one-way from the nerve cell to the axon terminal. The axon terminal is the point where the electrical charge being sent from a nerve cell is changed into a chemical signal.

Large axons are covered with a sheath of fatty material called myelin, giving them a white appearance. Myelin acts like an insulator and helps to speed up nerve impulses. There are breaks along the myelin sheath called nodes of Ranvier and these help to transmit the nerve impulse. Each nerve cell has only one axon, but the axon may have many branches.

NEURONE

There are three main types of neurones:

- *Sensory* or *afferent* neurones. These neurones are responsible for receiving stimuli from sensory organs and receptors. The impulse is then transmitted to the spinal cord and brain. Sensations transmitted by the sensory neurones include heat, cold, pain, taste, smell, sight and hearing.

 SmartScreen 305 Worksheet 11

- *Motor* or *efferent* neurones carry impulses away from the brain and the spinal cord taking messages to muscles and glands
- *Association* or *connecting* neurones connect sensory and motor neurones and are found in the brain and spinal cord.

THE ORGANISATION OF THE NERVOUS SYSTEM

The nervous system can be divided into two parts:

- the central nervous system
- the peripheral nervous.

THE CENTRAL NERVOUS SYSTEM

The central nervous system or CNS consists of two parts:

1 the brain

2 the spinal cord.

The brain

Our brains are our consciousness and intellect. Our memories are stored here and they are sure of our ability to think, judge and reason. The human brain is a mass of complex nervous tissue lying within the protection of the skull. There are over 12 billion neurons and 50 billion supporting glial cells. The average brain weighs less than 1.4kg. The brain is the central communication centre of the nervous system and its function is to receive all sensory information, process it and co-ordinate a response. This may be an instant reflex action or a slow thought process.

The outer surface of the cerebral cortex (cerebrum) consists of grey matter and this contains the cell bodies of the nerves. Under this is the white matter of our brains containing myelin-covered axons.

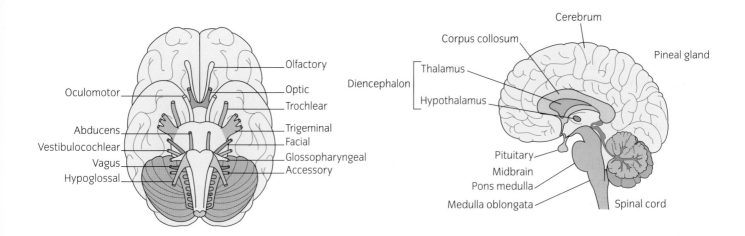

Structures in the brain

- *Cerebrum* – this is largest part of the brain and forms two distinct sections. The cerebrum is involved in mental activities such as those involving memory and is responsible for intelligence, sensory perception and voluntary movement.

- *Cerebellum* – this area of the brain is responsible for fine or precise movement, balance and posture.
- *Hypothalamus* – see endocrine system. This controls automatic body processes and is lined to the posterior lobe of the pituitary gland. It controls the hormones from both pituitary lobes to regulating the activity of other endocrine glands. The other functions of the hypothalamus include control of:

  - the autonomic nervous system
  - thirst and water balance
  - appetite and feeling of fullness
  - body temperature
  - emotions
  - biorhythms – sleeping and waking cycles.

- *Thalamus* – this acts like a relay station to sort, interpret and direct sensory information. It includes information about touch, pain, and temperature and from the other senses.
- *Brain stem* – contains centres that regulate many basic survival functions eg heartbeat, respiration, blood pressure, digestion and swallowing.
- *Cerebrospinal fluid* – a clear fluid which is produced and distributed all around the brain. It protects the brain from mechanical forces and infections.
- *Meninges* – these are a special tough membrane that cover and protect the brain and spinal cord.

The spinal cord

The spinal cord is an extension of the brain stem and extends from the base of the skull down to the lumbar vertebrae. The nerve cell bodies are grouped in the centre of the cord. Surrounding this are the axons running up and down the cord. Spinal nerves leave the cord to supply the body.

The functions of the spinal cord

- It relays impulses to and from the brain from both internal and external stimuli.
- It provides the communication link between the brain and the organs of the body.
- The spinal cord is the centre for reflex actions. Our reflex actions provide us with a very quick automatic response to external or internal stimuli, without involving the brain. They enable our body to respond extremely quickly without the need to think a process through, such as moving a hand away from a hot surface.

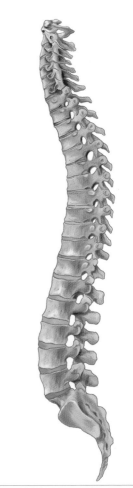

The spinal cord goes along the length of the spine

INDUSTRY TIP

The blood supply to the brain is extremely important. The brain only makes up 2% of the body's weight but has 20% of the body's blood circulating through it.

THE PERIPHERAL NERVOUS SYSTEM

The peripheral nervous system is composed of the parts of the nervous system outside the brain and the spinal cord. It consists of:

- 31 pairs of spinal nerves
- 12 pairs of cranial nerves
- the autonomic nervous system.

THE CRANIAL NERVES

There are 12 pairs of cranial nerves which connect directly to the brain and between them they provide a nerve supply to sensory organs, muscles and skin of the head and the neck.

The main facial nerves that you need to be aware of include the following:

- trigeminal nerves which are the chief sensory nerves for the face and head which includes the ophthalmic, maxillary and mandibular nerves
- facial nerves, which supply the facial muscles of expression
- olfactory nerves, which give us our sense of smell.

THE SPINAL NERVES

Spinal nerves receive sensory impulses from the body and transmit motor signals to specific regions of the body. Each spinal nerve passes out of the spinal cord to link with the autonomic nervous system. Each of the spinal nerves are numbered and named according to the level of the spinal column from which they pass out from:

- eight cervical
- 12 thoracic
- five lumbar
- five sacral
- one coccygeal.

ACTIVITY

Think of the last time you had a reflex action – write down what it was and how you responded.

Each spinal nerve divides into several branches to form a network of nerves, which serve different parts of the body.

THE SOMATIC NERVOUS SYSTEM

The somatic nervous system or voluntary nervous system is made up of nerve fibres that send information from the central nervous system to the muscles. It allows you to carry out voluntary actions (ie actions that you are aware of, such as picking up an object).

THE AUTONOMIC NERVOUS SYSTEM

This is the part of your nervous system that makes sure that all your internal organs (including the cardiac muscle) and your glands function smoothly. This allows your body to carry out involuntary actions (eg your heart beating). The autonomic system is divided into two parts:

- the sympathetic nervous system
- the parasympathetic nervous system.

The sympathetic and parasympathetic nervous systems work together to regulate and balance the internal workings of the body but have opposite effects. For example, the sympathetic nervous system might increase your heart rate and breathing rate in a stressful situation whereas the parasympathetic nervous system will try to maintain your heart rate and breathing at a low level in a stressful situation.

DISEASES AND DISORDERS OF THE NERVOUS SYSTEM

Disease	Description and cause	Contra-indications and general precautions	Advice for client
Epilepsy	Epilepsy can be described as uncontrolled electrical activity in the brain. This change can lead to a simple vacant expression with a lack of response or a grand mal seizure, which is when the individual becomes partially unconscious and suffers twitching and uncontrollable movements. Epilepsy often has no known cause but it can be triggered by a brain injury or a chemical imbalance. Some epileptics have seizures that are caused by flashing lights which is known as photosensitive epilepsy.	Not generally a contra-indication; however it is a contra-indication to any electrical treatment. You might want to refer the client to a medical practitioner for advice. If the client's condition is controlled and they know what triggers their seizures, so that they can avoid the trigger, there is no reason why they shouldn't have safe treatments. As a therapist you need to decide whether you can cope with the possibility of an epileptic client having a seizure. This might be a frightening experience but if you are aware, prepared and take the right precautions you can treat these clients.	Suggest the client seeks medical advice before considering any treatment.
Bell's palsy	Facial paralysis caused by compression of the facial nerve. Symptoms include drooping of the facial contours and paralysis of the facial muscles on one side of the face.	Recovery usually takes a few months. Suggest the client seeks medical advice before any treatment is given. Avoid the use of electrical treatments in the area especially if the cause is unknown.	Suggest the client seeks medical advice before treatment.
Cerebral palsy	Cerebral palsy can affect body movement, balance and posture. It is caused by brain damage or abnormal brain development. The condition makes it difficult to control and coordinate muscles. The disease does not affect mental ability but can affect communication.	Contra-indicated.	Suggest the client seeks medical advice before treatment.

Disease	Description and cause	Contra-indications and general precautions	Advice for client
Multiple sclerosis (MS)	A **neurological** condition that can affect memory and thinking. It can also have an impact on emotions. Symptoms include problems with vision, balance, muscle stiffness and spasms. The immune system attacks the substance that protects the nerve fibres. This damage causes scars or lesions on the nerve fibres.	Treatment might be possible in the early stages.	Suggest the client seeks medical advice before treatment.
Parkinson's disease	A progressive disease that affects the muscles. It causes a loss of muscle movement, ridged muscles and tremors that cannot be controlled. It is caused by a lack of nerve cells and dopamine in the brain. Dopamine transmits messages between the brain and the nervous system. Without dopamine, movement becomes slower and takes longer to perform.	Treatment with care might be possible in the early stages of the disease. As the disease progresses it will contra-indicate treatments.	Suggest the client seeks medical advice before treatment.

Neurological
Related to the nervous system

DIGESTIVE SYSTEM

Most of the nutrients we eat are made up of complex substances that need to be broken down into smaller molecules that can be used more easily. The digestive system breaks down food using both physical and chemical processes. The body needs a constant supply of nutrients to continue to function, grow and repair and these are obtained from the food we eat.

In this part of the chapter you will learn about:
- basic dietary requirements
- the structure of the digestive system
- the process of digestion
- diseases and disorders of the digestive system.

HANDY HINT

Food provides us with energy. We use energy even when we are resting to keep the body ticking over. The energy in food energy is measured in joules or calories.

BASIC DIETARY REQUIREMENTS
So that the body is provided with everything it needs to function and repair itself, we need to eat a balanced diet containing a variety of essential nutrients:
- water
- carbohydrates – including fibre (cellulose), sugar and starch

- proteins
- fats (or lipids)
- vitamins
- minerals.

CARBOHYDRATES

Carbohydrates take the form of sugars and starches. These provide the body with its main source of energy. There are two types of carbohydrate:

- Simple carbohydrates (or monosaccharides) – these are simple sugars that are easily absorbed in the bloodstream.
- Complex carbohydrates – these are more complex sugars (such as starch and cellulose (fibre)) that need to be broken down into simple sugars before they can be absorbed into the bloodstream. Cellulose and hemicelluloses form the main structure of plants' cell walls. Their fibrous structure gives the plants their ridged form. These are so complex that our digestive systems cannot break down these structures. Fibre has the ability to absorb water as it passes through the digestive system. This increases bulk in faeces and encourages the large intestine to function more easily. A diet with good cellulose content is essential to preventing many conditions and may help prevent constipation and some digestive problems, eg irritable bowel.

> **HANDY HINT**
>
> Many cells, such as brain cells, need a constant supply of glucose to survive as glucose is used immediately. This is why our thinking skills and reactions become slower if we haven't eaten for a long time.

> **INDUSTRY TIP**
>
> Most foods that are high in fibre are low in sugar and have little fat. Because fibre increases bulk it will reduce the space available and encourage a more satisfied feeling.

> **HANDY HINT**
>
> Unrefined foods such as wholemeal breads, cereals, grains, root vegetables and fruits can increase dietary fibre. Good sources are whole-grain flour, dried apricots and other dried fruit, peanuts, celery, peas (pulses), green beans, prunes, unrefined bran, potato skins.

ACTIVITY

Eat a piece of wholemeal bread and chew until it is really liquid in your mouth. Can you now taste the sweetness of the sugars being broken down?

> **INDUSTRY TIP**
>
> A drop in sugar levels causing you to feel hungry, irritable and light-headed causes many food cravings. Sugary foods increase the sugar levels rapidly but do not sustain them. Complex carbohydrates produce a slow release of sugars maintaining sugar levels, so it would be more beneficial to have a slice of wholemeal bread than a chocolate bar.

FATS (LIPIDS)

Fats have a number of functions in our diet. They:
- transport and supply fat-soluble vitamins around the body
- improve the flavour of food
- provide energy and warmth.

There are two main types of fat:
- saturated fat (solid at room temperature – eg cheese and butter)
- unsaturated fat (liquid at room temperature – eg olive oil).

When fat is digested, it is made into an **emulsion** by the action of bile from the intestine. The enzyme lipase is released by the pancreas and digests the fat. The lipase breaks the fat down into **fatty acids** and glycerol which are easily absorbed into the body.

Emulsion

Tiny droplets of one liquid in another

Fatty acids

Building blocks of fat for the body

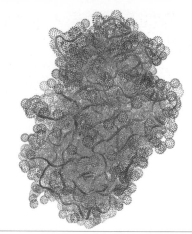

Pepsin – a protein molecule

PROTEIN

Proteins are necessary for the growth and repair of tissue. They are also used in the production of hormones and enzymes. Protein is found in fish, milk, meat and pulses.

During digestion proteins are broken down by the action of enzymes into amino acids. Protein is partly digested in the stomach. The enzyme pepsin breaks down large protein molecules into smaller ones. In the small intestine, other enzymes break the small proteins into amino acids. These are then absorbed into the bloodstream and transported to the tissues where they are rebuilt into another type of protein.

WATER

Water is an essential nutrient. Without it we would not survive more than a few days. Water is a major part of many foods and drinks. Water is essential in maintaining the body's fluid balance and for transporting fluids around the body.

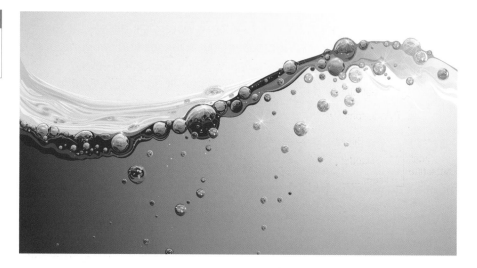

> **HANDY HINT**
>
> An average male adult needs 3.7 litres of water every day and a female adult needs 2.7 litres.

> **INDUSTRY TIP**
>
> Too much alcohol deprives the body of its vitamin reserves including vitamins C and B and causes dehydration.

VITAMINS

Vitamins are organic substances that are needed in small amounts:

- for normal functioning of the body
- to help the body's resistance to disease.

Vitamins are divided into two types:

- Fat-soluble vitamins include vitamins A, D, E, K. These vitamins are carried in fats and are absorbed from the fat in the intestine and are stored in the liver or fatty tissue.
- Water-soluble vitamins include vitamins B and C. The body has a limited ability to store water-soluble vitamins and gets rid of any excess vitamins in the urine.

Hyperkeratinisation

The excessive production of keratin in the epidermis causing an abnormal thickening of skin on the palms of the hands and soles of the feet

Scurvy

A disease cause by a lack of vitamin C. Vitamin C is needed to make collagen

> **INDUSTRY TIP**
>
> A deficiency in vitamin A can cause **hyperkeratinisation**.
>
> A deficiency in vitamin B causes nerve damage.
>
> A deficiency in vitamin B2 can cause cracks at the corner of the mouth.
>
> A deficiency in vitamin C can cause premature ageing and can make wounds slow to heal.
>
> A severe deficiency in vitamin C can cause **scurvy**.

MINERALS

Minerals have many functions and are vitally important in building bones and teeth. They also help to control the water balance within the cells and are also essential for the normal function of nerves and muscle tissue, gland secretion and enzyme activity.

WHY DON'T YOU ...
discuss in a small group how much fluid you drink daily and what form it takes (eg tea, coffee, water, fizzy drinks or squash). Review your fluid intake and discuss whether you think it is sufficient.

THE STRUCTURE OF THE DIGESTIVE SYSTEM AND THE PROCESS OF DIGESTION

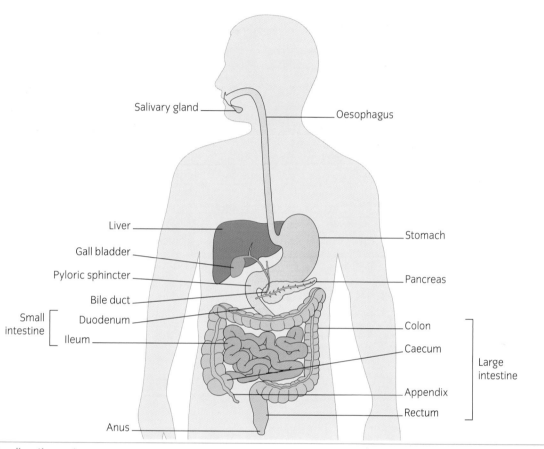

The digestive system

The alimentary canal is a long tube which is about 9m in length. It starts at the mouth and ends at the anus. It includes:

- the mouth
- the pharynx and oesophagus
- the stomach
- the small intestine – the duodenum, jejunum and ileum
- the large intestine – the caecum, appendix, colon, rectum and anus.

The digestive system has organs that work alongside the alimentary canal and these are known as accessory organs. They include:

- the liver
- the gall bladder
- the pancreas.

INDUSTRY TIP

The alimentary canal is also known as the gastrointestinal tract.

INDUSTRY TIP

Clients should be encouraged to drink liquids – water, fruit or herbal teas – following treatments to help aid the removal of waste from the body.

THE DIGESTIVE PROCESS

MOUTH

Digestion begins in the mouth where food is broken into smaller pieces, chewed, and ground down by the teeth. This process involves several muscles, one of which is the tongue which moves the food around the mouth and mixes it with saliva to form a soft mass called the bolus.

The salivary glands

There are three pairs of glands that connect to the mouth and produce saliva. Saliva is a digestive fluid and is released in response to sensory nerves in the mouth and by the sight and smell of food. Saliva moistens food and makes it easier to swallow. It begins the digestive process helping to start to break down food. It also plays a key role in oral hygiene removing food particles and pathogens.

Pharynx

This is commonly known as the throat; it extends from behind the nose, mouth and larynx and is about 12–14cm long.

Oesophagus

This passes through the diaphragm down to the stomach. It is about 25cm long. Food is moved along by special intermittent muscular contraction called peristalsis.

STOMACH

At the end of the oesophagus underneath the diaphragm sits the stomach. It is a is a J-shaped muscular bag that can extend and hold about 1.5 litres after a meal.

The main functions of the stomach are:

- to store food
- to begin protein digestion
- to control the entry of food into the duodenum. The stomach mixes food with gastric juices secreted by glands in the lining of the stomach to form chyme. It then churns this mixture of liquid and small particles.

Alcohol, water and glucose are absorbed into the blood directly from the stomach. After about four hours the partially digested food leaves the stomach and passes into the duodenum. Carbohydrates leave the stomach first, then proteins and finally fats.

SMALL INTESTINE

The part of the digestive system includes:

- the duodenum
- the jejunum
- the ileum.

The small intestine extends to about 7m in length and is about 4cm in diameter. The main functions of the small intestine is to carry out digestion and absorption absorbing some nutrients and water into the bloodstream. There are several digestive enzymes found in the small intestines and these include:

> **INDUSTRY TIP**
>
> Coeliac disease is an autoimmune disease caused by an extreme reaction to the protein found in grains called gluten. In this condition all the villi in the gut are destroyed.

- bile
- pancreatic juice
- intestinal juice.

The inner intestinal wall of the small intestine is covered by millions of tiny projections called villi which are essential for the absorption of fats and play a role within the lymphatic system.

Chyme leaving the stomach enters into the duodenum. This is the first part of the small intestine and it is shaped like a small C-shaped tube. Digestive fluids from the pancreas and bile from the gall bladder enter into the duodenum. From the duodenum the digestive processes continue into the middle part of the small intestine called the jejunum. Enzymes produced here complete the process of digestion before finally moving food into the last part of the small intestine called the ileum. The main function of the ileum is to absorb nutrients from the digested food.

Absorption of digested food

Absorption mainly takes place in the *ileum*. The inner surface area is greatly increased by tiny special projections called villi. These contain a network of capillaries and lymph vessels called lacteals. The ileum's specialised structure helps to increase the surface through which nutrients from digested foods can be absorbed into blood and lymph.

The contents that are left move through into the large intestine for the final part of the digestive journey. The large intestine is wider than the small intestine. Within the large intestine are the:

- caecum
- appendix
- colon
- sigmoid colon
- rectum
- anal canal.

The main function of the large intestines is to remove liquid from the contents to produce faeces. The caecum continues to become the ascending colon. At this point there is a junction called the ileocecal valve where the ileum feeds into the large intestine. At one end of the caecum is a fine tube that contains lymphoid tissue and is known as the appendix. Small amounts of digested food are still absorbed. The mucus produced in the large intestine helps to lubricate the movement of faeces. It also contains antibodies that help fight pathogens that may still be in the digested food. The colon also stores faeces until they are ready to be removed. Finally the faeces move into the last part of the large intestine – the rectum. This is a short space about 12.5cm long which holds faeces. When the muscles contract faeces are removed.

ACCESSORY ORGANS

THE LIVER

The liver is the second largest organ and the largest internal gland in the body. It is located in the upper right-hand side of the abdomen sitting under the diaphragm. The liver has many essential functions within the body.

Functions of the liver

- Regulation of carbohydrate metabolism – absorbs excess glucose and stores it as glycogen. Releases glucose if blood sugar levels falls.
- Regulation of fat metabolism – converts fats into a form that can be stored or broken down to release energy.
- Vitamin storage – several fat-soluble vitamins including A, D and B12.
- Mineral storage – iron and copper needed to make haemoglobin.
- Protein metabolism – amino acids are collected and used to make proteins. Surplus amino acids are broken down.
- Bile production – bile consists of water, mineral salts, mucus, bilirubin (pigments which give its colour), bile salts and cholesterol. It is alkaline and breaks up (emulsifies) fat droplets.
- Detoxification of toxic substances – toxic substances are changed where possible into safer substances.
- Hormone breakdown – liver removes hormones from the blood and breaks them down.
- Excretory function – breakdown of old red blood cells.
- Heat production – the activity of metabolism within the liver creates heat.
- Metabolises ethanol in alcohol.
- Breaks down erythrocytes once they are no longer productive.

GALL BLADDER

The gall bladder is a small pear-shaped muscular sac that is located underneath the liver. The gall bladder stores bile from the liver. When partly digested food enters the duodenum, the muscular **sphincter** at the opening of the bile duct relaxes and pumps bile into the duodenum. The functions of the gall bladder are to:

- store bile
- secret mucus into the bile
- release the stored bile through the pancreatic duct into the duodenum.

Sphincter
Circular muscle

THE PANCREAS

The pancreas is a pale grey-coloured gland, about 12–15cm long. It lies next to the duodenum and between the stomach, spleen and kidney. Its function is to produce pancreatic juices, which are rich in enzymes that break down carbohydrates, proteins and fats in the duodenum. These secretions together with those from the liver pass into the duodenum via the pancreatic duct. The pancreatic juices are alkaline and combined with those from the liver neutralise the acidic action of chyme.

The pancreas is also an endocrine gland and produces the hormones insulin and **glucagon**, which control the level of glucose in the blood.

Glucagon

A hormone released by the pancreas when the level of glucose in the blood becomes low. It has the effect of converting gylcogen to glucose so that more glucose is released.

DISEASES AND DISORDERS OF THE DIGESTIVE SYSTEM

There are many common digestive problems. Most of them are not a cause for concern. However, there are a few that you will need to be aware of because in their more inflammatory stages they will cause discomfort and it would be best to avoid treatment during these times. Always ask the client how they feel and their level of discomfort. Clients with contra-indications of the digestive system may prefer not to have the abdominal area treated – although some light soothing effleurage might be beneficial.

Disease	Description and cause	Contra-indications and general precautions	Advice for client
Crohn's disease	An inflammatory bowel disease. It affects the intestinal tract causing inflammation and ulcers in the layers of the intestinal walls. It might also affect the lymph nodes in relevant areas. Symptoms include abdominal pain, tiredness, diarrhoea and weight loss.	Treat abdominal areas with care and avoid if painful.	Suggest client seeks medical advice.
Gallstones	Tiny stones of cholesterol that form in the gall bladder. There may not be any symptoms. When they do occur, they include abdominal discomfort, bloatedness and sickness.	Avoid treatment in the abdominal area if the client has gallstones.	Suggest client seeks medical advice.
Hiatus hernia	Caused when the stomach pushes through the diaphragm where the oesophagus passes through it. Can cause a lot of internal discomfort and **acid reflux**.	Caution. Avoid pressure over the upper abdominal area.	Suggest client seeks medical advice.
Irritable bowel syndrome (IBS)	Affects the large intestine or bowel. It causes an urgent need to open the bowels with loose faeces and/or constipation. Symptoms also include pain, bloating, discomfort and tiredness. It is commonly linked with stress and diet.	Avoid the abdominal area. If constipation is a symptom, massage can be quite beneficial.	Suggest client seeks medical advice if there are any sudden changes in the body's functions.

Acid reflux

Stomach acid flows back up the oesophagus

ENDOCRINE SYSTEM

The endocrine system works alongside the nervous system to communicate, control and coordinate the body's activities. It produces hormones which control the body's metabolic processes.

Hormones are specialised chemical messengers that are stored and secreted by the endocrine glands. Hormones are transported to their target location via the bloodstream.

Hormones have an effect on or control the following bodily functions:

- emotions
- appetite
- sexual activity
- metabolism
- water (electrolyte) balance.

In this part of the chapter you will learn about:

- the location and function of the endocrine glands
- diseases and disorders of the endocrine system.

THE LOCATION AND FUNCTION OF THE ENDOCRINE GLANDS

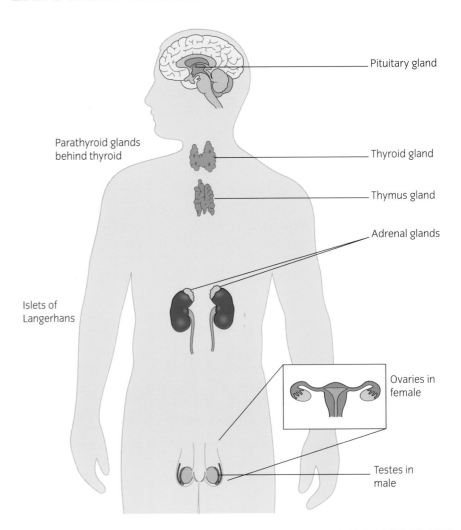

Parathyroid glands behind thyroid

Pituitary gland

Thyroid gland

Thymus gland

Adrenal glands

Islets of Langerhans

Ovaries in female

Testes in male

PITUITARY GLAND

The pituitary gland is found at the base of the skull and consists of two lobes:

- anterior
- posterior.

Anterior pituitary gland

Hormone(s) secreted	Action	Target tissue
Growth hormone (GH)	- Controls the growth of the skeleton and muscles. - Monitors chemical substances (minerals) necessary for growth.	Bones and skeleton Liver, intestines, pancreas
Thyroid stimulating hormone (TSH)	- Controls the thyroid gland. - Regulates metabolism.	Thyroid gland
Adrenocorticotrophic hormone (ACTH)	- Regulates the activity of the adrenal cortex and adrenal glands.	Adrenal cortex
Sex gland (gonad) hormones	- Control the development and function of the testes and ovaries.	Sexual organs
Female hormones		
Follicle stimulating hormone (FSH)	- Controls the secretion of oestrogen from ovarian follicles.	Ovarian follicles
Luteinising hormone (LH)	- An accute rise triggers ovulation.	Sexual organs
Prolactin	- Stimulates milk secretion from the breast following birth.	Breasts
Male hormones		
Follicle stimulating hormone (FSH)	- Stimulates the testes to produce sperm.	Testes
Luteinising hormone (LH)	- Acts on the testes to produce testosterone.	Testes

Posterior pituitary gland

Hormones secreted	Action	Target tissue
Anti-diuretic hormone (ADH) or vasopressin	- Controls the amount of water absorbed by the kidneys.	Kidneys
Oxytocin hormone	- Stimulates contraction of the uterus during childbirth. - Stimulates breast milk production for breastfeeding.	Uterus during and after childbirth, breasts

PINEAL GLAND

This small gland – about the size of a grain of rice – is located centrally within the brain. Its main function is to control our natural daily rhythms associated with sleep and being awake.

Hormone secreted	Action	Target tissue
Melatonin	■ Secretion is controlled by daylight. ■ Controls the natural **biorhythms** of the body (sleep/wake cycles). ■ Causes sleepiness. ■ Involved in sexual development.	General body tissues

HYPOTHALAMUS

Biorhythms

A recurring cycle in a living organism (eg daily cycle of sleeping and waking)

Negative feedback

A process that occurs in the body where hormones work together to maintain a balance. The rise in one hormone generates the release of another to balance the effect and maintain homeostasis

Hormones secreted	Action	Target organ
Growth hormone releasing hormone (GHRH)	■ Stimulates release of growth hormone from the pituitary gland.	Anterior pituitary gland
Growth hormone release inhibiting hormone – (GHRIH somatostatin)	■ Produced to reduce the release of growth hormone from the pituitary gland – **negative feedback**.	Anterior pituitary gland

THYROID GLAND

The thyroid gland is an h-shaped gland positioned at the front of the neck. It is has two lobes. The lobes lie on either side of the larynx and on top of the trachea.

Hormones secreted	Action	Target tissue
Thyroxine and triodothyronine	■ Stimulates metabolism in the tissues and is essential for normal growth and mental and physical development. ■ Keeps skin and hair healthy. ■ Controls the nerves and cardiovascular systems. ■ Stores iodine for the manufacture of thyroxine.	Cells and tissues within the body
Calcitonin	■ Reduces calcium levels in the blood when they get too high. ■ Controls storage of calcium – stores calcium in the bones and causes calcium to be reabsorbed by the kidneys when levels in the blood are low.	Kidneys, blood and bone tissue

SmartScreen 307 Worksheet 10

THE PARATHYROID GLANDS

There are four parathyroid glands that sit behind the thyroid gland.

Hormones secreted	Action	Target organ
Parathormone (PTH)	■ Controls the excretion of phosphate and levels of calcium. ■ When calcium levels fall, parathormone is released to increase the amount of calcium in the blood and bones.	Kidneys, blood and bones

ADRENAL GLANDS

There are two adrenal glands which can be found above each kidney. They are made up of two parts:

- the adrenal cortex – the outer part of the adrenal gland that secretes glucocorticoids, mineralocorticoids and sex hormones
- the adrenal medulla – the inner part of the adrenal gland that secretes adrenaline and noradrenaline.

Adrenal cortex

Hormones secreted	Action	Target tissue
Glucocorticoids (cortisone, cortisol and hydrocortisone)	■ Regulate the metabolism of proteins and carbohydrates and uses fats. ■ Control blood sugar level and increase during times of stress.	Liver, blood sugar
Mineralocorticoids (aldosterone)	■ Maintain the balance of essential electrolytes (salts) and water in the body. ■ Affects blood pressure.	Water content in tissues, renal tubes (ie in kidney)
Sex hormones (androgens)	■ Regulate the development and maintenance of the **secondary sex characteristics**.	Sex organs

Secondary sex characteristics
The features that distinguish the two sexes that appear at puberty. For example, male bodies become more muscular and a female's hips usually become wider than her shoulders

Adrenal medulla

The adrenal medulla secretes adrenaline and noradrenaline. In times of stress these hormones work together.

Hormones secreted	Action	Target tissue
Adrenaline	▪ Dilation of the arteries and increased blood circulation and heart rate. ▪ Dilation of bronchi which increases rate of breathing. ▪ Constriction of the blood vessels to the skin so that blood is diverted to the brain and muscles where it is needed. ▪ Increases glycogen for rapid muscle contraction. ▪ Increases activity of sweat glands.	Bronchi, blood vessels, muscles, sweat glands
Noradrenaline	▪ Constricts blood vessels resulting in increased blood pressure. ▪ Increases rate of breathing. ▪ Relaxes intestine and slows digestion.	Bronchi, blood vessels, intestine

PANCREAS

The pancreas has two functions:

▪ to aid digestion by secreting pancreatic juice (an exocrine function)
▪ secretion of insulin from the **islets of Langerhans**.

Islets of Langerhans
Cells within the pancreas that secrete the hormone insulin

Hormones secreted	Action	Target tissue
Insulin	▪ Reduces the level of glucose in the blood to maintain normal blood sugar levels. ▪ After a meal, sugar levels in the blood increase and insulin is produced to bring the levels down.	Bloodstream
Glucagon	▪ Raises the level of glucose in the blood if it is too low.	Bloodstream
Somatostatin	▪ Helps to control the release of glucagon and insulin. ▪ Helps to control secretion of pancreatic juice.	Pancreas

THYMUS

The thymus gland lies in the upper part of the chest behind the sternum. It extends up towards the base of the neck. It is very active during childhood and plays an important part in developing a child's immune system. It produces T-lymphocytes or T-cells (see page 85). After puberty it begins to shrink.

Hormones secreted	Action	Target tissue
Thymosin	▪ Stimulates the T-cells in the other lymphatic organs to mature to provide a defence mechanism against diseases.	Blood

SEX GLANDS

Ovaries

The two ovaries are the female sex glands and are found beneath the kidneys. They produce ova and oestrogen and progesterone. They are controlled by follicle-stimulating hormone (FSH) and luteinising hormone (LH).

Hormones secreted	Action	Target tissue
Oestrogen	▪ Controls the development and function of the female sex organs. ▪ Controls the development of secondary sexual characteristics.	Uterus, ovaries, anterior pituitary gland
Progesterone	▪ Prepares the uterus for pregnancy. ▪ Prepares breasts for milk secretion.	Uterus, anterior pituitary gland

Testes

The testes are the male sex glands. They are located in the groin area and produce sperm and secrete testosterone.

Hormones secreted	Action	Target tissue
Testosterone	▪ Produces male sexual characteristics. ▪ Controls the development and function of the male sex organs.	Testes
Androgens	▪ Controls the development of secondary sexual characteristics.	Various body tissues, muscles, skin etc

SmartScreen 307 Worksheet 9

DISEASES AND DISORDERS OF THE ENDOCRINE SYSTEM

Disease	Description	Contra-indications and general precautions	Advice to client
Thyroid gland			
Hypothyroidism (myxodema)	Underactive thyroid gland. Produces little or no thyroxine. Causes swelling of the thyroid gland because of iodine deficiency (goitre). Symptoms include reduced mental activity, tiredness and coarse dry skin and hair.	A common condition. Seek medical advice unless the condition has been stabilised with medication.	Suggest client seeks medical advice prior to treatment.
Hyperthyroidism (thyrotoxicosis)	Excess thyroxine hormone. Results in increased metabolism. Symptoms include increased mental and physical activity, overactive sweat glands, weight loss, raised pulse and protrusion of the eyeballs (exophthalmia). Sometimes the thyroid may be partly or fully removed to reduce the effects of over-stimulation and medication given to stop the thyroid gland producing excess amounts of thyroxine.	Seek medical advice unless the condition has been stabilised with medication.	Suggest client seeks medical advice prior to treatment.
Parathyroid gland			
Hyperparathyroidism	An excess of parathyroid hormone. Symptoms can include tiredness, nausea, vomiting, kidney stones and bone pains.	Do not treat clients with active kidney stones.	Suggest client seeks medical advice prior to treatment.
Adrenal glands			
Addison's disease	Insufficient secretion of cortisol and aldosterone from the adrenal cortex hormones. Symptoms include the need to urinate frequently, muscle weakness, weight loss, reduced metabolic rate, lack of energy, loss of body hair, low blood sugar and low blood pressure.	Contra-indicated.	Suggest client seeks medical advice prior to treatment.

Disease	Description	Contra-indications and general precautions	Advice to client
Cushing's syndrome	The adrenal cortex produces too much cortisol. It can also be caused by corticosteroid medication. Symptoms include weight gain on the chest, stomach and face, muscle weakness, kidney stones, high blood pressure (hypertension). It can also cause osteoporosis (brittle bones). Women may also experience hirsutism (excessive facial/body hair) and irregular periods.	Treat with caution following medical advice.	Suggest client seeks medical advice prior to treatment.
Pancreas			
Type 1 diabetes	This is a condition caused by a disorder of the pancreas gland (see page 120). In type 1 diabetes the body suffers a severe **deficiency** or total absence of insulin and is unable to control the metabolism of carbohydrates (sugars) and fat. Type 1 diabetes is treated with insulin injections.	There is no cure and diabetes can have many long-term side effects on many of the systems of the body. This is why diabetic clients should be treated with caution. If the client knows that they have problems with skin sensitivity (ie they are having tests to see if they can feel different sensations) you should not treat them until they have consulted their medical practitioner. As a therapist you need to be aware of some of the complications that can occur as the treatment might need to be adapted or restricted. A diabetic might develop changes to the small blood vessels which become weakened and blocked. The nerves might become affected causing numbness or pins and needles in the hands and feet, both of which will also reduce their sensory perception.	Ask the client to seek medical advice before treatment if you feel this is appropriate to the treatment the client is wishing to have.

Deficiency
A lack of something

Disease	Description	Contra-indications and general precautions	Advice to client
Type 2 diabetes	This the most common form of diabetes and about 90% of diabetics are type 2. There is a variety of causes but the most common is obesity. Insulin secretion might be below or above normal levels. Treatment might include changes to diet and the use of drugs to help control the condition. In some cases there might still be the need for insulin injections to control the symptoms.	There is no cure and diabetes can have many long-term side effects on many of the systems of the body. This is why diabetic clients should be treated with caution. As a therapist you need to be aware of some of the complications that can occur as the treatment might need to be adapted or restricted. A diabetic might develop changes to the small blood vessels which become weakened and blocked. The nerves might become affected causing numbness or pins and needles in the hands and feet, both of which will also reduce their sensory perception.	Ask the client to seek medical advice before treatment if you feel this is appropriate to the treatment the client is wishing to have.

HANDY HINT

Information on polycystic ovary syndrome can be found on page 134.

URINARY SYSTEM

The urinary system processes and gets rid of the body's normal metabolic waste. This waste includes excess water, urea, uric acid and mineral salts. The other main function of the urinary system is to maintain homeostasis in the body by controlling blood pressure and volume. Water is introduced into the body through digestion but also through cellular activity. It is removed from the body through urine, faeces, sweat and our breath. Too much or too little fluid in the body can cause a variety of medical conditions. Approximately 80% of our blood is water and if this changes it can have an effect on the heart as it makes the heart work harder.

In this part of the chapter you will learn about:

- the structure and function of the urinary system
- disorders of the urinary system.

THE STRUCTURE AND FUNCTION OF THE URINARY SYSTEM

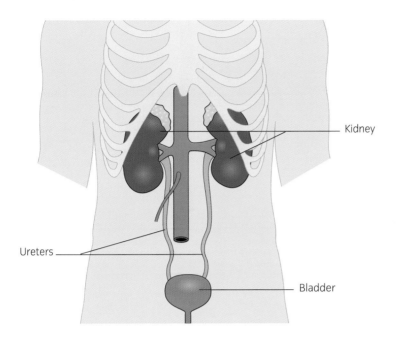

Kidney

Ureters

Bladder

The urinary system processes and eliminates normal metabolic waste. This includes excess water, urea, uric acid and mineral salts. Up to 60% of the human body is water. The main function of the urinary system is to regulate the amount of fluids that there are in the body and plays an essential role in maintaining homeostasis in the body. The amount of water intake and water removed must be equal in order to maintain homeostasis. Water is introduced to the body through digestion but also through cellular activity. Water is removed from the body through urine, **faeces**, sweat and our breath. If there is too much or too little fluid in the body it can cause a variety of medical conditions. Approximately 80% of our blood is water and if this changes it can have an effect on the heart as it makes the heart work harder.

Faeces

Waste that is removed via the digestive system through the bowel

In this section you will learn about:

- the basic function of regulation of body fluids
- the general structure of the urinary system
- the functions of the urinary system
- contra-indications associated with diseases of the urinary system.

The body will normally make changes to balance the fluid in the body such as making us go to the toilet to get rid of excess water or making us feel thirsty so that we replace the water we have lost. There is complex interaction between both the nervous and endocrine systems to maintain these levels.

The urinary system consists of the following:

- two kidneys, which secrete urine
- two ureters, which transport urine from the kidneys to the bladder
- the bladder, where urine collects and is temporarily stored
- the urethra, through which urine is removed from the bladder to the outside of the body.

THE KIDNEYS

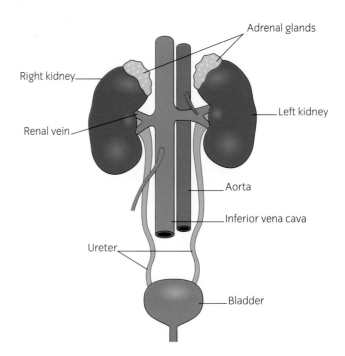

Adrenal glands

Right kidney

Left kidney

Renal vein

Aorta

Inferior vena cava

Ureter

Bladder

Electrolyte

A chemical (potassium, sodium) that ionises to produce an electrically conductive medium

Hypothalamus

Endocrine gland found in the head

Renal

Referring to the kidney

The kidney itself is a bean-shaped organ which lies on the posterior side of the body near the abdominal wall close between the twelfth thoracic and third lumbar vertebrae. The kidney is made up of a fibrous outer capsule made up of connective tissue where fluid is filtered from blood. The kidneys have the following functions:

- to filtrate impurities and metabolic waste from blood
- to regulate water and the salts in the body known as the **electrolyte** balance
- maintains the balance of fluid in the circulatory system
- to produce urine.

The kidneys are responsible for regulating the amount of water and chemical compounds contained within the blood. If you have an excess of water in the blood, the blood concentration will be dilute, and the nerve receptors in the hypothalamus will trigger the pituitary gland to secrete the hormone ADH (anti-diuretic hormone). This carries a message to the kidneys to produce more diluted urine. If the blood becomes concentrated and we become dehydrated, the nerve receptors in the **hypothalamus** trigger the pituitary gland to send a message to the kidneys to produce more concentrated urine and reabsorb more water back into the body. The blood must also be kept at a constant pH of between 7.35 and 7.45: the kidneys help to maintain the chemicals in the circulation to keep this within these narrow limits.

The kidney is composed of 1–2 million nephrons. Each nephron is an independent filtering and urine-processing unit. A nephron consists of:

- a **renal** corpuscle which acts as a filter
- a renal tubule which is a long tube which collects and processes the filtered fluid.

At the renal corpuscle a network of very tiny capillaries called the glomerulus makes contact with the closed end of the renal tubercle and acts as a sieve. The glomerus is made up of a semipermeable single layer of epithelial cells which allows selective molecules to move across from the blood supply by **osmosis** and filter into the kidney tubule to form urine.

Surrounding the glomerulus is the blind end of the tube, which forms a hollow cup-shaped structure called the glomerular capsule. There is a difference in pressure of the blood in the glomerulus and the filtrate now in the glomerular capsule and it is this difference in pressure which allows filtration under osmosis to take place. When blood pressure drops it affects this filtration process and the kidney function.

Osmosis

The movement of water molecules from a weaker or more diluted solution through a semi-permeable membrane

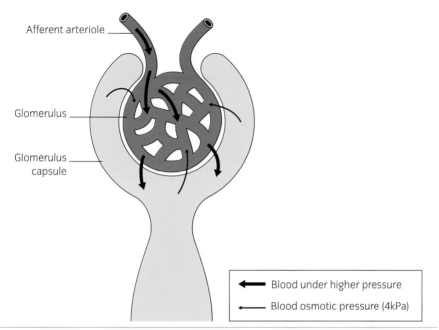

Filtration in the glomerulus

Legend:
← Blood under higher pressure
← Blood osmotic pressure (4kPa)

Labels: Afferent arteriole, Glomerulus, Glomerulus capsule

Urine is made of excess water, salt and protein waste. Urine has a pH of 4.5–7.8. The colour varies according to its concentration, composition and quantity; the amber colour is due to the presence of a pigment produced in bile by the liver. A healthy adult passes 1000–1500ml of urine per day.

As urine moves along the renal system is it further processed and selective substances (eg glucose, amino acids, mineral salts, vitamins and some water) that the body may need again are reabsorped back into the bloodstream via the renal vein.

Urine is the waste product of filtration produced by the kidney. It collects in a funnel-shaped structure called the renal pelvis. Eventually the urine flows into a small tube called the ureter and into the bladder.

ACTIVITY

Next time you go to the loo – think about the colour of your urine. Does it indicate concentrated or weak urine? When do you think urine will be at its most concentrated?

ACTIVITY

Discuss with your tutor how you think body treatments could affect urine output? In relation to the urinary system, what advice can you give your clients following body treatments and why will you give your clients this advice?

URETERS

The ureters are tubes made of smooth muscle fibers that transport urine from the kidneys to the bladder. Muscles in the ureter walls tighten and relax and force urine downwards from the kidneys to the bladder.

BLADDER

The bladder is a muscular balloon-shaped sac that is located in the pelvis. Its function is to store and remove urine through the urethra. In an adult, the bladder can hold up to 600ml of urine.

URETHRA

This is a tube connected to the bladder through which urine is released from the body. The urethra is shorter in women than in men. In men it also has a reproductive function.

DISORDERS OF THE URINARY SYSTEM

Disorder	Description and cause	Contra-indications and general precautions	Advice for client
Cystitis	An inflammation of the bladder. It can be caused by an infection or sensitivity to certain foods or chemicals. If it is not treated early enough it can travel up the ureter and infect the kidneys. Symptoms include a burning, stinging sensation or pain when passing urine and the urine may be dark and have a strong odour. There may also be discomfort in the lower back.	Contra-indicated for body treatments. Caution is required. If the client is having a body treatment, suggest that they rebook once the condition has been treated. Any body treatment that makes the body work hard to eliminate waste will have an effect on the kidney and bladder and may further irritate the condition.	Suggest client seeks medical advice.
Nephritis	Inflammation of one or both of the kidneys. It can be caused by an infection or may be an **autoimmune disease**. Symptoms include reduced urine output, fluid retention, high blood pressure, tiredness and nausea.	Contra-indicated. Any body treatment that makes the body work hard to eliminate waste will have an effect on the kidney and bladder and may further irritate the condition.	Suggest client seeks medical advice.

Autoimmune disease

A disease where the body's immune system attacks itself

REPRODUCTIVE SYSTEM

The reproductive system includes the internal and external organs that enable us to reproduce. There are very obvious different physical appearances between male and female organs. Adults produce specialised cells called gametes and in the male these are called spermatozoa and in the female the ova. They contain the genetic materials which we call our genes or DNA and these enable us to pass on our characteristics to the next generation.

THE MALE REPRODUCTIVE SYSTEM

THE SCROTUM

The scrotum is a sac made of fibrous and connective tissue along with muscle. There are two sections with one testis in each. The scrotum is suspended from the abdominal cavity and has a thin outer layer to keep the testis cool.

TESTES

These are the reproductive glands in the male. They are suspended in the scrotum by the spermatic cords. Each testis contains special lobules within each are germinal epithelia cells called seminiferous tubules. Between the tubes are cells that secrete testosterone after puberty. Blood and lymph pass to the testis in the spermatic cord.

Sperm or spermatozoa are produced in the seminiferous tubules. Once these are mature they pass to the epididymis and are stored.

URETHRA

The male urethra provides a pathway for both the flow of urine and semen.

THE PENIS

The penis has two parts: the root and body. It contains erectile tissue and smooth muscle and is supported by a rich blood supply. At the tip of the body is an expanded structure called the glans penis. During ejaculation semen is propelled by powerful contraction of the muscles from the epididymis and through the deferent duct and along the urethra.

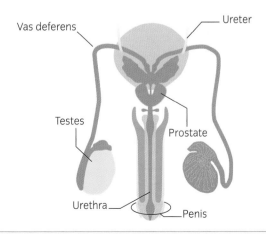

The male reproductive system

THE FEMALE REPRODUCTIVE ORGANS

FEMALE EXTERNAL GENTALIA

Female genitalia come in many shapes and forms, all of which are quite normal.

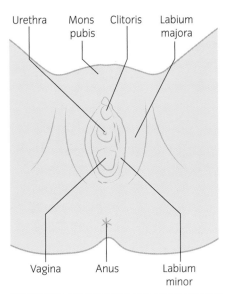

The external female genitalia

- Mons pubis or pubic mound – this is the padded area lying over the pubic bone where pubic hair grows.
- Vulva – this consists of the labia majora, labia minora, clitoris and vaginal orifice (opening).
- Clitoris – erectile tissue located above the opening of the vagina containing sensory nerve endings.
- Labia majora – two large folds encircling the vulva. The lateral sides are covered with pubic hair. They are composed of skin, fibrous tissue and fat and contain large numbers of sebaceous glands.
- Labia minora – two smaller folds of skin between the labia majora. The cleft between the labia minora is known as the vestibule.

FEMALE INTERNAL GENITALIA

Vagina

This is a muscular tube which extends from the external organs, to the internal opening of the neck of uterus called the cervix.

The uterus

This is a hollow muscular organ which lies in the pelvic cavity. Its function is to nourish the ovum and the developing embryo and foetus during the first few weeks of pregnancy. The uterus has a thick layer of muscle tissue, the inner layer of which is called the endometrium. This contains large numbers of mucus secretion glands and a rich blood supply. The outer layer of the endometrium is shed during menstruation.

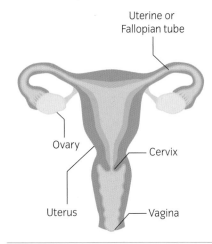

The female reproductive system

The uterine or Fallopian tubes

These extend from the uterus to the ovaries.

The ovaries

The ovaries are the female gonads. They are almond in shape and one lies on either side of the wall of the pelvis. Each ovary is attached to the uterus by the ovarian ligament and to the back by another ligament. The ovaries are composed of two parts: the medulla and the cortex. The cortex contains the ovarian follicles; each follicle contains an ovum or egg. Our ovaries contain thousands of immature ova.

PUBERTY

Puberty typically begins between the ages of 12 and 14 at which time the reproductive organs begin to change and mature. Puberty is the start of the reproductive years.

- The breasts develop.
- Pubic and axillary hair begins to grow.
- The uterus, Fallopian tubes and ovaries mature.
- The menstrual cycle begins to occur at regular intervals.

- Ovulation begins.
- The pelvis changes shape and there are increased deposits of fat around the buttocks and hips.

INDUSTRY TIP

The average women can expect to have approximately 35 reproductive years.

MENSTRUAL CYCLE

During the menstrual cycle one ovum begins to mature and rise to the surface of the ovary. The ovum is contained in a follicle which eventually ruptures and releases the ovum into the Fallopian tube. The ovaries are stimulated by the gonadotrophins from the anterior pituitary gland, FSH (follicle-stimulating hormone) and LH (luteinising hormone).

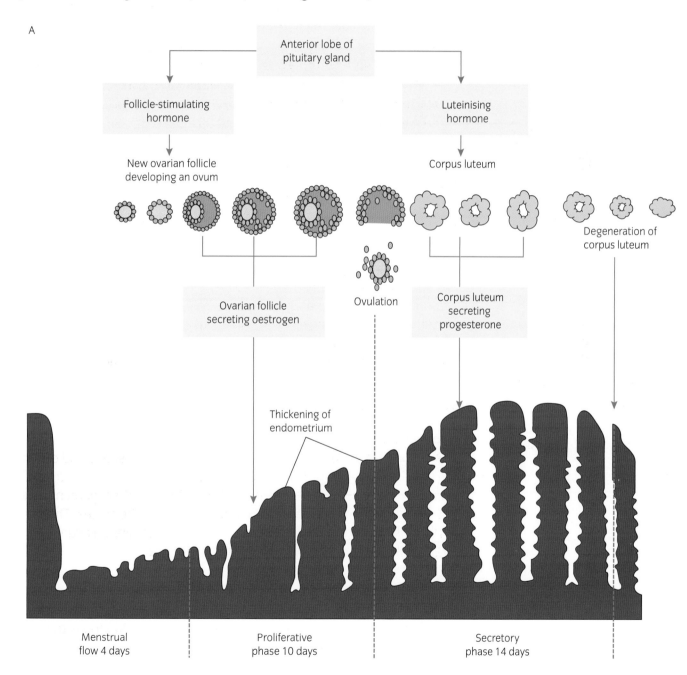

A

Anterior lobe of pituitary gland

Follicle-stimulating hormone

Luteinising hormone

New ovarian follicle developing an ovum

Corpus luteum

Degeneration of corpus luteum

Ovarian follicle secreting oestrogen

Ovulation

Corpus luteum secreting progesterone

Thickening of endometrium

Menstrual flow 4 days

Proliferative phase 10 days

Secretory phase 14 days

The menstrual cycle usually occurs regularly in females in 23–35 day cycles. It consists of three stages:

1 The first (follicular or proliferative) phase lasts ten days.
  - The ovarian follicle is stimulated by FSH.
  - Several follicles develop each with an egg; however usually only one develops to maturity.
  - The ovarian follicle produces oestrogen preparing the wall of the uterus.
  - LH surges triggering ovulation.

2 The second (luteal or secretory) phase lasts 14 days:
  - Ovulation occurs.
  - LH stimulates the egg to burst out of the follicle. The corpus luteum is what is left of the follicle once the egg is released.
  - The corpus luteum secretes the hormone progesterone. Progesterone causes the uterus to become thick, vascular and ready for an egg to implant.
  - Each egg is capable of being fertilised only for a very short time.

3 The third and final phase is the menstrual phase, lasting four days on average:
  - High levels of progesterone in the blood prevent the activity of the pituitary gland and the production of LH is reduced.
  - The lack of LH hormone causes the corpus luteum and progesterone to decrease.
  - The uterus begins to degenerate and the menstrual flow begins.

The anterior pituitary glands secrete FSH following menstruation causing the following:
- New follicles develop in the ovary.
- The ovary secretes oestrogen.
- The walls of the uterus are repaired following menstruation.
- Oestrogen begins to build up until it reaches a peak about two weeks following menstruation stimulating the anterior pituitary to produce LH.

If the egg is fertilised, the corpus luteum the embryo starts to produce the hormone hCG. hCG tells the corpus luteum to continue producing progesterone. The corpus luteum disintegrates after about ten weeks. Progesterone continues to be produced after this time but by the placenta during the pregnancy.

MENOPAUSE

The menopause marks the end of the fertile years. It is a natural progression and part of the ageing process. Menopausal symptoms start between around the ages of 45 and 55 and may be experienced for several years.

Hormone levels change and the ovaries become less responsive to FSH and LH. Eventually the ovaries become inactive and eventually the menstrual cycle ceases.

INDUSTRY TIP

Even if the cycle is irregular ovulation occurs on average 14 days between ovulation and the next menstrual cycle. This is the luteal phase and remains constant from cycle to cycle.

INDUSTRY TIP

Be aware that ladies in their forties and fifties may get very hot very quickly during treatment. Be careful not to make them too cozy during treatment and allow easy removal of covers during treatment. Be particularly aware of this if applying any kind of heat treatment.

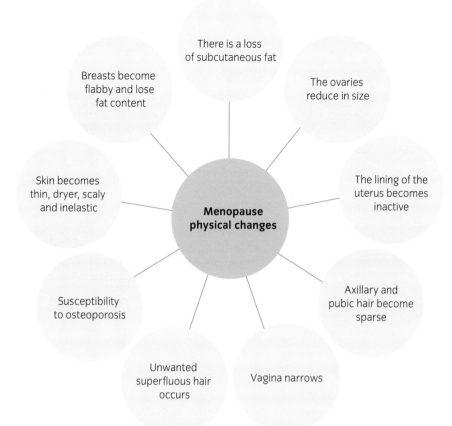

Menopause physical changes

- Breasts become flabby and lose fat content
- There is a loss of subcutaneous fat
- The ovaries reduce in size
- The lining of the uterus becomes inactive
- Skin becomes thin, dryer, scaly and inelastic
- Axillary and pubic hair become sparse
- Susceptibility to osteoporosis
- Unwanted superfluous hair occurs
- Vagina narrows

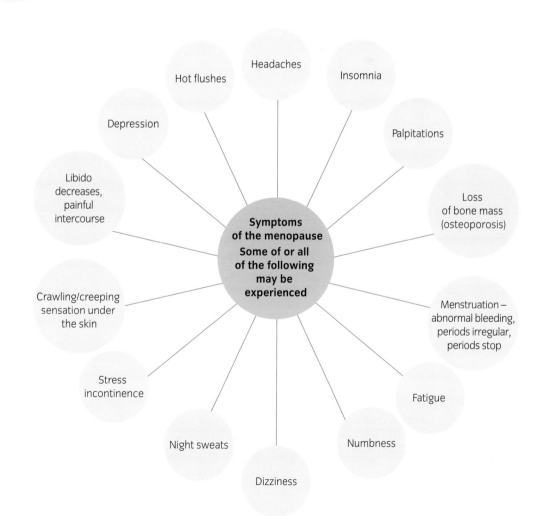

Symptoms of the menopause
Some of or all of the following may be experienced

- Hot flushes
- Headaches
- Insomnia
- Depression
- Palpitations
- Libido decreases, painful intercourse
- Loss of bone mass (osteoporosis)
- Crawling/creeping sensation under the skin
- Menstruation – abnormal bleeding, periods irregular, periods stop
- Stress incontinence
- Fatigue
- Night sweats
- Numbness
- Dizziness

HORMONES

DISEASES AND DISORDERS OF THE REPRODUCTIVE SYSTEM

Disease	Description	Contra-indications and general precautions	Advice to client
Genital herpes	Itching or irritation in the genitals or surrounding areas. Develops into painful red blisters that burst to leave open sores. Transferred from mouth to genitals during oral sex and vice versa.	Contra-indicated as it is a highly contagious condition. Treatments in the pelvic/abdominal area could be very painful and could lead to bleeding.	Suggest client seeks medical advice.
Polycystic ovary syndrome	Cysts develop around the edge of the ovaries. The cysts may be caused by the failure of the ovary to release an egg during ovulation or higher than average levels of male hormones. Symptoms include an increase in hair growth (hirsutism) with growth particularly around the lower face and jaw, irregular and/or light menstruation, infertility, thinning of hair on the scalp, acne and an increase in weight.	Carry out treatment with caution. Clients with excessive hair growth will benefit from epilation.	Suggest client seeks medical advice before treatment if they are concerned.
Thrush	A yeast infection, caused by a yeast-like fungus called Candida albicans that affects the mucous membranes, eg vagina and other areas of moist skin causing intense itching, irritation. Candida is naturally present in the body, but changes in the body's pH can upset the body's natural balance. Symptoms include vaginal discharge, some discomfort when urinating, a red rash with flaky white patches (similar to nappy rash). Can occur after a course of antibiotics which destroy too many of the body's good bacteria causing a change in the pH.	Carry out treatment with caution. Avoid the area to prevent further irritation and cross-infection.	Suggest client seeks medical advice from a GP or pharmacist.
Endometriosis	A condition where the endometrial tissue grows outside of the uterus. This could be in the ovaries, Fallopian tubes and other pelvic organs. The endometrial tissue still behaves in the same way as the tissue that lines the uterus and responds to changing hormones at different times in the menstrual cycle (ie it grows during the menstrual cycle and bleeds). The endometrial tissue has no way of leaving the body which causes pain and swelling. Pain can be mild to severe. The condition can lead to infertility.	Carry out treatment with caution. A common condition and symptoms vary. Treatment over the abdomen should be avoided if there is discomfort.	Suggest client seeks medical advice before treatment if they are concerned.

CHAPTER SUMMARY

Now you have reached the end of the chapter, check the following list to see if you feel confident in all the areas covered. If there are still any areas you are unsure of, go back over them in your book and ask your manager for additional support:

- cells, tissues and organs
- skin, hair and nails
- the skeletal system
- the muscular system
- the cardiovascular system
- the lymphatic system
- the respiratory system
- the nervous system
- the digestive system
- the endocrine system
- the urinary system
- the reproductive system.

TEST YOUR KNOWLEDGE

Use the questions below to test your knowledge of the Anatomy and Physiology chapter to see how much information you have retained. These questions will help you revise what you have learnt in this chapter.

Turn to page 499 for the answers.

1 What is the name of the chemical released by the body that causes vasodilation?
   a Histamine
   b Erythrocyte
   c Macrophage
   d Pathogen

2 Which **one** of the following is not found in the acid mantle?
   a Urea
   b Water
   c Sweat
   d Sebum

3 Which **one** of the following is produced by fibroblasts?
   a Histamine
   b Collagen
   c Pathogens
   d Papillae

4 Meissner's corpuscles are nerve endings that are able to sense which one of the following?
   a Pressure
   b Pain
   c Touch
   d Temperature

5 The depth of skin colour is dependent on which of the following?
   a How melanin is structured
   b More active melanocytes
   c The amount of melanin in the melanosomes
   d How melanosomes are distributed

6 Which **one** of the following is a bacterial infection?
   a Impetigo
   b Shingles
   c Milia
   d Urticaria

7 What is psoriasis often caused by?
   a Bacteria
   b Virus
   c Fungus
   d Stress

8 What is the outer layer of the hair called?
   a Medulla
   b Shaft
   c Cortex
   d Cuticle

9 How many cervical bones are there?
   a 4
   b 5
   c 7
   d 12

10 Which **one** of the following is a characteristic of veins?
   a They carry oxygenated blood
   b Blood flow is under pressure
   c The vessels have a thick layer of muscle
   d The vessels have valves

11 Which **one** of the following is involved in the blood clotting process?
   a Thrombocytes
   b Leucocytes
   c Erythrocytes
   d Granulocytes

12 Which area does the thoracic duct not drain lymph from?
   a Both legs
   b Abdominal cavities
   c Neck and left arm
   d Thorax and right arm

13 What is the name of the blood vessel that carries blood to the kidney?

a Renal artery

b Renal vein

c Aorta

d Vena cava

14 How much urine is held in the bladder before the normal sensation to urinate occurs?

a 100–200ml

b 200–300ml

c 300–400ml

d 400–500ml

15 Which of the following parts of the cell is commonly referred to as the 'powerhouse of the cell'?

a Mitochondria

b Liposomes

c Cytoplasm

d Ribosome

16 Which **one** of the following occurs to skin cells during mitosis?

a An exact replica of the original cell is produced

b Two new but different cells are produced

c Two new identical cells are produced

d One new but different cell is produced

17 Which **one** of the following hormones regulates the metabolism?

a Thyroid-stimulating hormone

b Insulin

c Glucagon

d Adrenocorticotrophic hormone

18 Which **one** of the following hormones reduces the level of glucose and nutrients in the blood?

a Insulin

b Glucagon

c Adrenaline

d Thyroxine

19 Which **one** of the following hormones prepares the uterus for pregnancy?

a Oxytocin

b Progesterone

c Oestrogen

d Androgen

20 How many pairs of cranial nerves are there?

a 8

b 10

c 12

d 14

21 Which **one** of the following would happen in response to the parasympathetic nervous system?

a Dilation of the bronchi

b Decreased urine secretion

c Increased cardiac output

d Constriction of the blood vessels

22 What are fats made up of?

a Monoglycerides

b Diglycerides

c Triglycerides

d Polyglycerides

23 In which part of the digestive system are villi found?

a Stomach

b Large intestine

c Small intestine

d Colon

24 Which of the following occurs during inspiration?

a Air is breathed out, diaphragm and intercostal muscles contract

b Air is breathed out, diaphragm and intercostal muscles relax

c Air is breathed in, diaphragm and intercostal muscles contract

d Air is breathed in, diaphragm and intercostal muscles relax

25 Which **one** of the following is not caused by a viral infection?

a Influenza

b Sinusitis

c Asthma

d Bronchitis

LEGISLATION

This chapter will help you to learn about **legislation**. Legislation means laws (**Acts** or **regulations**) that are set and passed by the government. They consist of a set of rules or guidelines that must be followed for legal reasons. While they apply to all businesses we will be looking at how these Acts and regulations are important to the beauty and nail industries. Failure to meet legal requirements can result in a fine and, in very serious cases, the loss of the business and possibly imprisonment. In the beauty and nail industries you must make sure you follow the relevant legislation to show you are acting professionally and following expected industry standards.

In this chapter you will learn about:

- laws relating to health and safety
- laws relating to **consumer** protection
- other relevant legislation.

You will need to use this chapter in conjunction with all the other chapters and refer back to it.

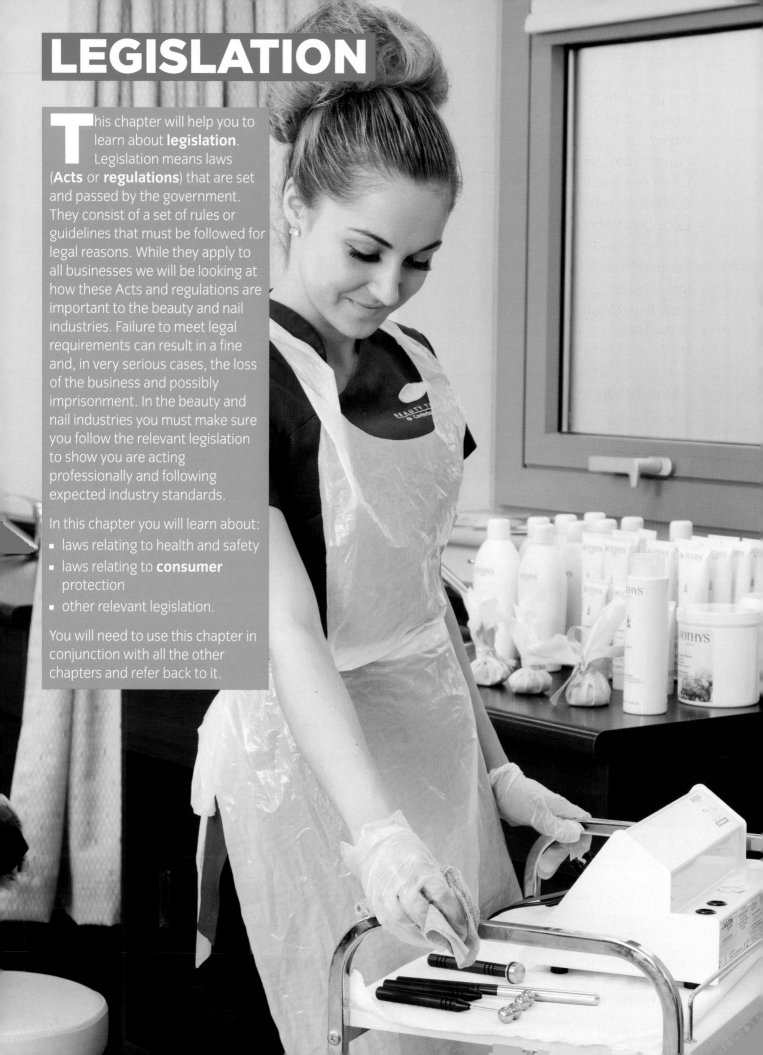

LAWS RELATING TO HEALTH AND SAFETY

In this part of the chapter you will learn about the:

- Health and Safety at Work Act
- Workplace (Health, Safety and Welfare) Regulations
- Provision and Use of Work Equipment Regulations
- Local Government Miscellaneous Provisions Act
- Control of Substances Hazardous to Health Regulations
- Electricity at Work Regulations
- The Regulatory Reform (Fire Safety) Order (RRO)
- Personal Protective Equipment (PPE) at Work Regulations
- Manual Handling Operations Regulations
- Reporting of Injuries, Diseases and Dangerous Occurences Regulations
- Health and Safety (First Aid) Regulations
- Health and Safety (Display Screen Equipment) Regulations
- Environmental Protection Act
- EU Directive – Amendment Number/EU to Cosmetic Products Directive.

ACTIVITY

Use this table to help you remember the initials of some of the legislation you must learn.

Initials	Legislation name in full
HASAWA	Health and Safety at Work Act
COSHH	Control of Substances Hazardous to Health
PPE	Personal Protective Equipment at Work Regulations
RIDDOR	Reporting of Injuries, Diseases and Dangerous Occurrences Regulations
PUWER	Provision and Use of Work Equipment Regulations
EAWR	Electricity at Work Regulations
DPA	Data Protection Act
	Equality Act

HEALTH AND SAFETY AT WORK ACT

The Health and Safety at Work Act (HASAWA) imposes duties on employers to ensure that they provide a safe place of work for everybody affected by their activities. This Act also imposes a duty on employees to ensure that they comply with the employers' safety arrangements and do not behave in a way that endangers others. The Act applies to people who are self-employed too.

The HASAWA is an enabling Act that allows the government to make further laws known as 'regulations' with attached approved codes of practices (ACOP) that detail how employers must comply with them. The various health and safety regulations include guidelines on:

Legislation
Laws that are made or passed by Parliament

Act
A law

Regulations
The rules of the Act

Consumer
Someone who pays for goods or a service

HANDY HINT
Sometimes you might be asked which year an Act was passed. These dates are on the HASAWA data sheet which needs to be displayed in a salon. You could answer this question by saying that Acts are dated when they are passed but as they are reviewed and have changes made they then get a revised date.

HANDY HINT
Trading Standards is a local authority service that enforces a range of legislation. Approximately 100 Acts and 600 regulations are enforced by Trading Standards officers.

HANDY HINT
Acts are dated when they are passed, but as they are reviewed and have changes made, they get a revised date. Many Acts are reviewed and amended regularly as laws change.

 SmartScreen 305 Handout 4

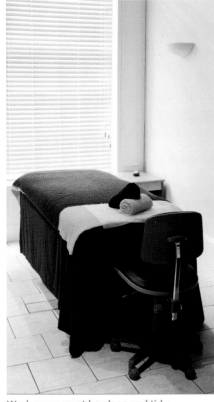

Work areas must be clean and tidy

- health and safety policies
- risk assessments
- hygiene, cleanliness and disposal of waste
- heating, lighting and ventilation
- work facilities and maintaining a safe and healthy work environment
- safe use of chemicals
- personal protective equipment (PPE)
- fire safety
- safe use and maintenance of work equipment
- manual handling (lifting and carrying).

ACTIVITY

Discuss with your tutor how the salon would be affected if the guidelines and rules of the HASAWA were not followed. What could happen?

THE MAIN LEGISLATION UNDER THE UMBRELLA OF THE HASAWA

The HASAWA is an umbrella for all other legislation relating to health and safety in the workplace.

EMPLOYER'S RESPONSIBILITIES

Under the HASAWA and other regulations, your employer is not just responsible for the health and safety of their clients but also the staff and any visitors (such as product representatives, area managers and tradespeople). Your employer must:

- maintain the workplace and make sure it is safe to work in
- give staff appropriate training and supervision
- keep access and exit points clear and free from hazards at all times
- provide a suitable working environment and facilities that comply with the HASAWA
- make sure the salon's health and safety systems are reviewed and updated.

EMPLOYEE'S RESPONSIBILITIES

Your responsibilities under the HASAWA are to yourself, your colleagues and your clients. You must:

- maintain the health and safety of yourself and others who might be affected by your actions
- work together and communicate with your employer about health and safety issues, so your employer can keep within the law.

Who is the person responsible for reporting health and safety matters? YOU are! If you see a health and safety problem, you must deal with it or report it. Everyone is responsible for maintaining a safe place of work.

WORKPLACE (HEALTH, SAFETY AND WELFARE) REGULATIONS

The Workplace (Health, Safety and Welfare) Regulations require everyone in the workplace to help maintain a safe and healthy working environment. You and your employer should follow **environmentally friendly** working practices.

EMPLOYER'S RESPONSIBILITIES

Your employer's responsibilities under the regulations are to:

- maintain equipment and the workplace
- regulate temperatures
- make sure working conditions and the size and shape of the room suit the number of staff employed
- make sure there is sufficient lighting and ventilation
- make sure all walkways are clear of hazards
- provide toilets and washing facilities
- provide drinking water and facilities for staff to rest, eat meals and change clothing
- provide secure areas or lockers for employees' clothing and property
- make sure all lights above the stairways and at fire exits are working.

Environmentally friendly

Safe for or good for the environment

HANDY HINT

The number of toilet and washing facilities must be sufficient for the the number of employees and customers using the premises.

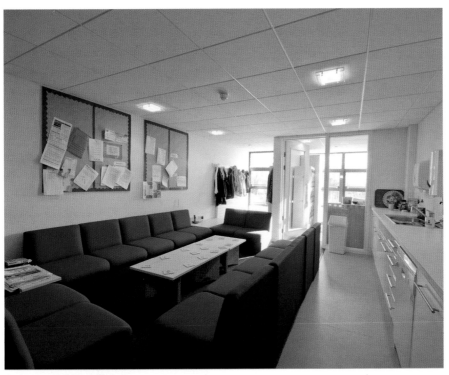

A clean and tidy staff room

Obstruction

Something that blocks your path

Evacuation

Leaving an area because of fire

Contamination

The presence of something unwanted that might be harmful

Greenhouse gas emissions

The release of gases into the atmosphere that absorb infra-red radiation. These gases contribute to the greenhouse effect and global warming

EMPLOYEE'S RESPONSIBILITIES

Your responsibilities under the regulations are to:

- make sure all doors, fire exits and stairways are kept free of **obstructions** and hazards
- make sure you know the fire **evacuation** procedure
- prevent infection and **contamination** by keeping the salon's workstations, mirrors, floors, gowns, towels, equipment and tools clean
- keep the salon tidy to prevent accidents, such as tripping over trailing electrical wires
- clean up spillages immediately to prevent slippery surfaces
- report any problems that you are unable to deal with to your employer.

PROVISION AND USE OF WORK EQUIPMENT REGULATIONS

The Provision and Use of Work Equipment Regulations (PUWER) require that all the equipment in the salon (both new and second-hand) must be used for its intended purpose only and kept in good working condition.

EMPLOYER'S RESPONSIBILITIES

Your employer's responsibilities under the regulations are:

- to provide you with training to use the equipment as it is intended
- to make sure that the equipment is properly built and fit for use
- to ensure all work equipment is properly maintained including equipment supplied by employees.

EMPLOYEE'S RESPONSIBILITIES

Your responsibilities under the regulations are:

- to make sure you know how to use the equipment in the salon properly and safely
- to use equipment only for its intended purpose (eg do not use a warm wax heater for heating paraffin wax).

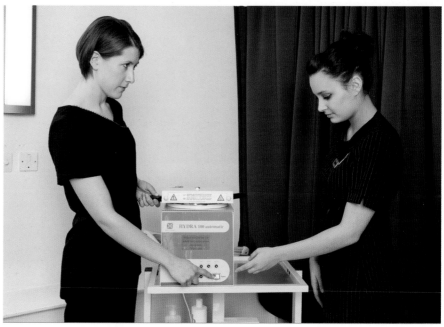

Therapist instructing a colleague

LOCAL GOVERNMENT MISCELLANEOUS PROVISIONS ACT

The Local Government Miscellaneous Provisions Act requires all businesses to be registered with the local authority, first so that the government knows they exist and second so that they can be **monitored** and regulated. Your employer must make sure they take the relevant steps to register for the services they are offering.

A business must show that its standards meet the rules and regulations set out in the local council's **by-laws**. By-laws are a set of local laws that deal with local issues and tell a business how it must act with regards to health and safety, hygiene and cleanliness. Specific by-laws relate to specific business practices (eg ear piercing and electrolysis). Some councils have a downloadable copy of their by-laws on their website.

This Act also gives local authorities the power to inspect business premises and to act if something falls below the required standard.

CONTROL OF SUBSTANCES HAZARDOUS TO HEALTH REGULATIONS

Various chemicals are seen as hazardous (eg cleaning substances and bleach). The Control of Substances Hazardous to Health (COSHH) Regulations identify dangerous chemicals. Hazardous substances can enter the body through **ingestion**, **absorption** or **inhalation**. A hazardous substance in the workplace can put a person's health at risk and cause disease or injury, such as asthma, cancer or dermatitis.

Hazardous substances must be **identified** by specific symbols which you should be able to recognise. All suppliers must legally provide guidelines on how their materials should be stored and used. All products identified as hazardous must by law be listed and a COSHH risk assessment must be **accessible**. Be aware that substances that seem to be harmless can be hazardous if used or stored incorrectly. A risk assessment should be carried out for each substance used in the salon.

Low-risk products should be used instead of high-risk products wherever there is an **alternative**. For example, a low-risk product would be tinting peroxide (10 volume or 3 per cent) that had already been diluted and packaged for the purpose. Using a higher concentration of peroxide (30 volume or 9 per cent) that needed to be diluted in the salon would be high risk.

Under COSHH you must make sure that any hazardous substances are stored, handled, used and disposed of correctly and safely. The best way of remembering this is by following **SHUD**:

- **S**torage: keep in a locked cupboard at room temperature when not in use, ideally this cupboard should also be **fire retardant**.
- **H**andling: wear appropriate personal protective equipment (PPE) such as gloves, mask and apron.
- **U**sage: use according to the manufacturer's instructions or workplace guidelines.

Monitored
Kept an eye on

By-law
A local council rule

Ingestion
Taking food into the mouth and digestive system

Absorption
The process whereby nutrients enter the bloodstream via the stomach or intestines

Inhalation
Breathing in

Identified
Recognised or pointed out

Accessible
Easy to get to

Alternative
A different possible choice or outcome

Fire retardant
Made of a material used to slow down the spread of fire

Incinerate
To burn something to ashes

Environment
This can be both the natural world around us as well as the things that have an effect on you

Disposed of
Got rid of something that is no longer wanted or needed

WHY DON'T YOU...
make a list of all the items in your salon that would come under COSHH – everything from washing powder to peroxide. Ask your tutor or manager to check your list.

■ **D**isposal: make sure you dispose of all hazardous waste in a hazardous waste bag; the local authority or a private company will collect the waste and **incinerate** it. This usually consists of tissues, cotton wool and wax strips that have been in contact with bodily fluids (eg blood).

The manufacturer's instructions will explain how to store, handle, use and dispose of chemicals or substances. The local by-laws will tell you how to dispose of them, be considerate to the **environment** and follow the local authority's guidelines on waste and refuse. Your salon's policy will explain where to store and mix the chemicals and where to dispose of them in the workplace.

EMPLOYER'S RESPONSIBILITIES
Your employer's responsibilities under the regulations are:
■ to make sure COSHH health and safety information sheets are available for substances and chemicals in the workplace
■ to make sure chemicals are **disposed of** according to local by-laws and with respect to the environment
■ to ensure that a COSHH risk assessment is undertaken.

EMPLOYEE'S RESPONSIBILITIES
Your responsibilities under the regulations are:
■ to follow SHUD
■ to read and follow the manufacturer's instructions, local by-laws and your salon's policy
■ to know where to find the COSHH information sheets.

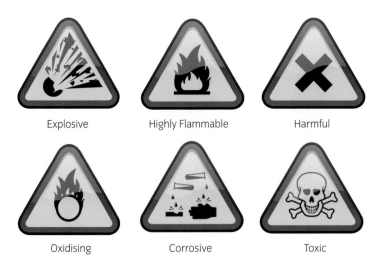

| Explosive | Highly Flammable | Harmful |

| Oxidising | Corrosive | Toxic |

Hazard labels

ELECTRICITY AT WORK REGULATIONS
The Electricity at Work Regulations (EAWR) require all electrical **appliances** to be used with caution and handled correctly. Electrical equipment must be *maintained in a condition suitable for use*, checked and tested on a routine basis.

Appliance
A device or piece of equipment made to perform a specific task

EMPLOYER'S RESPONSIBILITIES

Your employer's responsibilities under the regulations are to make sure that all electrical equipment:

- is in a safe working condition
- is portable appliance tested (PAT) by a qualified electrician at least once a year (some appliances might need checking more frequently). This means anything that has a cable and a plug must be tested. A record must be kept. Insurance companies require all electrical equipment to be routinely tested
- is visually checked by salon employees routinely and frequently.

EMPLOYEE'S RESPONSIBILITIES

Your responsibilities under the regulations are to:

- not use electrical appliances until you have been trained
- use appliances correctly and to switch them off after use
- carry out routine visual checks. These could be done in the morning when equipment is switched on or at the end of the day when equipment is switched off. You must check any electrical appliance you use for faults or problems (eg frayed or loose cables or flexes, broken plugs or damage to the external casing)
- not overload plug sockets
- report any faults immediately to your supervisor or manager and to label the item as faulty. The label should be clear and secure. Write down what the problem or fault is and include the date. Remove the equipment from the working area if possible until it can be repaired or disposed of
- not use faulty equipment.

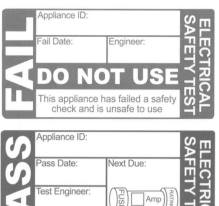

PAT testing stickers/labels

LEGISLATION

HANDY HINT

Fixed wiring such as plug sockets and fuse (distribution) boards should be tested every five years as recommended.

WHY DON'T YOU...
make a list of the electrical checks that a therapist should carry out routinely. Discuss the list with your tutor or manager.

ACTIVITY

Can you see evidence of PAT testing having taken place in your salon? What date did it take place? When is the next test due?

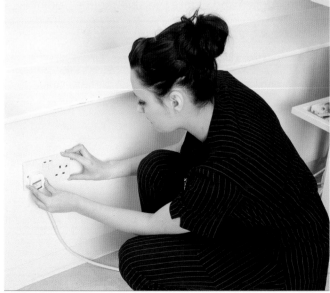

Therapist checking a plug

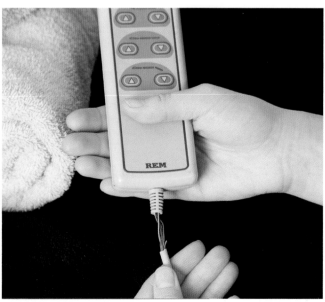

Faulty wiring

145

Emergency exit route
The safest route by which staff, clients and visitors can escape a building

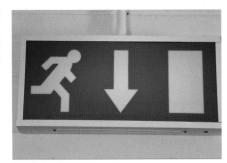

Fire exit sign

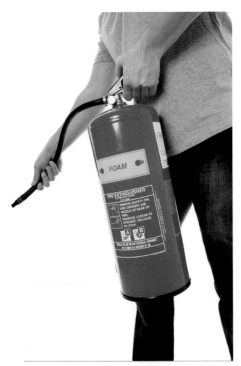

A foam extinguisher used for putting out class B fires involving flammable liquids (except cooking oils)

THE REGULATORY REFORM (FIRE SAFETY) ORDER (RRO)

The RRO requires all premises to have basic standards of fire prevention and control and an **emergency exit route**.

Every business must carry out a fire risk assessment which should be reviewed annually or following any changes. It assesses how to prevent a fire and in the event of a fire how to control it.

A fire safety risk assessment must:

- identify fire hazards
- identify people at risk
- evaluate, remove or reduce risks and protect staff, clients and visitors from risk
- record, plan, inform, instruct and train staff
- be reviewed.

EMPLOYER'S RESPONSIBILITIES

Your employer's responsibilities under the order are to:

- carry out a full fire risk assessment, even if the workplace is covered by a fire certificate
- make sure all fire exits are unlocked, have fire exit signs and are easy to access
- train staff in fire evacuation procedures so that they know what is expected if there is an emergency – procedures should be practised so that all staff know what to do
- supply suitable fire-fighting equipment, such as fire extinguishers and fire blankets and to make sure they are maintained.

EMPLOYEE'S RESPONSIBILITIES

Your responsibilities under the Act and the regulations are to:

- know where the fire extinguishers and blankets are located in the salon
- know which fire extinguishers can be used on different fires
- know the evacuation procedure and where the safe meeting point is for salon staff and clients.

HANDY HINT

Further information on which extinguishers can be used on different fires can be found in Chapter 302.

PERSONAL PROTECTIVE EQUIPMENT (PPE) AT WORK REGULATIONS

Gloves, aprons, masks and eye protection for salon employees as well as your uniform and shoes all come under the Personal Protective Equipment (PPE) at Work Regulations. Protective equipment used for the client is not covered by these regulations. It is important that you wear the appropriate PPE to protect yourself from harm when you are working with chemicals and to minimise cross-infection.

EMPLOYER'S RESPONSIBILITIES

Your employer's responsibilities under the regulations are to:

- supply free of charge any PPE required for you to carry out your job
- maintain supplies of PPE so that they are always accessible
- train staff how to use PPE appropriately
- carry out risk assessments and to recommend when to use PPE.

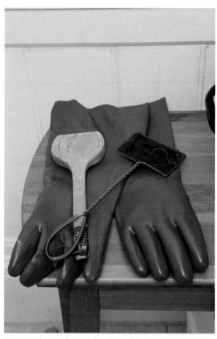

Heavy-duty gloves for handling hot stones during massage

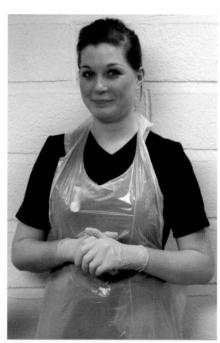

Wearing disposable gloves and apron

EMPLOYEE'S RESPONSIBILITIES

Your responsibilities under the regulations are to:

- wear PPE when you are mixing, handling and using chemicals or substances
- report any shortages of PPE to the relevant person so that additional stock can be ordered.

MANUAL HANDLING OPERATIONS REGULATIONS

You are sometimes required to move equipment and stock around the salon and this is called manual handling. Always follow the Manual Handling Operations Regulations. There are correct ways to lift objects so you do not injure yourself.

WHY DON'T YOU...
make a list of all the occasions when you know you will need to wear PPE and what PPE you will need. Review the list with your tutor or manager.

According to the Health and Safety Executive (HSE), more than a third of all injuries resulting in over three days' absence from work are caused by manual handling. A recent survey showed that over 12.3 million working days are lost each year due to work-related **musculoskeletal disorders** that have been caused or made worse by poor manual handling.

ACTIVITY

Write a list of problems or disorders that might affect a therapist's muscles and bones if they do not follow manual handling guidelines.

EMPLOYER'S RESPONSIBILITIES

Your employer's responsibility under the regulations is to carry out risk assessments on all employees for manual lifting to make sure they are able to lift boxes and other heavy objects without causing injury.

EMPLOYEE'S RESPONSIBILITIES

Your responsibility under the regulations is to always ask yourself: 'Can I lift this?' If the answer is 'no', then don't! Ask for help. If the answer is 'yes', remember to bend your knees and keep your back straight. Lift the weight with your thigh muscles not your back and keep the item you are lifting close to your body. Even if a box is light, you should ask for help if it obscures your view.

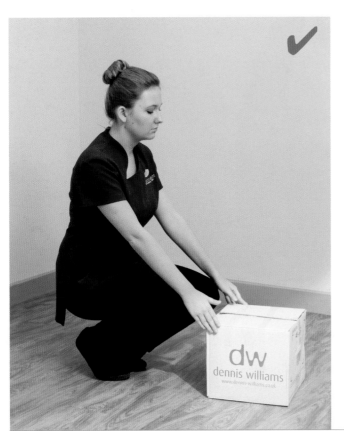 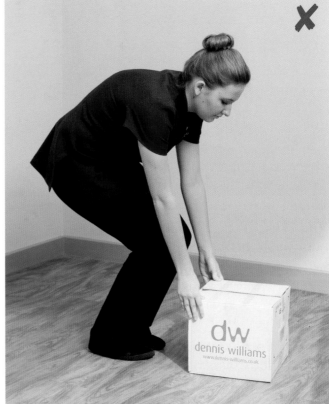

The picture on the left shows the correct lifting technique; the lifting technique on the right is incorrect. The technique on the right will put pressure on the spine and could lead to injury

THE CITY & GUILDS TEXTBOOK

REPORTING OF INJURIES, DISEASES AND DANGEROUS OCCURRENCES REGULATIONS

The Reporting of Injuries, Diseases and Dangerous Occurrences Regulations (RIDDOR) require the following occurrences to be reported to the HSE immediately by telephone and then in writing within ten days of the incident:

- injuries resulting in over seven days' loss of work (including non-working days)
- injuries (eg falls) sustained by you, your colleagues, clients or visitors in the workplace that result in three or more days off work
- major injuries, such as amputation, dislocation, fractures (not fingers or toes), loss of sight and any other eye injuries
- any work-related incident where a person has had to spend more than 24 hours in hospital
- accidents and injuries sustained from violence in the workplace
- death in the workplace
- diseases, such as **occupational** dermatitis or work-related asthma
- dangerous occurrences (eg a gas leak) even if they occur outside working hours and no one is injured.

Occupational
Relating to a job

EMPLOYER'S RESPONSIBILITIES

Your employer's responsibility under the regulations is to report any of the above **occurrences** and make sure that information about the occurrence has been recorded.

Occurence
Something that happens

EMPLOYEE'S RESPONSIBILITIES

Your responsibilities under the regulations are to:

- report any work-related diseases to the person responsible for health and safety
- prevent any work-related diseases by wearing PPE
- report any accidents or injuries that happen to you at work
- prevent accidents or injuries by following safe working guidelines and maintaining a tidy environment.

ACTIVITY

Which work-related diseases might you be exposed to? Make a list. Discuss your list with your manager and colleagues.

HANDY HINT
Make sure you know where the business keeps their health and safety policies as these should all be accessible.

HEALTH AND SAFETY (FIRST AID) REGULATIONS

The Health and Safety (First Aid) Regulations apply to all workplaces in Great Britain – including those with fewer than five employees and those with self-employed staff. The regulations require the protection of everyone in the workplace by making sure risk assessments are carried out to prevent accidents and injuries at work. It is **advisable** that at least one person has undertaken first-aid training.

HANDY HINT
Know where your first-aid box is kept just in case you need to access it.

Advisable
Suggested that you should

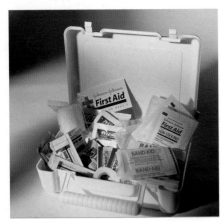

First-aid box

A basic first-aid box or container should include:

- a leaflet giving general guidance on first aid (eg HSE's leaflet *Basic advice on first aid at work*)
- 20 individually wrapped sterile plasters (assorted sizes), appropriate to the type of work (**hypoallergenic** plasters can be provided, if necessary)
- two sterile eye pads
- four individually wrapped triangular bandages, preferably sterile
- six safety pins
- two large sterile individually wrapped unmedicated wound dressings
- six medium-sized individually wrapped unmedicated wound dressings
- a pair of disposable gloves
- eyewash kits, because of the chemicals used in salons.

The appointed person should check the contents of the first-aid container frequently and make sure it is restocked if anything is used. They should ensure the safe disposal of items when they reach their expiry date.

EMPLOYER'S RESPONSIBILITIES

Your employer's responsibilities under the regulations are to:

- take immediate action if employees are injured or taken ill at work
- consider providing a first aider
- choose an appointed person to be responsible for first-aid arrangements
- provide a well-stocked first-aid container
- make sure all staff know who the appointed first aider is (if appropriate).

EMPLOYEE'S RESPONSIBILITIES

Your responsibilities under the regulations are to:

- avoid taking any unnecessary risks that might put you or others in danger
- report to your appointed person any first-aid supply shortages
- record any accidents in an accident book. Make a note of who had the accident, the date and time of the accident and what action was taken. Record the name of any witnesses and who else was present at the time of the accident. The accident book should be kept in a central location in the salon.

HEALTH AND SAFETY (DISPLAY SCREEN EQUIPMENT) REGULATIONS

The Health and Safety (Display Screen Equipment) Regulations protect the health of people who work with display screen equipment (DSE). This includes computer workstations or visual display units (VDU) (ie computer screens). It applies to people, such as salon receptionists, who use display screen equipment for long periods at a time as part of their job. It does not apply to occasional use, such as making appointments. Long-term use is often associated with neck, shoulder, back or arm pain, fatigue and eyestrain. Display screen equipment work is not risky but users need to follow good practice, such as setting up their workstations well and taking **periodic** breaks.

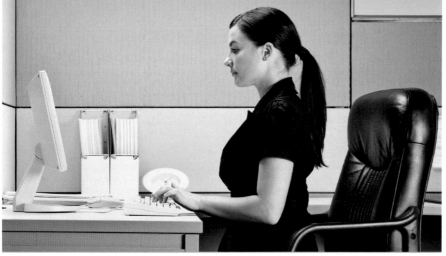

Good posture when sitting at a computer

EMPLOYER'S RESPONSIBILITIES

Your employer's responsibilities under the regulations are to:

- carry out risk assessments on new workstations or make changes to current workstations
- re-assess workstations if staff suffer from any discomfort
- train employees in good practice for working with display screen equipment
- plan scheduling of work, regular breaks and changes of activity
- pay for employees to have eyesight tests if required.

EMPLOYEE'S RESPONSIBILITIES

Your responsibilities under the regulations are to:

- make sure you maintain good posture. Keep your back straight when you work and do not slouch. Keep your feet flat on the floor when sitting
- take regular breaks if you are using display screen equipment for long periods of time and to change activity. If you are a receptionist change to a different task, such as filing
- organise your desk space effectively
- keep your 'mouse arm' straight and rest it lightly on the mouse
- use a wrist support
- keep your keyboard close to your body and do not over-stretch
- adjust the screen or lighting position where possible to suit your personal needs.

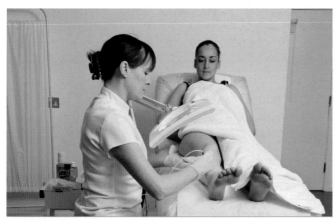

Both therapist and client must be comfortable

ENVIRONMENTAL PROTECTION ACT

Any waste products from the salon must be disposed of correctly so you do not pollute the environment or harm others. You must always dispose of products by following the MFIs and local by-laws. All staff must be trained and be made aware of how to dispose of waste in a safe way.

LAWS RELATING TO CONSUMER PROTECTION

In this part of the chapter you will learn about the:

- Data Protection Act
- Consumer Protection Act
- Consumer Protection (Distance Selling) Regulations
- Supply of Goods and Services Act
- Sale of Goods Act
- Sale and Supply of Goods Act
- Trade Descriptions Acts
- Prices Act.

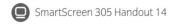

SmartScreen 305 Handout 14

DATA PROTECTION ACT

Clients give you their personal information, such as their addresses and phone numbers, because they trust you and the salon to use it correctly. Clients' information must be protected and you must always follow the Data Protection Act.

The Information Commissioner's Office is the UK's independent authority set up to uphold information rights in the public's interest. It sets the rules for the Data Protection Act, which protects people's rights to confidentiality and privacy. When completing client record cards and taking contact details at reception, you must make sure you follow the requirements of the Data Protection Act. Under the Data Protection Act, businesses must register if they keep client data on a computer. There are several principles to the Data Protection Act.

EMPLOYER'S RESPONSIBILITIES

Your employer's responsibilities under the Act are to:

- keep only information that is needed for the business
- keep records as accurate as possible and up to date
- dispose of information carefully (eg shred paper documents) when it is no longer required
- never pass on any information to a **third party**
- limit access to records to only those employees who need it for their work.

Third party

Another person who is not directly involved but has connections with the business

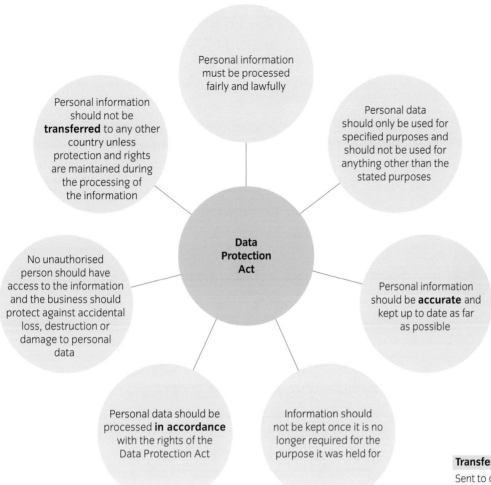

Personal information must be processed fairly and lawfully

Personal information should not be **transferred** to any other country unless protection and rights are maintained during the processing of the information

Personal data should only be used for specified purposes and should not be used for anything other than the stated purposes

Data Protection Act

No unauthorised person should have access to the information and the business should protect against accidental loss, destruction or damage to personal data

Personal information should be **accurate** and kept up to date as far as possible

Personal data should be processed **in accordance** with the rights of the Data Protection Act

Information should not be kept once it is no longer required for the purpose it was held for

Transferred
Sent to or shared with

In accordance
Consistent with

Accurate
Correct and true

EMPLOYEE'S RESPONSIBILITIES

The Data Protection Act protects you and all the data stored about you, whether it is held on paper or on a computer. This includes medical and dental records, bank records and employment and college records. You have a right to access this information if and when you want to and you should expect it to be kept confidential. Remember this and be professional with any information you record regarding any individual.

You must keep records as accurately as you can and keep information confidential. You must not pass on any information about your clients to a third party, whether that is personal details, services that they have had or products that they have bought.

Failing to keep client confidentiality could mean losing clients and gaining a poor reputation. A client could sue the business in which case the guilty employee could be given a warning or lose their job for **gross misconduct**.

> **HANDY HINT**
> Make sure you are familiar with how the law affects you as you do not want your reputation as well as that of the business to be affected.

Gross misconduct
Very bad, unacceptable behaviour

Unethical
Immoral or unacceptable behaviour

> **HANDY HINT**
> Never give clients personal information, such as your address or phone number. It is **unethical** and might put you at risk. Your contract of employment might also forbid this – for example, to prevent staff from encouraging clients to have their treatments done privately in their homes.

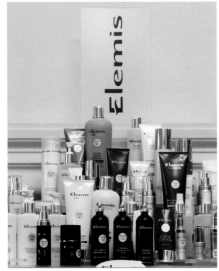

A product range

Negligent

Failing to take proper care

SmartScreen 304 Worksheet 5

Incurred

Acquired or come into

CONSUMER PROTECTION ACT

In the salon, we are exposed daily to different products and we have a right to expect those products to be as safe as possible. The Consumer Protection Act safeguards staff and clients from products that do not reach a reasonable level of safety.

It is now possible to sue a supplier even without proof of the supplier being **negligent** under the Sale of Goods Act (see page 157). A therapist using the product in the salon can sue if a product is faulty (even though your employer purchased it).

The Consumer Protection Act also covers:

- misleading prices, services or facilities
- price comparisons
- inaccurate conditions attached to the price.

HANDY HINT

Do you know where to find the product price lists, if there is a price query?

EMPLOYER'S RESPONSIBILITIES

The employer's responsibilities under this Act are to:

- have clear prices for products and services. The client should be able to tell exactly how much something will cost
- not make false claims about a product or service nor mislead a client
- not attach conditions of sale for either a product or service that are inaccurate or misleading.

EMPLOYEE'S RESPONSIBILITIES

Your responsibilities under the Act are to:

- give clients clear prices for products and services
- be honest when you are promoting or selling a product or treatment. Do not say a product or treatment does something if it does not.

CONSUMER PROTECTION (DISTANCE SELLING) REGULATIONS

The Consumer Protection (Distance Selling) Regulations make sure that when goods are purchased over the phone, from the Internet or by mail order the consumer has the right to receive a refund. If there was a delivery charge this must also be refunded. However, costs **incurred** by the client to return the item are not included.

If you need to return something you must check the contract information, which will include the name and address of the supplier, a description and details of the goods or services and the price paid.

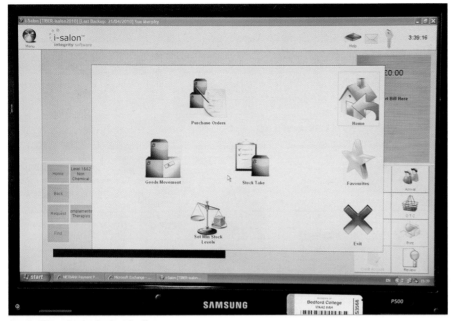

Controlling stock electronically

EMPLOYER'S RESPONSIBILITIES

The employer's responsibilities under the regulations are:

- to give clients a refund if they are unhappy with a product but not to cover the cost of the postage to return the item
- to display **contractual** information on the website with clear terms and conditions of sale.

Contractual
Agreed in a contract

EMPLOYEE'S RESPONSIBILITIES

Your responsibility under the regulations is to offer and process a refund if a client wants to return a product.

SUPPLY OF GOODS AND SERVICES ACT

Services, faulty goods and materials provided with those services or treatments are covered within the Supply of Goods and Services Act. The Act makes sure that:

- a treatment is carried out with skill and reasonable care
- a treatment is carried out within a reasonable amount of time
- a treatment meets what it claims to do
- the charge for the service is reasonable
- any goods supplied in the course of the treatments are of a satisfactory quality and fit for the purpose
- a consumer has the right to have goods replaced, repaired or compensated if they are of poor quality or are not fit for the purpose for which they have been supplied.

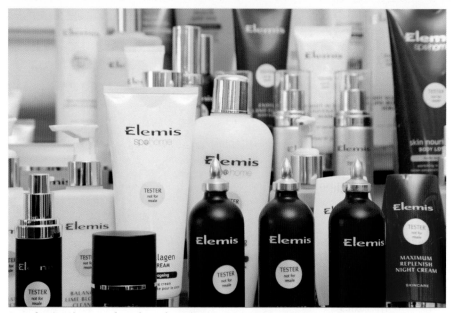

A professional range of products for sale

EMPLOYER'S RESPONSIBILITIES

The employer's responsibilities under the Act are to:

- make sure staff are **adequately** trained
- make sure employees are aware of their responsibilities and what is expected of them during their working hours
- charge a reasonable price for a treatment service
- have clear treatment/service times and make sure therapists know and work to the treatment/service times
- state exactly what a treatment does
- make sure that the goods that the business supplies are of a good quality and fit for the purpose they are sold for
- replace products which are faulty or not fit for the purpose for which they were sold
- **compensate** a client if a service is of a poor quality.

EMPLOYEE'S RESPONSIBILITIES

Your responsibilities under the Act are to:

- carry out services professionally with skill and care and to offer only those treatments for which you are trained
- charge a reasonable price for services
- know and work to the service times of the salon
- state only what a treatment does (do not make up information)
- retail only products of a good quality and fit for the purpose for which they are being sold
- refer any complaint regarding faulty goods or services to a manager to action a refund or compensation.

Adequately

To a suitable or acceptable standard

Compensate

To give someone their money back

HANDY HINT

Always check that the products you are using are in date. If they are out of date let your manager know so that they can be replaced.

SALE OF GOODS ACT AND SALE AND SUPPLY OF GOODS ACT

The Sale of Goods Act and the Sale and Supply of Goods Act cover consumer rights including:

- goods being of satisfactory quality
- the conditions under which goods might be returned after purchase
- whether the goods are fit for their intended purpose
- goods being free from faults or defects.

If these are not followed the consumer has the right to a replacement or refund.

EMPLOYER'S RESPONSIBILITIES

The employer's responsibilities under the Acts are to:

- check that goods being ordered are of a satisfactory condition and free from faults
- have a clear conditions of sale policy that states when products can be returned.

EMPLOYEE'S RESPONSIBILITIES

Your responsibilities under the Acts are to:

- check stock being delivered for damage or faults and to make sure it meets **expectations**
- check stock before retailing to make sure it is in good condition and has not passed its shelf life
- accept returns within the return period and to offer a replacement or refund.

Expectations
A strong belief that something will happen

TRADE DESCRIPTIONS ACTS

The Trade Descriptions Acts prevent services or products:

- being falsely described or false claims being made
- giving false information, including quality, price or purpose
- being falsely advertised, displayed or described.

EMPLOYER'S RESPONSIBILITIES

The employer's responsibility under the Acts is to make sure that all staff are properly trained and understand the products they are using and the services they are giving.

EMPLOYEE'S RESPONSIBILITIES

Your responsibilities under the Acts are to:

- describe treatment and products accurately. You need to know your product information well so that you can do this
- not make any false claims about a treatment or product.

ACTIVITY

Make a list of the different ways products could be priced incorrectly or advertised to give a misleading impression. Discuss with your colleagues.

ACTIVITY

Discuss with your colleagues offers that you have been interested in only to discover hidden costs. How did it make you feel?

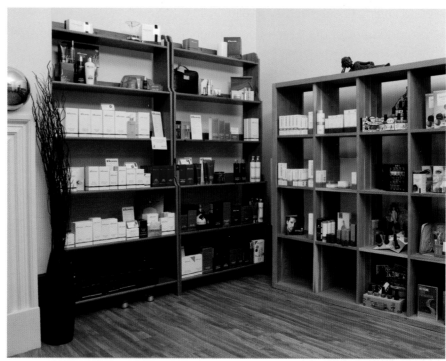

Retail products with prices displayed

PRICES ACT

The Prices Act requires the price of products or services to be displayed clearly. A treatment price list needs to be visible and product prices need to be clearly marked either on the item or on the shelf where they are displayed.

Liability

Responsibility for something that has been done wrong

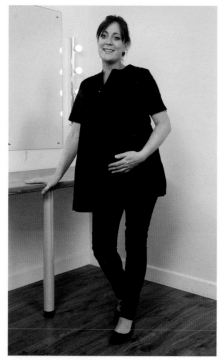

Pregnant therapist

OTHER RELEVANT LEGISLATION

In this part of the chapter you will learn about the:

- Equality Act
- Employers' **Liability** (Compulsory Insurance) Act
- Copyright, Designs and Patent Act.

EQUALITY ACT

The Equality Act lays down laws to prevent discrimination against anyone on the grounds of:

- race or ethnic origin
- sexual orientation
- marriage or civil partnership status
- pregnancy
- religion

- beliefs
- age
- disability.

The Equality Act has replaced these older regulations:

- Sex Discrimination Act
- Race Relations Act
- Race Relations Act (Amendment) Regulations
- Equal Pay Act
- Disability Discrimination Act
- Employment Equality Regulations.

The Equality Act applies to both the employer and the employees within a business so it is important that everyone understands the effects of not adhering to it as they could be held liable. The Act includes protection against intimidation and bullying through **victimisation** and **harassment**.

Victimisation
When a person is treated less favourably than others

Harassment
Unwanted behaviour towards someone

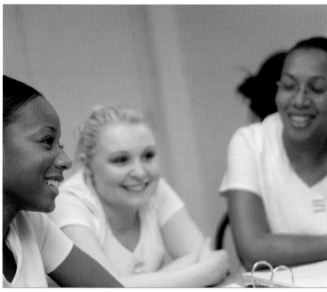

Beauty and nail therapy is multicultural

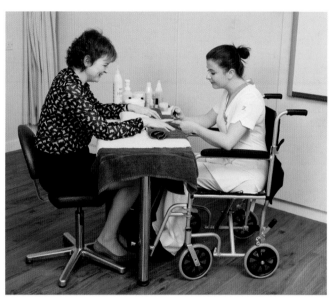

Disabled therapist at work

EMPLOYERS' LIABILITY (COMPULSORY INSURANCE) ACT

If a business has employees it must have employers' liability insurance to comply with the Employers' Liability (Compulsory Insurance) Act. If an employee becomes injured or ill as a result of their work they have the right to claim compensation from their employer. Employers must have adequate insurance to cover any possible insurance claims. Most businesses would be unable to pay a claim so insurance is taken out to cover potential payments. The insurance must be with an **authorised** insurance provider. It might be part of a wider insurance package to meet the other liabilities, such as professional **indemnity** and public liability insurance.

Authorised
When a person or company has official power

Indemnity
Insurance against damage or loss

Ambience

The character and atmosphere of a place

WHY DON'T YOU...

find out more about the PRS by looking at its website: www.prsformusic.com. Click on the link 'Become licensed to play music at work'.

HANDY HINT

Look for the most recent amendment date (change) for the most up-to-date law if you need to check any legislation.

HANDY HINT

Treat everyone as you would want to be treated – we all have the right to be treated fairly.

COPYRIGHT, DESIGNS AND PATENT ACT

Music being played in the salon can help to create the right atmosphere and **ambience**. Music can create an upbeat feel to a room or help listeners to feel calm and relaxed. In order to play music in the salon you need to hold a special licence to comply with the Copyright, Designs and Patent Act.

When we play music (even the radio in the staff room) it becomes a public performance. Your employer must purchase a licence from the Performing Rights Society Ltd (PRS) in order to play music in the salon using a radio, TV, CD or MP3 player. The PRS works on behalf of artists, writers and publishers to collect and distribute a fee for a licence as royalties.

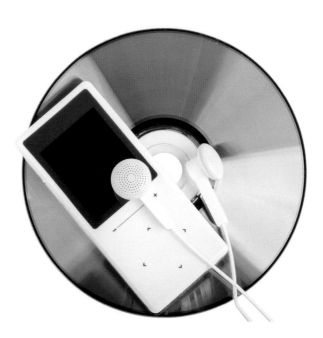

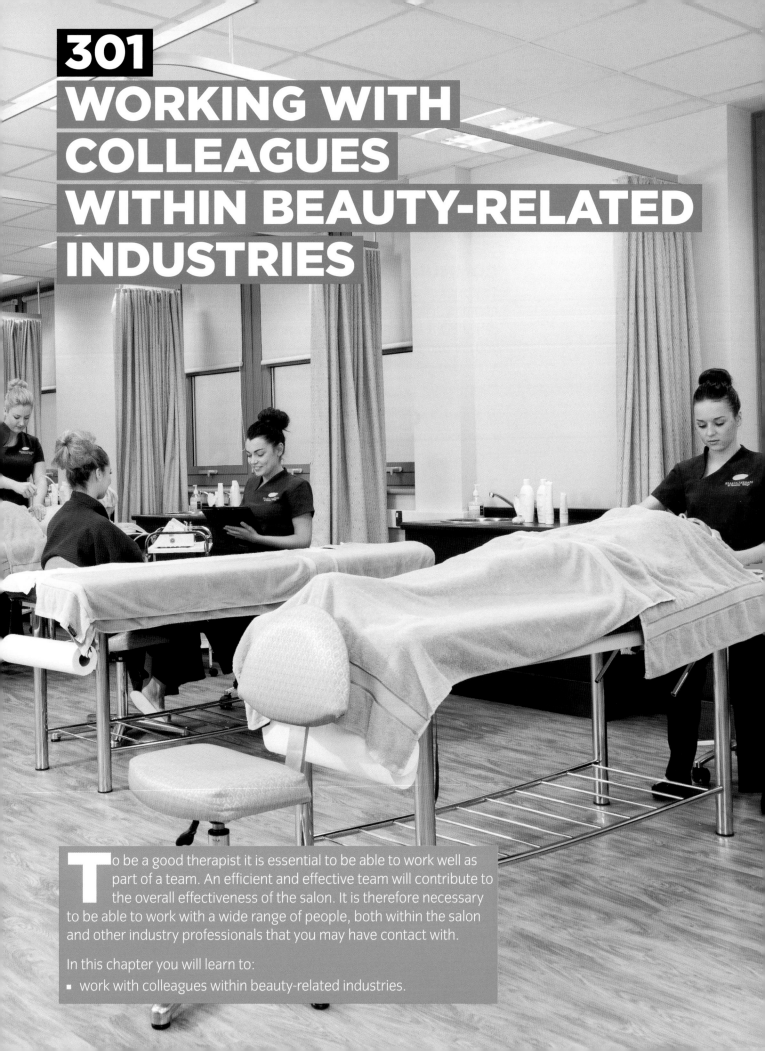

301
WORKING WITH COLLEAGUES WITHIN BEAUTY-RELATED INDUSTRIES

To be a good therapist it is essential to be able to work well as part of a team. An efficient and effective team will contribute to the overall effectiveness of the salon. It is therefore necessary to be able to work with a wide range of people, both within the salon and other industry professionals that you may have contact with.

In this chapter you will learn to:
- work with colleagues within beauty-related industries.

WORKING WITH COLLEAGUES WITHIN BEAUTY-RELATED INDUSTRIES

In order to be an effective therapist you will need to work well with your colleagues. Colleagues can be:

- internal colleagues: other people within your salon whom you work with directly
- external colleagues: people whom you do not work with directly but whom you need to communicate with on a regular basis (eg account managers and maintenance contractors).

COMMUNICATION

To work well with all your colleagues, good communication skills are essential. The ways in which you communicate are judged by others and can affect the way in which colleagues see you and act towards you. If you communicate poorly with your colleagues, it may cause problems, such as anger and annoyance, and create a difficult working environment.

There are three different ways in which we communicate:

- verbal communication
- non-verbal communication
- listening skills.

VERBAL COMMUNICATION

Verbal communication is any communication that is spoken and includes sounds such as laughing or any noises we may make to agree something or confirm a decision (eg 'uh-huh'). How we communicate verbally is important. You must:

- be aware of how you speak to people
- make sure you are not aggressive
- speak clearly and calmly
- avoid using technical jargon unless it is necessary.

During conversation:

- only 7% of what we are communicating comes from the words we use
- 38% of what we are communicating comes from our tone of voice
- 55% of what we are communicating comes from our body language or non-verbal communication.

You can see how important body language and tone of voice are.

For further information on verbal communication refer to Chapter 303, page 207.

HANDY HINT

When addressing your colleagues and clients you will not speak to them in the same way you would to your friends. You need to speak to colleagues in a more formal and professional manner.

 SmartScreen 301 Worksheet 2

NON-VERBAL COMMUNICATION

Non-verbal communication includes:

- written communication
- body language.

Written communication

Written communication is anything that includes written words:

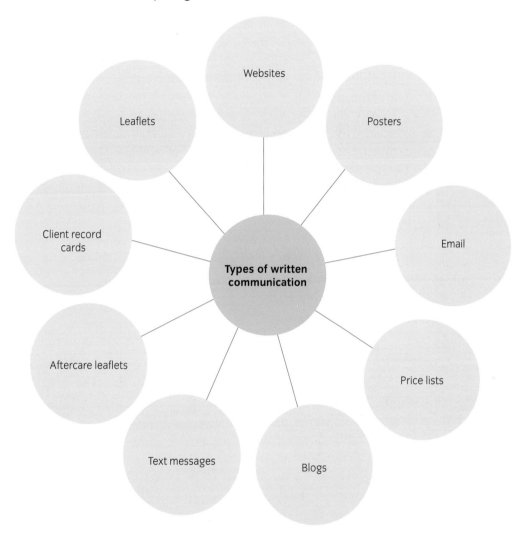

Any written information relating to the salon or spa should be clear and concise. You should proofread, spell check and check the grammar in any material before it is issued as it is a representation of your salon or spa and it reflects on your professional image.

Reading is an important means of communication for gathering and sharing information. For example you might read instructions to understand how to use a product or you might read them aloud to share the information with other people.

HANDY HINT

Think about your body language when you are communicating face to face and think about the tone of your voice when you are on the phone.

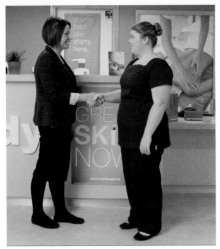

A therapist showing open body language when greeting a client

Body language

Body language is the way in which we use our bodies to communicate. Body language can be positive or negative depending on the way in which it is used.

Examples of positive and negative body language include:

Good body language	Negative body language
Smiling	Frowning
Arms uncrossed	Arms crossed
Good posture (eg sat upright/ stood upright)	Slouched
Making eye contact	Staring or looking away
Subtle mirroring of other person's body language	Yawning

A therapist showing negative body language

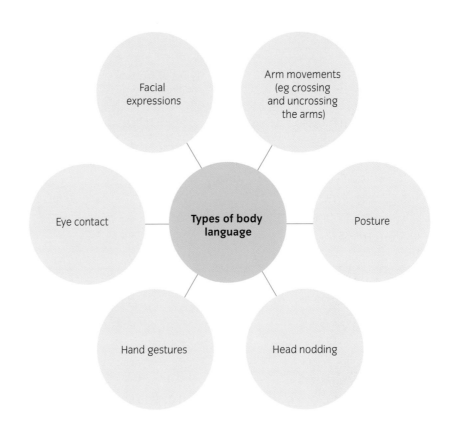

Facial expressions

Arm movements (eg crossing and uncrossing the arms)

Eye contact

Types of body language

Posture

Hand gestures

Head nodding

HANDY HINT

When reading something aloud it is important that you pronounce words clearly and do not read too fast.

HANDY HINT

Whether you are speaking or listening, it is important to maintain eye contact with the other person. This shows that you are paying attention to them and that you are not distracted. When maintaining eye contact it is important not to stare at the other person as this can be unnerving, particularly if it is a situation in which a complaint or problem is being dealt with.

Visual aids

Using visual aids can help you to communicate with your colleagues more effectively, especially if the instructions are complicated. It is often easier to understand something if you are able to look at it in action. Visual aids may include:

- magazines
- videos/DVDs
- photographs
- charts
- instruction booklets.

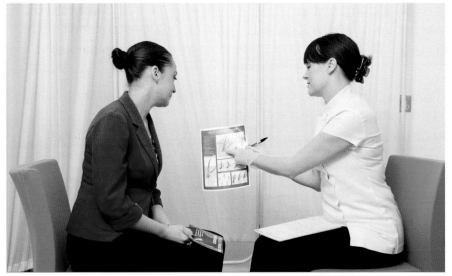
A therapist using a visual aid with a client to explain a treatment procedure

ACTIVITY

Think of your salon. What visual aids do you have there to help you communicate with colleagues and what makes these effective?

LISTENING SKILLS

When someone else is talking to you, you should make sure you listen. Do not interrupt them by talking over them. You need to develop your listening skills so that you gather valuable information (eg information related to a task that you need to carry out). Listening also shows that you are interested in what your colleagues have to say and that what they have to say is important. When listening to instructions it is a good idea to repeat back the important points to make sure that you have fully understood the information. This is known as 'summarising and confirming'.

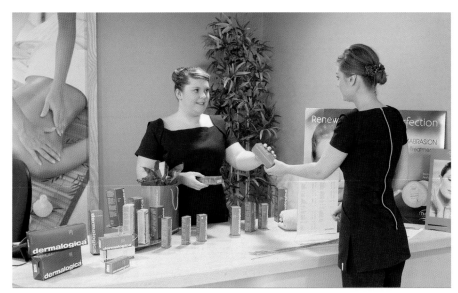
A therapist listening to a colleague explain a new product range

GIVING AND FOLLOWING INSTRUCTIONS

Another aspect of effective communication is giving and following instructions. Clear instructions avoid lost time, frustration, confusion and poor service.

It is very important when you have been given instructions verbally or when you have read instructions that to make sure you understand them. If you are unsure, make sure you clarify the instructions with the person who has given them to you.

If you are giving instructions, make sure they are clear and easy to understand. Instructions need to be:

- clear
- brief
- broken down into easy-to-follow segments
- clarified (ie ask for the instructions to be repeated back to you so that you can make sure everyone is aware of what is needed).

HANDY HINT

When giving instructions, think KISS – Keep It Simple Stupid! Use terminology that is relevant to the task and easy to understand. Do not use technical jargon if it is not necessary as this may lead to confusion, especially with more junior members of staff.

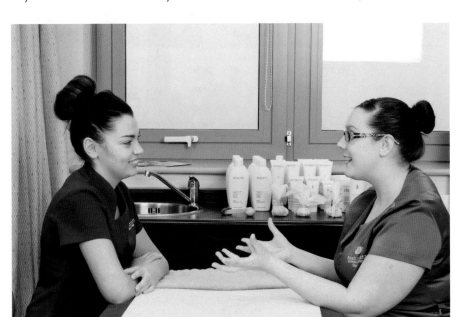

A therapist receiving instructions from a manager

ACTIVITY

Give your colleagues a pen and some paper:

- Tell them they are going to draw a picture but do not tell them what the picture is.
- Think of a picture.
- Do not look at your colleagues; turn your back to them.
- With your back turned, describe the picture. Mumble the instructions by putting your hand in front of your mouth.
- Describe the whole picture in one go (ie don't break it down into steps).
- Finally ask your colleagues to show you the pictures they have drawn. Do they resemble the picture you described?

HANDY HINT

Instructions are best given in small segments so that they aren't too complicated.

PROFESSIONAL BEHAVIOUR

It is important to be professional at all times, both in the salon environment and outside of the salon. It is important when wearing your uniform outside of the salon that you remain professional as people may recognise where you work or you may be seen by clients. The way in which a person behaves reflects on the image of the salon.

Acting in a professional way gives out the message that you are a dependable and responsible person. It also gives people confidence in your ability to do your job well.

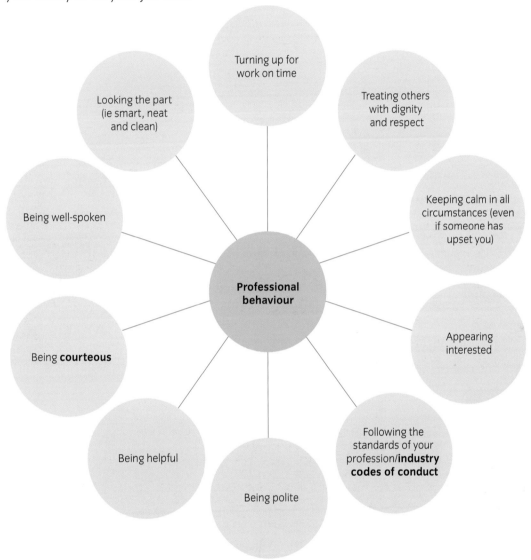

- Turning up for work on time
- Treating others with dignity and respect
- Keeping calm in all circumstances (even if someone has upset you)
- Appearing interested
- Following the standards of your profession/**industry codes of conduct**
- Being polite
- Being helpful
- Being **courteous**
- Being well-spoken
- Looking the part (ie smart, neat and clean)

Professional behaviour

NEGATIVE BEHAVIOUR

If you don't act in a professional way it can lead to friction and unrest within the workplace. Negative behaviour will often have an impact on everyone within the working environment.

Negative behaviour will have an impact on everyone you work with including both internal and external colleagues. Negativity is stressful for everyone. It can create a poor working environment and can lead to conflict within the team.

Negative behaviour must be addressed and dealt with quickly and effectively.

Courteous

Considerate

Industry codes of conduct

A written set of rules/guidelines for everyone in the profession to follow

Pessimistic

Seeing the negative in everything

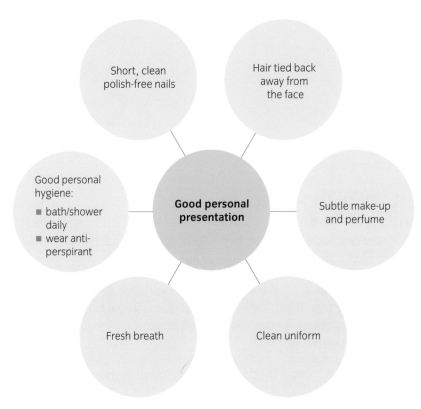

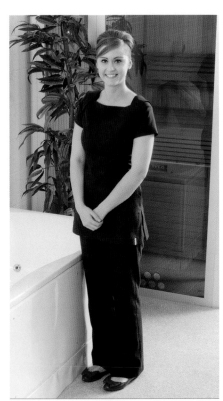

A well-presented therapist

FOLLOWING SAFE AND HYGIENIC WORKING PRACTICES

Being professional also includes following safe and hygienic working practices in line with legislation.

PERSONAL PRESENTATION

It is important that you have a professional appearance at all times. This will give clients confidence in you.

TREATMENTS

When carrying out treatments, it is essential that you follow good hygiene and safety practices.

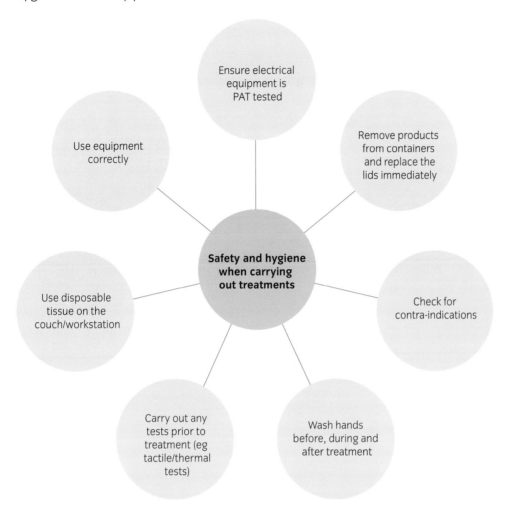

Ensure electrical equipment is PAT tested

Remove products from containers and replace the lids immediately

Use equipment correctly

Safety and hygiene when carrying out treatments

Check for contra-indications

Use disposable tissue on the couch/workstation

Carry out any tests prior to treatment (eg tactile/thermal tests)

Wash hands before, during and after treatment

THE WORK AREA

Your work area also needs to be safe, clean and hygienic.

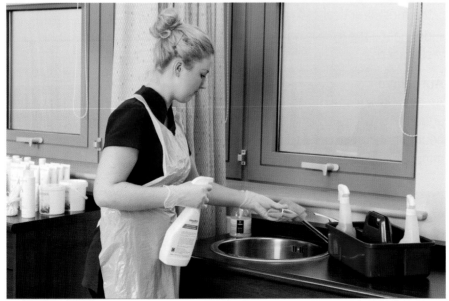

A therapist cleaning a work area

By following hygienic working practices and keeping the work environment clean and tidy it means that equipment and work areas are ready to be used at all times. It only takes one person to not clear away and it can cause disruption to the rest of the salon and possible conflict with the rest of the team.

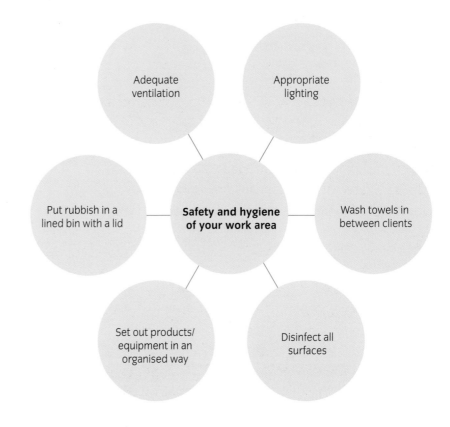

- Adequate ventilation
- Appropriate lighting
- Put rubbish in a lined bin with a lid
- **Safety and hygiene of your work area**
- Wash towels in between clients
- Set out products/equipment in an organised way
- Disinfect all surfaces

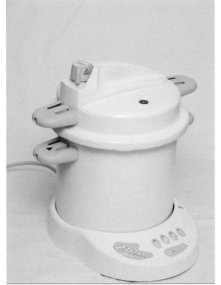

An autoclave

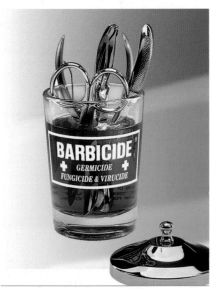

Barbicide is one method of disinfection used in the beauty industry

STERILISATION

Sterilisation is the total removal or destruction of *all* living micro-organisms including their spores.

Sterilisation is done by using heat:

- moist heat – steam or boiling water. Steaming using an autoclave is the most practical and most effective method
- dry heat – the item is baked using a high heat (eg in a glass bead steriliser).

Autoclave

An autoclave is the most effective method of sterilisation. It heats water under pressure to around 126°C. The steam created is used to sterilise equipment (small metal tools). The sterilisation cycle takes about 20 minutes.

DISINFECTION

Disinfection is the destruction of micro-organisms but *not* their spores. Disinfection is less effective than sterilisation. Disinfection can be carried out by the use of:

- UV (ultraviolet) radiation
- chemicals.

UV cabinet

A UV cabinet uses ultraviolet radiation to kill bacteria. Tools need to be cleaned with an alcohol-based product before being placed in the UV cabinet. Only the surface areas of objects that the rays come into contact with (ie the cleaned areas) will be disinfected. This means that the items need to turned over after about 20 minutes to make sure that all surfaces are disinfected.

Chemicals

These tend to be concentrated solutions which are placed in jars or containers into which tools can be placed (eg Barbicide). These solutions need to be diluted according to the manufacturer's instructions before being poured into a jar or container. The tools must be fully submerged to be disinfected effectively.

Examples of chemicals used for disinfection are:

- QUATS – quaternary ammonium compounds
- hypochlorite – a form of chlorine (eg Milton Sterilising Fluid)
- bleach – most bleach contains chlorine which makes It unsuitable for disinfecting equipment. It should only be used for cleaning toilets, surfaces, sinks etc
- glutaraldehyde – an organic compound (eg Cidex)
- alcohol – available in a number of forms including surgical spirit, isopropyl alcohol and ethyl alcohol. It is suitable for wiping tools.

DISPOSAL OF CONTAMINATED WASTE

In addition to cleaning equipment, it is necessary to ensure that all waste is removed from your work area and disposed of appropriately. Some treatments can produce **contaminated waste** or waste that poses a high risk (eg **sharps**). These types of waste must be disposed of in the correct way. You must not put yourself or your colleagues at risk of cross-contamination.

All general waste should be placed in a lined bin with a lid to avoid the spread of micro-organisms. This is put out with the main bin.

All contaminated waste or sharps waste needs to be disposed of in either a yellow sharps bin liner or a sharps container. When the sharps container is full, it is usually collected by a specialist collector who will **incinerate** the contents.

> **INDUSTRY TIP**
>
> Each council has its own local by-laws. You therefore need to check with your local council what their policy is with regards to the collection of sharps.

> **INDUSTRY TIP**
>
> If it is not possible to fully submerge your tools in a chemical solution, use a chemical spray or wipe to clean the equipment instead.

> **INDUSTRY TIP**
>
> Do not mix chemicals together as they may react together.

> **HANDY HINT**
>
> Further information on sterilisation and disinfection can be found in Chapter 302 on page 193.

 SmartScreen 301 Worksheet 3

Contaminated waste
Waste containing human tissue (eg blood)

Sharps
Any sharp object that might have become contaminated during use, including electrolysis needles

Incinerate
To destroy something by burning it

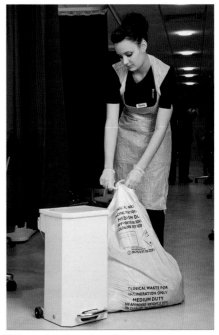

A therapist disposing of waste

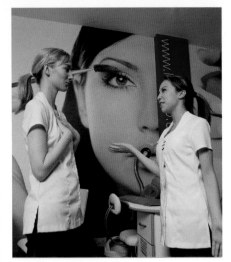

Problems between colleagues must be dealt with quickly

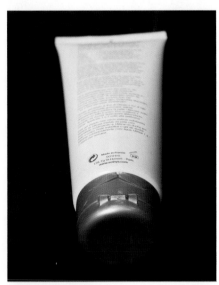

Companies that fail to replace faulty products once you have purchased them are in breach of the Sale and Supply of Goods Act

DEALING WITH PROBLEMS

When there is a problem or conflict within the salon, it needs to be dealt with quickly. Stay positive as this will help when trying to come up with a solution to the problem.

You may need to start by asking a more senior member of staff such as a senior beauty therapist/senior nail technician for help.

UNDERSTANDING THE PROBLEM

First of all you need to understand the problem so that you can deal with it in the best possible way. Ask yourself the following questions:

- What is the problem? – Identify the problem.
- Who is involved? – Is the problem with a client or a colleague?
- Why has it happened? – Is it a one-off incident or has it been building up for a while?
- When did it happen or is it ongoing? – Was it recent or was it a while ago?
- Where has it happened/where is it happening? – Did it take place on or off the premises?

Once you have answers to these questions then you can begin to work out a solution. You may need to get the input of a more senior person to help you answer some of the questions and to help you work towards a solution.

DEALING WITH THE PROBLEM

It is essential that any problems or conflicts are dealt with immediately and in a courteous manner:

1 Approach the person involved and discuss the problem with them in a polite, truthful and non-aggressive way. This should be done in private away from other colleagues and clients.

2 If the problem continues, speak to your manager and ask them to help. A good manager will speak to everyone involved to get their side of the story and they will be objective. They will also help to find a solution to the problem.

3 If after you have spoken to your manager and the problem continues, make a complaint in writing. This is a more formal way of complaining and it will be taken more seriously. Ask for a written response that explains what is going to be done about the problem.

4 Finally, if your manager does not deal with the problem, it may be necessary to make an appointment to speak to someone more senior (eg an area manager or the salon owner) to find a solution.

The above steps can also be used to deal with problems with external colleagues. However, if you aren't able to reach a solution then the salon may need to consider taking legal action. For example, if a supplier has sold the salon a box of cleansers that are faulty, then you should approach the company and ask them to replace the faulty items. If they are unwilling to replace them, they will have breached the Sale and Supply of Goods Act. Threatening them with legal action will quite often resolve the problem quickly.

EFFECTIVE TEAMWORK

Good teamwork leads to a happy working environment. Usually behind every successful business is a good team. A successful team needs to communicate clearly and work well together. The keys to a successful team are:

- good leaders – good leaders will help to give the team direction and they will ensure that everyone has a role
- communication – a good team needs to communicate well, either in writing or verbally
- setting objectives – setting objectives gives a team something to aim for and achieve – objectives can be fun things (eg open evenings, marketing events and special events where staff dress up)
- up-to-date skills and techniques – members of the team need to continually update their skills and techniques and share their skills and knowledge with the team
- achievement of targets – sales targets should be specific, achievable and realistic and should be raised if the team achieves them easily.

TEAM MEETINGS

Team meetings are an excellent way of encouraging communication and creating a sense of belonging within a team. Regular team meetings provide an opportunity for new ideas to be exchanged. It is important that everyone is given an opportunity to take part and that everyone's ideas are considered. Never dismiss someone's ideas as this will cause negativity. Team meetings provide an opportunity to ensure that the workplace is a happy place to be by discussing a range of ideas and issues (eg about treatments, treatment areas, staff areas, policies and social events etc).

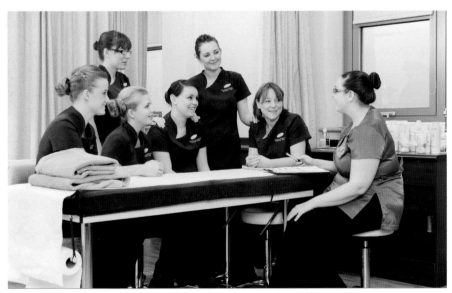

A team of therapists in a meeting with their manager

AN INEFFECTIVE TEAM

Poor communication can lead to misunderstandings and a breakdown in communication. If this isn't resolved, it can result in an unhappy workplace. This in turn might lead to a high turnover of staff and cost the business money. A high turnover of staff would result in the salon having to train new staff and it would make the clients feel unsettled as they would constantly be having to build new relationships with new therapists/technicians. An unhappy team is likely to result in loss of business and loss of revenue. In severe cases, it may even result in the closure of the business.

ACTIVITY

Working with your colleagues, make a list of things that would help to make your workplace a better environment. Make suggestions about how these can be put into action.

ROLES AND RESPONSIBILITIES OF TEAM MEMBERS WITHIN BEAUTY-RELATED INDUSTRIES

ROLES AND RESPONSIBILITIES OF INDIVIDUAL TEAM MEMBERS

Every person within the salon needs to know their role and responsibilities so that they know what is required of them. Each member of staff should receive a job description which gives details of:

- their job title
- the tasks they are required to perform
- the people they are responsible for (ie the people they manage)
- the areas they are responsible for (eg, spa area, reception, nail bar)
- any procedures and policies they need to follow
- who their manager is.

Having a job description makes sure that each member of staff is aware of their responsibilities. It will also ensure that therapists know which tasks they need to carry out so that there isn't any doubling-up of tasks and so that tasks don't get missed accidentally. It also ensures that workload is shared out evenly.

REFERRING PROBLEMS TO SOMEONE MORE SENIOR

It is important to remember that you must work within the limitations of your job role. If your role is that of a junior therapist then you do not have the authority to deal with certain situations. There are certain situations which need the manager's involvement. For example, if a client is very unhappy with a service they have received, you should ask a manager to help you. Only the manager can authorise refunds, free treatments and resolve problems. Likewise, a receptionist will not usually deal with account handlers who visit the premises to sell products. This would be done by the manager.

INDUSTRY TIP

Even though you might have specific tasks as set out in your job description, you might need to help out other team members from time to time. For example, if you have no client booked in and another therapist is very busy, offer to prepare their treatment room for them as they meet and greet their next client.

DIFFERENT JOB ROLES WITHIN A SALON

Salon or spa manager

A salon or spa manager is responsible for managing the day-to-day running of the business. They need to be experienced, organised and able to **delegate** work to ensure the smooth running of the business. Their role might include supervising staff, controlling stock levels and cashing up at the end of the working day.

Delegate

Pass work to someone else

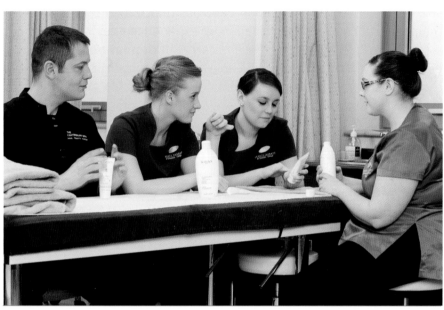

A salon manager telling therapists about a new product

Salon owner

A salon owner owns the business. They have overall responsibility for the day-to-day running of the business and the final say in how the business is run. The salon owner might have built the business from scratch or they might have bought it as a **going concern**. It might also be a **franchise**.

Going concern

An existing business that is making a profit

Franchise

Where an individual or group of salons have been given the right to trade under an existing brand and use and sell that company's goods or services. An example of a franchise in the beauty industry is Saks

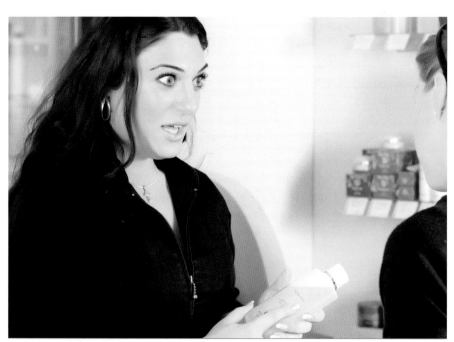

A salon manager talking to a client about a product

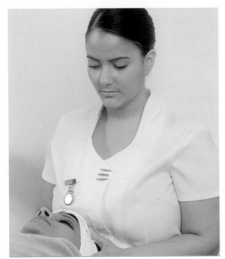

Beauty therapist

Depilation
Hair removal

Holistic
Looking at the person as a whole

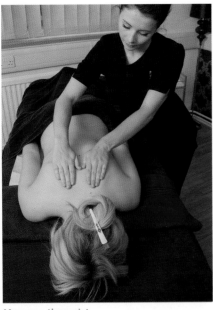

Massage therapist

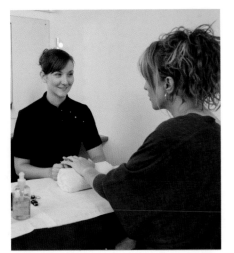

Nail technician

Beauty therapist

Depending on experience, there will be different levels of beauty therapist within a salon (ie from a newly qualified junior therapist to an experienced senior therapist). Therapists will offer a selection of beauty therapy treatments working on the body, hands, feet and face. The exact treatments will vary depending on their qualification level.

A junior therapist (ie a recently qualified therapist with little commercial salon experience) will offer support and assistance to the more senior therapists. Once they have gained more experience, they will usually work on the face, hands and feet and carry out **depilation**. If they qualify to Level 3, they will also be able to offer a range of full-body treatments. Some of these treatments, such as microdermabrasion and electrolysis, might involve the use of electrical equipment.

A spa therapist is more likely to provide **holistic**, slimming and detoxifying treatments (eg massage, body wraps and body scrubs). A spa is a large establishment that usually offers spa treatments and water treatments that work alongside the spa treatments.

Massage therapist

A massage therapist is trained in the art of massage. This may be in one or more of the following types of massage:

- Swedish massage
- Thai massage
- Balinese massage
- Lomi Lomi massage
- hot stone massage
- Shiatsu
- aromatherapy massage.

Nail technician

A nail technician specialises in nail treatments and nail enhancements. This includes manicures, pedicures, nail art and the application of nail enhancements (ie gel, acrylic or fibreglass enhancements). Nail technicians may work in nail bars or studios rather than in beauty salons.

Receptionist

The reception is the focal point of any business and the receptionist is the first point of contact for the client. Receptionists need to be welcoming, confident and knowledgeable about the services offered. They are responsible for making appointments, taking telephone calls, reading and responding to emails, passing on messages to colleagues, taking payments, filing or monitoring treatment information and organising treatment rooms.

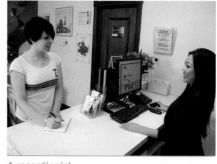
A receptionist

Make-up artist

A make-up artist works specifically to create an image, which may be used for red carpet events, theatre, TV/film, and photographic make-up. They may also be qualified in hairdressing, wig-making, prosthetics application and theatre make-up. Working as a make-up artist is usually freelance and will take place in a variety of settings such as photographic studios for still images, film sets (film, advertising, music etc), wedding or special event work, cat walk and fashion studios.

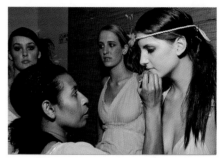
A make-up artist

Complementary therapist

This therapist specialises in treatments which include a range of holistic treatments including body massage, reflexology and aromatherapy. They may work independently or within a more complementary setting such as a spa, clinic or hospice.

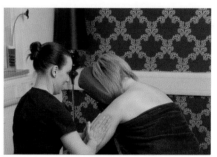
A complementary therapist providing an Indian head massage treatment

Cosmetic consultant

Cosmetic consultants tend to be situated within department stores. They are often brand specific, which means they will have had training in one particular skincare or make-up range; they are then responsible for retailing, demonstrating and advising customers on it.

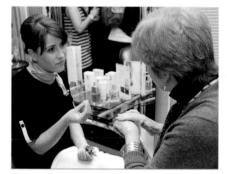
A cosmetics consultant

Trainer

A trainer works within a specific company to train therapists or technicians in treatment techniques and or product knowledge. The trainer may be based at the company head office and train there or provide onsite training at the business location.

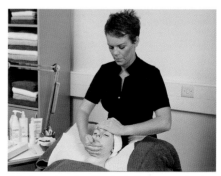
A trainer showing the techniques required for a facial skincare treatment

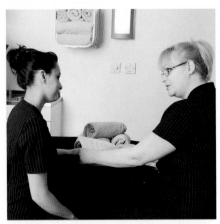
A teacher, lecturer or assessor

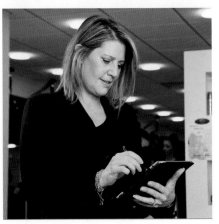
An account manager

Teacher, lecturer or assessor

This role could be within a private training provider or in a further education or higher education college. It involves training people to achieve a specific qualification, eg nail technician, Level 3 beauty therapist. The teacher assesses the students according to the awarding body requirements of the qualification, eg practical assessments, written assignments or questions. The teacher needs to be knowledgeable and approachable with occupational experience. As a student you need to be confident that you are being taught from experience and expertise, not from a textbook or handouts.

Sales/account manager

A sales manager visits salons, spas, training environments to show and tell people about the product or equipment they are selling for a specific company. The role involves travelling, developing new business, managing business accounts, organising stock orders and promotions for salons, as well as working at trade shows to promote to the industry.

Internal Quality Assurer

An Internal Quality Assurer (IQA) or Quality Assurance Co-ordinator is the usual progression route for an assessor. They are responsible for checking on the quality of the training and that it has been assessed fairly meeting the standards set by the awarding body. The IQA also offers guidance and support to assessors by providing them with constructive feedback after checking their practical assessments and marking of written work/tests.

Awarding Organisation Moderator or Consultant

Formally called an External Verifier, the role of the External Quality Assurer (EQA) is to visit training establishments on behalf of the qualification awarding body and make sure that the assessment and internal verification that takes place meets their standards. They also offer guidance and support to the training establishments and assist with any problems they may encounter.

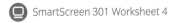
SmartScreen 301 Worksheet 4

GIVING SUPPORT, GUIDANCE AND FEEDBACK

Giving and receiving feedback is important for lots of reasons. Feedback helps to offer guidance and support for performance reviews, appraisals and during problems and conflicts amongst others and helps to improve performance.

Feedback should be **constructive**. It should therefore include both positive and negative comments. However, it should also be balanced, so every negative comment should be balanced with a positive comment. This will help to encourage people instead of making them feel inadequate. When providing constructive feedback you should also provide guidance to support the feedback. For example, when giving feedback on performance you should provide guidance on how areas of work may be improved.

Constructive
Beneficial

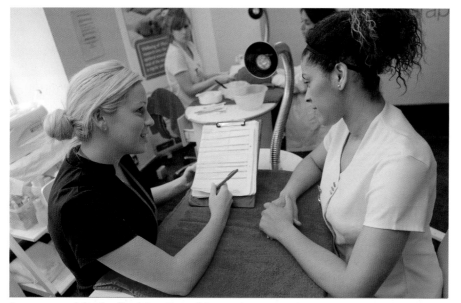
An assessor giving feedback to a therapist

Feedback can be both written and verbal. It can be obtained from a variety of sources:

- clients
- colleagues
- management
- publicity for the business
- questionnaires.

If a person has completed a task which needs feedback it should be provided as soon as possible. Any delay in providing feedback will mean that it will lose its impact.

GIVING POSITIVE FEEDBACK

Feedback meetings need to be held in a private area, away from other team members.

- Be clear about what you need to say and why.
- Sit up straight and maintain good eye contact.
- Ask the person you are giving feedback to for their evaluation of the situation or behaviour.
- Ask the person you are giving feedback to how they feel.
- Be positive but assertive in your praise and opinions.
- Back up what you need to say with facts (eg if you are feeding back about good performance back it up with some client feedback – *'Mrs Brown was very pleased with her treatment that you did on Tuesday morning. She is going to recommend you to her friends'*).

GIVING NEGATIVE FEEDBACK

Meetings need to be held in a private area, away from other team members.

- Be clear about what has gone wrong and why.
- Be objective, not personal. Talk about the situation rather than blame the person directly (eg *'It is not ideal that Mrs Brown's got massage*

medium in her hair during her massage treatment. What can be done to make sure this doesn't happen again?') By phrasing a negative situation in this way, you are giving the person the opportunity to think about what they have done and what they need to do to make sure it does not happen again. This may help identify training needs.

- Do not allow negative or defensive body language to put you off giving your feedback.
- Sit up straight and maintain good eye contact.
- Be positive and assertive when you express your negative opinions. Be clear and unmistakable.
- Back up what you need to say with facts or examples.

HANDY HINT

When you are providing guidance and feedback, use the opportunity to address any training needs and make people aware of their strengths and weaknesses. People can be very good at thinking about their weaknesses. Make sure you have some positive feedback for them.

TEST YOUR KNOWLEDGE

Use the questions below to test your knowledge of Chapter 301 to see how much information you have retained. These questions will help you revise what you have learnt in this chapter.

Turn to page 499 for the answers.

1 A mentor is:
  a A client
  b Another member of staff
  c An external trainer
  d A member of the public

2 Which **one** of the following is an example of positive body language?
  a Frowning
  b Folded arms
  c Smiling
  d Slouching

3 Which **one** of the following does a job description tell you?
  a How many hours you work
  b How much you get paid
  c When you start and finish
  d What your responsibilities are

4 What is the purpose of a code of conduct?
  a It says what you should do
  b It shows you how to perform treatments
  c It sets out professional standards and expected behaviour
  d It states how many hours a therapist should work

5 When giving negative feedback you must always:
  a Go to a private area
  b Give the feedback in front of other staff members
  c Go off the premises
  d Give the feedback in front of the client

6 A junior member of staff is responsible for:
  a Following their job description.
  b Managing staff rotas
  c Training new staff
  d Mentoring

7 Which **one** of the following is an example of verbal communication?
  a Talking
  b Writing
  c Body language
  d Making eye contact

8 Which **one** of the following is an example of negative behaviour?
  a Being polite
  b Being helpful
  c Being happy
  d Being angry

9 You are a beauty therapist working within a salon. Which of the following is an example of an external colleague?
  a The receptionist
  b The manager of the salon
  c One of the other therapists
  d An account handler for a product supplier

10 An internal colleague is someone who works:
  a In another salon
  b In your workplace
  c At the suppliers
  d At a previous workplace

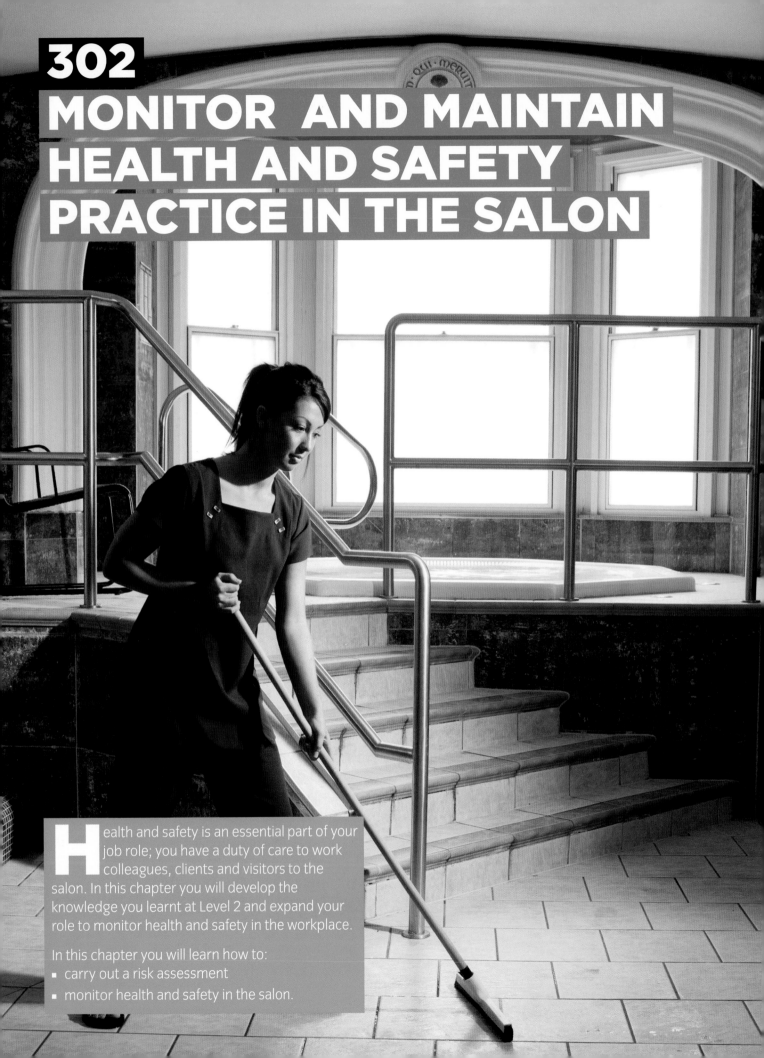

302
MONITOR AND MAINTAIN HEALTH AND SAFETY PRACTICE IN THE SALON

Health and safety is an essential part of your job role; you have a duty of care to work colleagues, clients and visitors to the salon. In this chapter you will develop the knowledge you learnt at Level 2 and expand your role to monitor health and safety in the workplace.

In this chapter you will learn how to:
- carry out a risk assessment
- monitor health and safety in the salon.

HEALTH AND SAFETY LEGISLATION

In order to make sure you are following health and safety regulations, you need to be familiar with all the legislation that is relevant to the workplace. This information can be found in the Legislation chapter on pages 139–152. Make sure you have a good understanding of each Act and how it will affect you in the workplace. The Acts you should be familiar with are the:

- Health and Safety at Work Act (HASAWA)
- Workplace (Health, Safety and Welfare) Regulations
- Provision and Use of Work Equipment Regulations (PUWER)
- Environmental Protection Act
- Local Government Miscellaneous Provisions Act
- Control of Substances Hazardous to Health (COSHH) Regulations
- Electricity at Work Regulations (EAWR)
- Regulatory Reform (RRO) (Fire Safety) Order
- Personal Protective Equipment (PPE) at Work Regulations
- Reporting of Injuries, Diseases and Dangerous Occurrences Regulations (RIDDOR)
- Manual Handling Operations Regulations
- Health and Safety (First Aid) Regulations
- Health and Safety (Display Screen Equipment) Regulations.

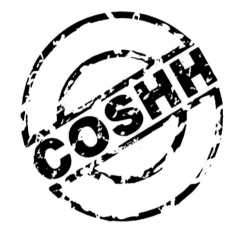

CARRY OUT A RISK ASSESSMENT

A risk assessment is a process carried out within the salon to review and report any potential **risks**. A risk assessment helps you protect your work colleagues, clients and visitors to the salon. Remember, a **hazard** has the potential to cause harm. You are not expected to remove all risks from the salon but you are expected to protect people as far as is **reasonably practicable**. People entering the salon have a right to be protected from harm. Failure to follow procedures can result in legal action and loss of business. If your salon employs five or more people you are required under the Health and Safety at Work Act (HASAWA) to record the findings of a risk assessment.

There are five steps to a risk assessment:

1 Identify the hazards.
2 Identify the risks by deciding who might be harmed and how.
3 Evaluate the risks and decide on precautions.
4 Record your findings and identify who should **implement** them.
5 Review your assessment and update if necessary.

Risk
The likelihood of a hazard causing harm

Hazard
Something that can cause harm

Reasonably practicable
The balance between the risk and the time, effort and cost of reducing the risk (eg if a risk is small but the cost of removing it is high, it may be decided that it would be too costly to remove it)

Implement
To put in place

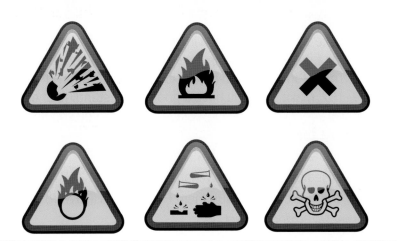

Hazard labels

LEVEL OF RISK

A hazard may not necessarily become a risk. You need to assess a risk based on the likelihood of it occurring. This will allow you to decide on the level of risk. The level of risk is worked out using the following calculation:

Risk level = consequence of exposure x likelihood of occurrence

CONSEQUENCE

- 1 – very unlikely
- 2 – minor injury
- 3 – moderate injury
- 4 – major injury
- 5 – injury resulting in death.

LIKELIHOOD

- 1 – very unlikely
- 2 – unlikely
- 3 – possible
- 4 – likely
- 5 – almost certain.

RISK LEVEL

- 1–3 = low risk
- 4–6 = medium risk
- 8–12 = high risk
- 15–25 = extremely high risk.

The result of this calculation will allow you to evaluate the level of risk and make suitable decisions about how to manage it.

The following table gives some examples of low-level risks and high-level risks.

Hazard	Low-level risk	High-level risk
Trailing wires 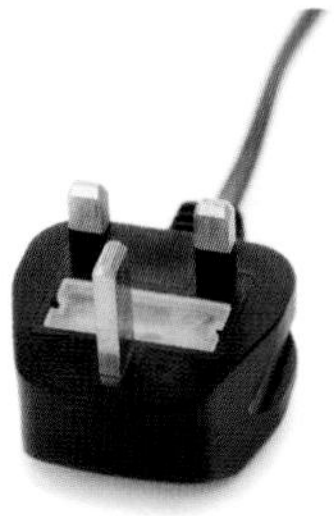	▪ At the back of the treatment area out of the way.	▪ Trailing across the treatment area.
Blown bulb 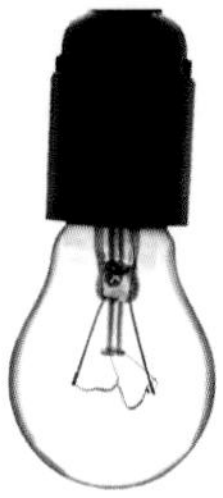	▪ If good natural light. ▪ During daytime.	▪ In a dark stairway – a risk of tripping and falling.
Stock delivery 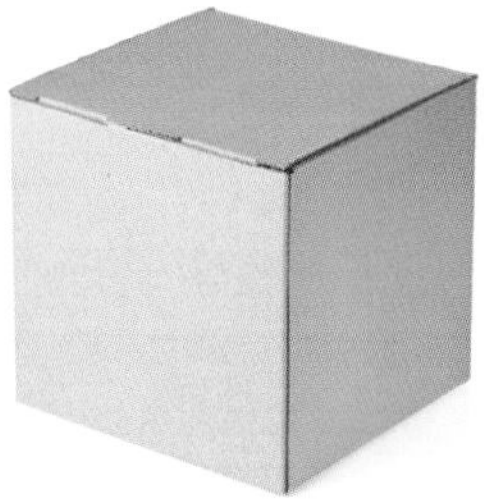	▪ Left in the corner of the stock room.	▪ In the middle of a walkway – a risk of tripping over it and injury.
Chemical hazards 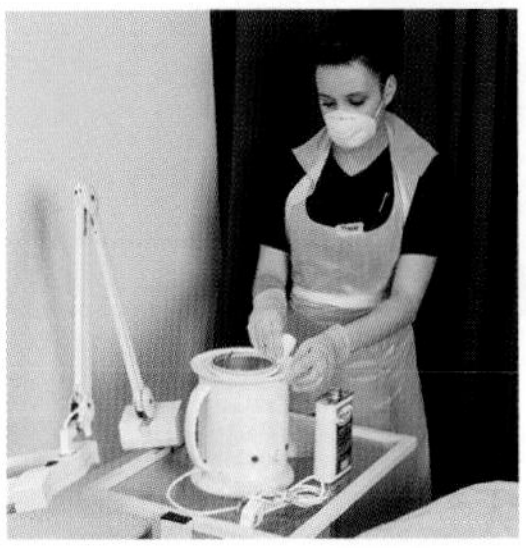	▪ Stored and handled correctly using the manufacturers' instructions.	▪ Stored in incorrect conditions (eg products may be flammable). ▪ Used incorrectly without referring to manufacturers' instructions.

INDUSTRY TIP

In winter months it is often dark while we are at work so lights bulbs should be tested regularly to ensure that they are working and available when needed to make sure that the risk is reduced.

INDUSTRY TIP

Any item blocking a fire exit is a high-level hazard.

INDUSTRY TIP

Products containing chemicals are widely used in beauty and spa therapy. You must always read and follow the manufacturers' instructions. Products should be stored safely and in line with the manufacturers' instructions. The stock storage area of the salon should only be accessible to authorised members of staff.

When using chemicals, remember SHUD:

▪ **S**tore
▪ **H**andle
▪ **U**se
▪ **D**ispose.

WHY AND WHEN A RISK ASSESSMENT SHOULD BE CARRIED OUT

A risk assessment should be carried out to ensure safety in the salon. Almost anything in the salon can be a hazard and become a risk. It is therefore your responsibility, along with your employer, to prevent these hazards from becoming risks to the safety of yourself and others.

A risk assessment must be carried out as a result of:

- a change to the salon environment
- the introduction of new treatments or products
- a change in personal circumstances.

CHANGES TO THE SALON ENVIRONMENT

A change to the salon environment could mean a total salon refit or something small, such as the installation of a ramp for disabled access. Whatever the change within the salon, the impact on the staff and people visiting the salon must be considered. Even a new shelving system in the stock cupboard or dispensary may need a risk assessment to work out where is the safest place to store certain items.

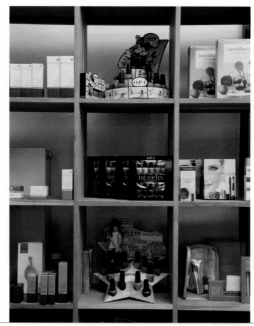

A risk assessment may need to be carried out for a new shelving system in the salon

ACTIVITY

Think of the way products and equipment are stored in your salon. List where you would put the following items so that they were stored safely and correctly:

- talc
- massage oil
- lash glue
- eye make-up remover
- epilation needles
- water testing kit.

INTRODUCTION OF NEW TREATMENTS OR PRODUCTS

It is always exciting to get brand-new products and offer your clients a new treatment. Before you start to use new products or introduce new treatments you must understand the risk they could pose to the client and the therapist carrying out the treatment. For example, if your salon was introducing a new skincare range and you were to put the products on clients' skin without reading the manufacturer's instructions, what could happen?

WHY DON'T YOU
look at a new product you have in the salon. Read the manufacturer's instructions to find out the possible hazards and risks.

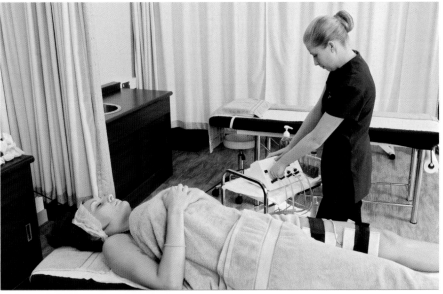

A new treatment

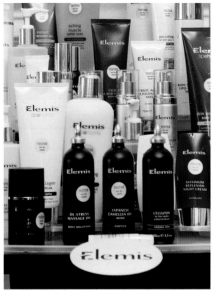

A new product range for a salon

INDUSTRY TIP

If your salon is going to offer a new treatment, such as body electrotherapy, you will need to check with your insurance company to make sure you are insured to offer this treatment.

A CHANGE IN PERSONAL CIRCUMSTANCES

Therapists' circumstances may change during the time that they are employed at a salon. For example, a work colleague may announce that she is pregnant. A risk assessment would therefore need to be carried out to identify any areas of her work she might no longer be able to participate in. The salon may also take on a new member of staff who is too tall or too short to use the salon's couches. A risk assessment would need to be carried out to prevent injury or long-term damage to them from poor posture.

ACTIVITY

If you or a work colleague becomes pregnant, you will have to carry out a risk assessment. Look on the Health and Safety Executive's (HSE's) website, www.hse.gov.uk/mothers/index.htm, for more information. List five main points you need to consider when carrying out a risk assessment for a pregnant colleague.

NECESSARY ACTIONS

The salon has many potential hazards. If you notice a hazard, it is your responsibility to report it and carry out a risk assessment before it becomes a risk and an injury occurs. When you have carried out a risk assessment and identified the possibility of a risk, you must decide on the necessary actions to take. You will need to:

- record the risk assessment
- report the risk to the salon manager or owner
- update risk assessment information
- inform staff.

RECORDING THE RISK ASSESSMENT

A risk assessment can be recorded in a number of different ways:

- a checklist
- a report
- a form or table.

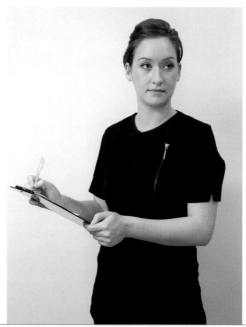

A therapist using a checklist to carry out a risk assessment

Once you have decided the way in which you are going to report your risk assessment, you need to think about the information that needs to be included:

- What are the hazards?
- Who might be harmed?
- What steps are already in place to manage the risk?
- What additional or follow-up action needs to be taken and by whom?
- How will follow-up actions be put into place?
- What is the level of the risk?
- What is the target date for putting into place follow-up action?
- The completion date for follow-up action.

An example of a risk assessment is shown in the following table:

Hazard (details of equipment or activity)	Who might be harmed?	What additional action needs to be taken?	How will additional actions be put into place?	Level of risk	Likelihood of risk	Target date	Completion date
Sharps (such as epilation needles): ■ cross-infection ■ needle-stick injuries. 	■ Staff ■ Clients	■ Clients: To sit or lie correctly on a treatment couch. ■ Staff: Dispose of sharps in sharps box to avoid needle-stick injuries, cross-contamination of blood.	■ Check all clients are positioned correctly prior to treatment that involves sharps (eg electrolysis). ■ Demonstrate correct posture for sitting at staff meetings. ■ Sterilise equipment. ■ Nominate a member of staff to be responsible for the sharps bin. ■ First-aid training.			22/4/14	26/5/14
Water: ■ skin irritations from contact with water. 	■ Staff	■ Wear **PPE** as needed. ■ Dry and moisturise hands correctly.	■ Check hands daily for signs of dermatitis. ■ Inform staff of risk of dermatitis and signs of dermatitis at regular meetings and new staff induction. ■ Get information leaflets from the HSE. ■ Monitor PPE.			16/5/14	3/6/14
Products and chemicals: ■ incorrect usage ■ client skin sensitivities. 	■ Staff ■ Clients	■ Clients: Always carry out a skin test on clients when using products (eg self-tan) with active ingredients. ■ Staff: Read and follow manufacturers' instructions. ■ Follow COSHH.	■ Staff must always use previous record cards to check for skin sensitivities and carry out patch tests. ■ Update all record cards.			27/5/14	1/6/14

Hazard (details of equipment or activity)	Who might be harmed?	What additional action needs to be taken?	How will additional actions be put into place?	Level of risk	Likelihood of risk	Target date	Completion date
Electricity ■ faulty equipment ■ dangerous positioning and storage of equipment ■ incorrect usage.	■ Staff	■ Visually check all equipment prior to use. ■ Clean all equipment. ■ Store equipment away from water. ■ Follow Electricity at Work Regulations	■ Make sure equipment is **PAT tested** and working correctly. ■ Staff must follow manufacturers' instructions.			12/4/14	31/5/14
Posture: ■ musculoskeletal injuries (eg neck and back pain) from standing for long periods.	■ Staff	■ Staff should make sure they stand at the correct height. ■ Staff to take regular breaks.	■ Employer to provide suitable stools and couches. ■ Employer to make sure staff wear sensible footwear.			25/5/14	1/6/14

PPE

Personal protective equipment

PAT tested

Portable appliance tested. Appliances need to be checked by a qualified electrician at least once a year

REPORTING THE RISK ASSESSMENT

It is important you report the findings of a risk assessment to your manager or the salon owner. They need to be informed of your findings to be able to make the necessary improvements or changes. Once you have completed the risk assessment you will need to make an action plan. Your action plan will need to include:

- long-term actions to ensure that the risks are dealt with and continue to be managed (eg routinely checking a piece of fixed equipment to make sure the same fault does not happen again)
- training for employees (eg a health and safety course and relevant information for staff to read)
- regular checks that will need to take place to make sure that the hazards and risks identified by the risk assessment are controlled
- staff responsibilities for maintaining and preventing the hazards and risks that you identified.

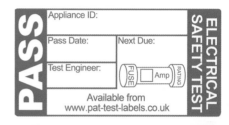

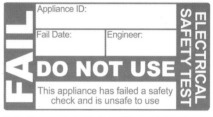

PAT test pass and fail labels

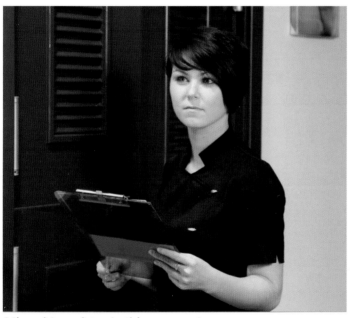

A therapist carrying out a risk assessment

INFORMING STAFF

Once you have completed a risk assessment, it is important that everyone working on the premises or anyone entering the premises is informed of any changes to procedures or policies as quickly as possible. Staff can be notified of any changes at staff meetings. For clients and visitors to the salon you can put a notice up or advise them verbally (eg 'we now have a new ramp so it is easier if you find the steps to the treatment rooms difficult'. Whichever way you decide is best to communicate this information, make sure everyone is aware and informed.

UPDATE RISK ASSESSMENT INFORMATION

It is important to revisit your risk assessments to check if documentation needs to be updated. If you think that something does need amending, make sure that all staff and anyone entering the premises is aware of this.

MONITOR HEALTH AND SAFETY IN THE SALON

When you work in a busy salon, you don't always have time for formal talks to discuss health and safety. However, it is vitally important that staff are aware of health and safety at all times and that information and updates are passed on to them.

Even when you have worked in the salon for a long time, you must not take health and safety for granted. Just because there has never been an injury before, doesn't mean there never will.

As well as being aware of new health and safety requirements, you must make sure you are familiar with existing requirements and the latest information about products, chemicals or work-related diseases (eg dermatitis). It is also important to remember the basic industry requirements for health and safety.

In this part of the chapter you will learn about:
- the health and safety support that should be provided to staff
- procedures for dealing with different types of security breaches
- the need for insurance.

HEALTH AND SAFETY SUPPORT

At Level 3, you will be expanding your role to monitor health and safety in the workplace and you will be supporting others to ensure all health and safety requirements are met. This will include regular monitoring and reviewing of the following key hazards and risks, so that they can be controlled and managed:
- sterilisation and disinfection
- work-related diseases (ie dermatitis)
- slips, trips and falls.

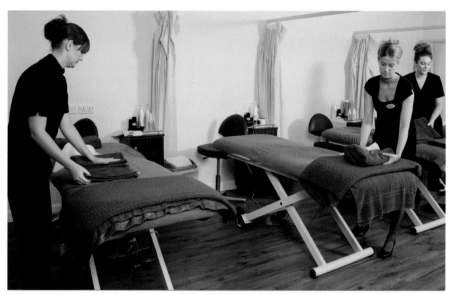

A tidy salon reduces the risk of falls and slips

INDUSTRY TIP

If you have new information regarding health and safety, it is your responsibility to pass it on!

HANDY HINT

Health and safety laws are always changing and being updated to help protect you. Always check the HSE's website (www.hse.gov.uk) for the most up-to-date information.

HANDY HINT

It is always beneficial to revise the regulations that relate to your work environment and keep up to date with changes. Within your working day you deal with more health and safety regulations than you realise!

HANDY HINT

Make sure that you recap your knowledge of health and safety requirements and the health and safety issues you covered at Level 2.

STERILISATION AND DISINFECTION

Sterilisation and **disinfection** are key areas where you can control risks to prevent harm to yourself and others. The consequences of not carrying out sterilisation and disinfection could be:

- loss of business
- creating an unprofessional image (eg because of a dirty, unhygienic couch or broken and dirty equipment)
- legal action from clients or colleagues (eg because of cross-infection or cross-contamination from unclean equipment and tools)

To prevent this you must:

- make sure you are fully trained and understand how the equipment for sterilisation and disinfection works
- always follow the manufacturers' instructions to give you the maximum level of sterilisation or disinfection.

Methods of sterilisation and disinfection

Sterilisation

The total removal or destruction of *all* living micro-organisms, including their spores

Disinfection

The destruction of micro-organisms but *not* their spores. Disinfection is less effective than sterilisation

INDUSTRY TIP

Check which methods of sterilisation your salon uses.

HANDY HINT

Remember, the autoclave is the *only* method that sterilises equipment. Other methods only disinfect.

 SmartScreen 302 Worksheet 2

Methods of sterilisation and disinfection

Autoclave:
- Only for sterilising metal and glass.
- Uses steam to sterilise.
- Heats water under pressure to 120°C.
- Only method of sterilisation in the salon.
- Kills organisms within 20 minutes.

Ultraviolet (UV) cabinet:
- Objects are exposed to ultraviolet rays.
- Only disinfects tools.
- Not suitable for tools with unexposed surfaces.
- Takes at least 15 minutes.

Chemicals (eg Barbicide):
- Only disinfects tools.
- Tools must be fully immersed.
- Tools need to be left in solution for recommended time.

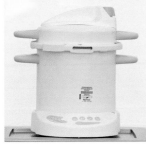

Autoclave

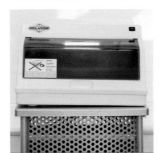

UV cabinet

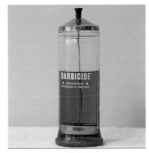

Barbicide

HANDY HINT

Chemical solutions lose their effectiveness over time so they need to be changed regularly.

HANDY HINT

Disinfecting spray or wipes can be used on certain tools and equipment.

INDUSTRY TIP

Objects need to be turned over in a UV cabinet to make sure that all surfaces are exposed to the rays and are disinfected.

INDUSTRY TIP

UV cabinets are good for storing sterilised instruments to keep them sterile.

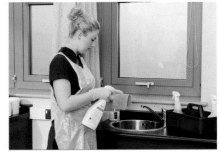

A therapist disinfecting a sink

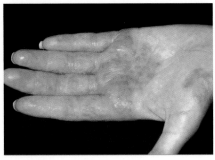

Dermatitis

DERMATITIS

It is important to protect your hands with gloves to avoid dermatitis. Dermatitis is a skin condition affecting the epidermis and dermis. It is caused by the skin coming into contact with substances that can irritate it and cause allergies. The skin becomes sore, dry, red and cracked with blisters. Dermatitis is not contagious but can spread on your own skin. Beauty therapists and hairdressers are more likely to get dermatitis because of the need to wash their hands regularly and because of exposure to products that may become irritants.

COMMON WORKPLACE INJURIES

Slips, trips and falls

Slips and trips are the most common cause of injury in the workplace. You must stay alert to the dangers of slips, trips and falls. They can cause serious injury and may end in legal action. You need to be alert to the causes of slips, trips and falls and try to prevent them.

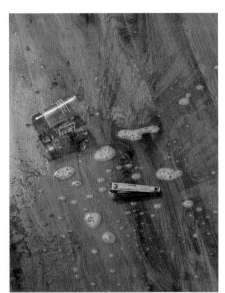

Liquids spilt on the floor are a slip hazard

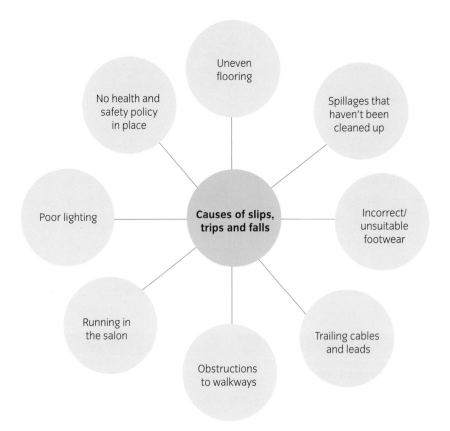

Uneven flooring

Spillages that haven't been cleaned up

No health and safety policy in place

Causes of slips, trips and falls

Incorrect/ unsuitable footwear

Poor lighting

Running in the salon

Obstructions to walkways

Trailing cables and leads

INDUCTION OF NEW STAFF

Whenever you start a new job, you will receive a staff induction, or you could be involved in carrying out the induction of new staff to the salon you already work in. New staff must have a staff induction to provide them with all the health and safety information they need to carry out their job safely. The induction should include information and training on:

- fire safety procedures
- disposal and storage of chemicals
- personal protective equipment (PPE)
- ergonomics
- safe use of equipment.

Toilets

New staff should be shown where the toilets and staffroom are located as part of their induction.

Fire safety procedures

Under the Regulatory Reform (Fire Safety) Order, new staff must be informed of fire safety procedures:

- what to do if the fire alarm sounds
- how to raise the alarm
- safe evacuation procedures
- fire assembly points.

All staff need to know where the fire extinguishers and blankets are located and which fire extinguishers can be used on different fires. The table below shows the different classes of fires and which extinguisher should be used in each case.

Class of fire	Uses	Type of extinguisher
A	Wood, paper, hair or textiles	Water extinguisher, foam extinguisher, dry powder extinguisher, wet chemical extinguisher
B	Flammable liquids	Foam extinguisher, dry powder extinguisher, CO_2 extinguisher
C	Flammable gases	Dry powder extinguisher, CO_2 extinguisher
D	Flammable metals	Specially formulated dry powder extinguisher
E	Electrical fires	CO_2, dry powder extinguisher
F	Cooking oils	Wet chemical extinguisher, fire blanket

INDUSTRY TIP

A fire risk assessment must also be carried out by employers for the premises and there should be equipment provided for detecting and fighting different types of fire in the workplace.

INDUSTRY TIP

Everyone entering and working in the salon must know the means of escape in case of fire and the designated assembly point.

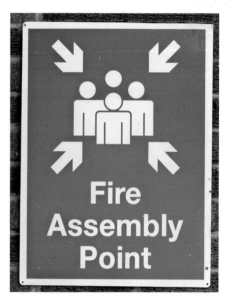

Fire Assembly Point

HANDY HINT

It is a legal requirement to have the fire exits and escape routes clearly marked in all areas of the salon.

SmartScreen 302 Worksheet 3

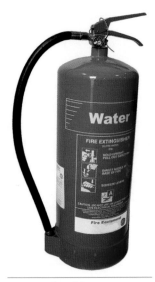

Water extinguisher

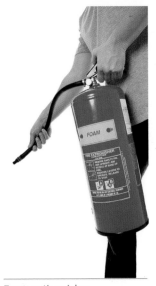

Foam extinguisher

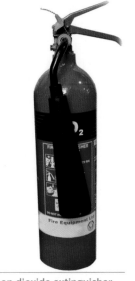

Carbon dioxide extinguisher

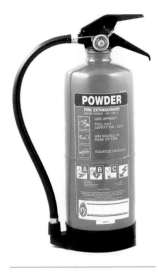

Dry powder extinguisher

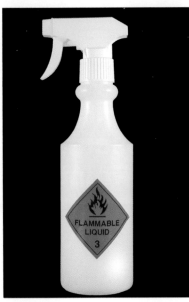

A warning label

Disposal and storage of chemicals

The COSHH Regulations cover the storage and disposal of chemicals. COSHH requires that all chemicals have a warning label.

It is vital that new staff:

- understand the hazard warning symbols
- are aware of how to store and dispose of hazardous chemicals safely.

Personal protective equipment (PPE)

Under the Personal Protective Equipment at Work Regulations, an employer must provide all **PPE** free of charge. They must give employees training on how to use PPE and how to protect themselves properly.

PPE

Equipment that should be worn by a person at work to protect them against a health or safety risk. PPE within the beauty industry includes:

- gloves
- eye protection
- aprons
- face masks.

INDUSTRY TIP

If you are given PPE to wear by your employer you must use and store it correctly as instructed.

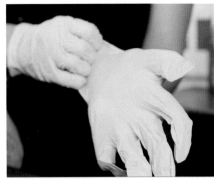

Gloves

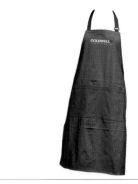

Apron

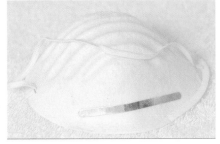

Face mask

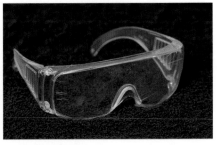

Protective glasses

Ergonomics

Ergonomics is covered by the Workplace (Health, Safety and Welfare) Regulations (see pages 141–142). **Ergonomics** relates to the way you work within your workplace and is about creating an efficient working environment. In a salon ergonomics would be considered when using adjustable couches. For some treatments, such as massage, you will have to take into account the client's body size and weight which will have an effect on how high or low you want your client positioned on the couch. Working with a client at an unsuitable height or on a poorly designed couch can result in **musculoskeletal** disorders, when problems occur with your back, neck and arms. This can lead to injury and in the longer term **work-related upper limb disorders (WRULD)** and back injuries.

Safe use of equipment

The safe use of equipment is covered by the Provision and Use of Work Equipment Regulations (PUWER) (see page 142). New employees need to be trained in the safe use of machinery, appliances or tools that they will use in the workplace, such as:

- electrotherapy equipment
- spa facilities
- epilation equipment.

ACTIVITY

Make a list of any other important areas that should be included within an induction for a beauty salon/spa facility.

UPDATING OF INFORMATION

The staffroom noticeboard should be used for updating information relating to health and safety (eg posters and notices). Any new information should be put in a place that is easy to spot. If you are responsible for the health and safety of others in your salon, It is very important that you make other members of staff aware of any updates to information. When you receive notifications of updates from suppliers or the HSE, the easiest way of passing that information on to staff is at a staff meeting. If you are chairing the staff meeting you need to make sure that all staff are informed of the date and time of the meeting. The meeting should be minuted and a copy of the meeting minutes should be given to all members of staff. If it is someone's day off, make sure you book a separate time when you can update them on any health and safety requirements.

HANDY HINT

Always attend staff meetings as this is the best place to get up-to-date information on the latest health and safety requirements from your manager or the salon owner.

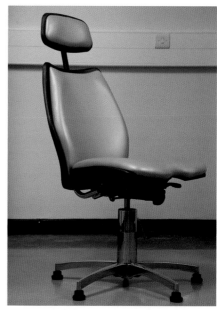

Ergonomic chair

Ergonomics

The creation of an efficient relationship between workers and their working environment (ie having things placed in such a way as to avoid unnecessary movement which may cause injury)

Musculoskeletal

Referring to muscles, ligaments, tendons, joints and bones

Work-related upper limb disorder (WRULD)

A general term that covers a number of musculoskeletal conditions that affect the shoulder, elbow, forearm, wrist or hand

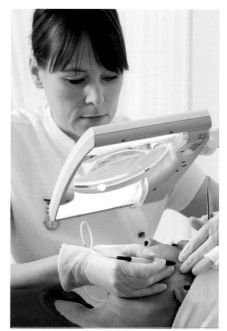

New employees will need to be trained in electrolysis

SPECIFIC TRAINING

According to the HSE, a salon is considered to be a medium risk environment. Even so, there should be at least one appointed person in every salon who is trained to deal with emergency incidents.

An appointed person does not have to be trained in first aid, but they do need to be able to think quickly and not panic in emergency situations. The role of the appointed person includes:

- looking after first-aid equipment
- restocking the first-aid box
- calling the emergency services when required
- evacuating the building in case of fire
- dealing with security incidents.

First aid

Your workplace must have first-aid arrangements in place. Even though a trained first-aider isn't required by law, it is good practice to have someone working in the salon who holds a recognised first-aid certificate. If you do have a trained first aider in the salon, it is necessary for them to renew their certificate every three years, although an annual refresher course is recommended.

DEALING WITH SECURITY BREACHES

It is important for employees to consider both their own security and the security of their clients. Employees should be aware of how to prevent breaches of security and deal with them if they occur.

DATA PROTECTION

Salons hold personal data about clients on record cards and on computer. This information may include the client's name, address, telephone number and medical information.

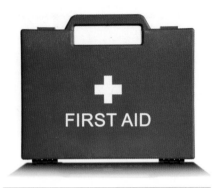

The first-aid box in a salon must be restocked by an appointed member of staff

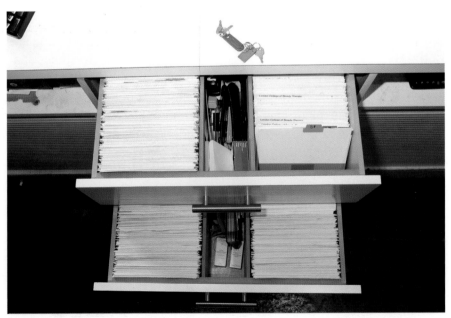

Secure cabinet with clients' files

Under the Data Protection Act, employees must:

- never give out information about clients to a **third party**
- keep information in a secure place
- maintain client confidentiality
- keep records as accurately as possible
- keep records as up to date as possible.

If the information is stored on a computer it must be registered with the Information Commissioner's Office. The Information Commissioner is responsible for ensuring that companies follow the rules of the Data Protection Act.

Under the Act, employers must:

- only keep information that is needed by the business
- keep records as accurately as possible
- keep records as up to date as possible
- dispose of information that is no longer needed
- never pass on information to a third party
- limit access to records to only those employees who need it.

It is important not to breach the Data Protection Act. Failure to keep client information confidential is a criminal offence. It could result in damage to the business's reputation, possible legal action from the client and the employee losing their job.

STOCK DISPLAYS

A salon stocks expensive items which are on display and can be tempting to thieves. Thieves will look out for opportunities (eg where stock is easily accessible and areas that are not always manned). Stock and product displays are usually found in the reception area as this is where the till is located.

If possible, products and stock displays should be kept in locked cabinets so they aren't easily accessible. Any products on display should be dummy products (ie empty containers).

Third party

Anyone other than the client or someone working in the salon

HANDY HINT

Further information about the Data Protection Act can be found on pages 152–153.

INDUSTRY TIP

Loss of stock from theft can cost a business a lot of money through lost income and the cost of replacing the stock.

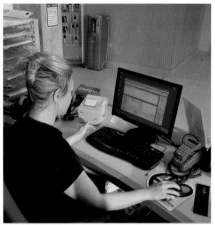

A computer being used to manage clients' records

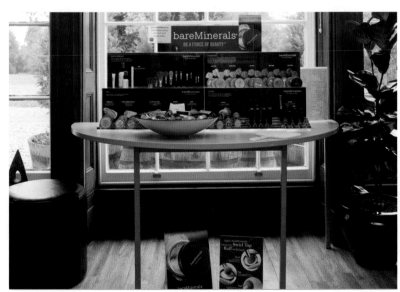

Dummy products on display

HANDY HINT
Don't bring expensive items to work with you.

INDUSTRY TIP
Make sure clients' bags are out of your way when you are working. Otherwise they could become a trip hazard.

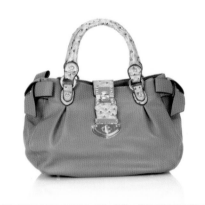

Ask clients to put their valuables away in their bags to make sure that they are secure

 SmartScreen 302 Worksheet 4

HANDY HINT
If you spot a thief, do not tackle them yourself. Get help. Dial 999.

PERSONAL BELONGINGS
Personal belongings may also provide an opportunity for a thief. The salon should provide lockers or safe storage areas for employees' belongings.

CLIENTS' BELONGINGS
When seating clients in the treatment area make sure their bags are stored away safely and that clients know where they are.

If a client removes their jewellery for a treatment, ask them to put it in their bag for safekeeping, so that you are not responsible for it. Your salon might have small plastic sealable bags that you can give clients so the item does not become lost or damaged in their bag.

When taking a client's coat to hang in a coat room, ask the client to remove all valuables and keep them in their bag.

TILLS
If too much money is stored in the till, this could become a security risk. Make sure that the till is locked at all times and that the reception area is manned. Never leave large sums of notes in the till; remove them regularly and put them in a safe place. When emptying the till, leave it open so that would-be thieves can see that it is empty.

HANDY HINT
Good practice security checklist:
- Never keep large sums of money in the till.
- Keep the till locked and the reception area manned.
- Keep tip boxes out of sight; store under the reception desk.
- When taking a client's coat, ask them if there is anything valuable in their pockets they wish to remove.
- Make sure a client keeps their personal belongings and clothing with them at all times, but make sure they are put away safely and securely when carrying out the treatment.
- Keep your personal belongings in your locker or a secure area.
- Don't leave any personal valuables in the salon overnight.
- Ensure windows and doors are locked when you leave the salon.
- Make sure product displays are dummies (ie use empty products when displaying in accessible areas).
- If you notice anything suspicious, inform your supervisor or manager: do not ignore it!

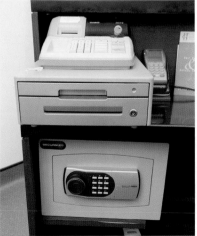

A salon till and safe

INSURANCE

Within the hair and beauty industry there are three types of **insurance** that an employer must have:

- public **liability** insurance
- employer's liability insurance
- product and professional treatment liability insurance.

Insurance provides protection both for the employer and the employee. It provides protection for the employer if a claim is made against them and they need to pay out compensation. It also provides protection for employees and visitors while they are on the premises.

PUBLIC LIABILITY INSURANCE

Public liability insurance is not compulsory but is highly recommended when dealing with the public, especially in a salon environment. It covers claims made by members of the public or other businesses. For example, if a client injures themselves on the premises or is injured by a member of staff during a treatment, they can make a claim against the salon's public liability insurance.

EMPLOYER'S LIABILITY INSURANCE

By law, employers are responsible for the health and safety of their staff. Employer's liability insurance is a legal requirement for all businesses. It protects the employer against claims by **employees** for illnesses and injuries related to their work at the salon. It covers all members of staff who have a contract of employment, including apprentices.

If an existing employee suffers an injury or an illness associated with their work, such as an allergic reaction or a trip or fall, they might try to make a claim against the salon if they think the salon was responsible. The salon would be covered by its employer's liability insurance. If an employee has left the salon and becomes ill at a later date and believes their illness was caused by their work in the salon, they might also make a claim. Again, the salon would be covered by its employer's liability insurance.

> **Insurance**
> Every year a business pays an amount to an insurance company who will pay out **compensation** if a claim is made against the business

> **Compensation**
> Money paid out to someone as a result of illness or injury

> **Liability**
> Legal responsibility

> **Employee**
> Someone is considered to be an employee if:
> - national insurance and income tax are deducted by the employer from the money they are paid
> - the employer controls where and when they work
> - the employer supplies work materials and equipment
> - any profit made by the employee belongs to the employer
> - they are treated the same way as other employees – for example, they do the same work under the same conditions as someone else

> **INDUSTRY TIP**
> Currently, the minimum cover available is £1 million, but the recommended amount to cover compensation costs is £2 million.

> **HANDY HINT**
> If the salon employs self-employed contractors, then it needs to check with its insurance provider whether separate personal cover is needed.

> **INDUSTRY TIP**
> Legally, businesses must be insured for at least £5 million. However, the industry standard is £10 million.

PRODUCT AND PROFESSIONAL TREATMENT LIABILITY INSURANCE

Product and professional treatment liability insurance protects the employer and employee against claims from clients for injury or damage caused by treatments or products. It covers treatments and products that you provide to your clients. Even if you have carried out a treatment correctly, you may still be held responsible for damages and injuries that result from products you use. For example, if you do not carry out a skin test on a client prior to a self-tanning treatment and they then suffer an allergic reaction, you will be held responsible.

ACTIVITY

Look at the different treatments offered by your salon and identify any risks that need to be covered by insurance. For each of the risks explain why insurance is necessary. If you work in a salon that offers other services, such as hairdressing and nail services, include these areas too.

ACTIVITY

Research the different professional beauty therapy organisations that offer product and professional treatment liability insurance. Find out the cost of the insurance, the amount of cover and what treatments are covered.

TEST YOUR KNOWLEDGE

Use the questions below to test your knowledge of Chapter 302 to see how much information you have retained. These questions will help you revise what you have learnt in this chapter.

Turn to page 499 for the answers.

1 When should a risk assessment be carried out?

    a Every day

    b Annually

    c For each new client

    d Before using a new product or piece of equipment

2 What is the correct sequence for carrying out a risk assessment?

    a Decide who might be harmed, decide on precautions, identify hazards, implement, record findings, review assessment

    b Identify hazards, decide who might be harmed, decide on precautions, record findings, implement, review assessment

    c Identify hazards, record findings, decide on precautions, decide who might be harmed, implement, review assessment

    d Review assessment, identify hazards, record findings, decide who might be harmed, decide on precautions, implement

3 Which one of the following is not good security practice?

    a Keeping the till locked and the reception area manned

    b Keeping your personal belongings in your locker or a secure area

    c Ensuring that windows and doors are locked when you leave the salon

    d Leaving valuables in the salon overnight

4 Statement 1

An obstruction to a fire exit is a hazard, but the risk of endangering someone's life is low.

Statement 2

Faulty electrical equipment poses a high risk to clients and staff.

Which one of the following is correct for the above statements?

	Statement 1	Statement 2
a	True	True
b	True	False
c	False	True
d	False	False

5 Statement 1

A risk assessment identifies potential hazards and assesses the risks arising from these. Risks are categorised as high, medium or low.

Statement 2

A risk assessment is carried out to identify and minimise the impact of hazards.

Which one of the following is correct for the above statements?

	Statement 1	Statement 2
a	True	True
b	True	False
c	False	True
d	False	False

6 Which one of the following identifies the best course of action to take to lower the risk of contact dermatitis to staff?

    a Use aprons when in contact with chemicals

    b Take regular breaks when standing for long periods

    c Carry out a PAT test before microdermabrasion treatments

    d Use gloves when carrying out body wrap treatments

7 An action plan arising from a risk assessment in the salon may contain which two of the following?

1 Training needs for staff members

2 An outline of staff responsibilities

3 Pay scales for staff members

4 Disciplinary proceedings for staff

a 1 and 2

b 2 and 3

c 3 and 4

d 1 and 4

8 Which one of the following laws is concerned with the use of chemicals in the workplace?

a The Management of Health and Safety at Work Regulations

b The Workplace (Health, Safety and Welfare) Regulations

c The Control of Substances Hazardous to Health Regulations

d Reporting of Injuries, Diseases and Dangerous Occurrences Regulations

9 Which one of the following is the legislation that requires the salon employer to carry out a risk assessment?

a The Health and Safety (Information for Employees) Regulations

b The Management of Health and Safety at Work Regulations

c The Workplace (Health, Safety and Welfare) Regulations

d The Health and Safety (First Aid) Regulations

10 Poor posture can lead to which one of the following?

a Infections

b Infestations

c Contact dermatitis

d Musculoskeletal disorders

303
CLIENT CARE AND COMMUNICATION IN BEAUTY-RELATED INDUSTRIES

It is important to make clients feel special. Your clients are your business and so you need to take care of them. Good client care will contribute to the success of the business and so it is important that clients feel valued and want to return to the salon for further treatments.

Good communication and a professional approach are essential parts of good client care. Good communication skills and a professional approach can make the difference between a good customer experience and a bad one. Managing client expectations is also an important part of client care so that the client knows what to expect and isn't disappointed.

In this chapter you will learn how to:

- communicate and behave in a professional manner when dealing with clients
- manage client expectations.

COMMUNICATE AND BEHAVE IN A PROFESSIONAL MANNER WHEN DEALING WITH CLIENTS

Excellent communication skills are essential within beauty-related industries. Clients will expect to receive a professional service and communication is an essential part of this. Good communication will make the client feel confident, valued and special.

In this part of the chapter you will learn about:

- communication techniques
- behaving in a professional manner within the workplace
- personal space
- using effective consultation techniques to identify treatment objectives.

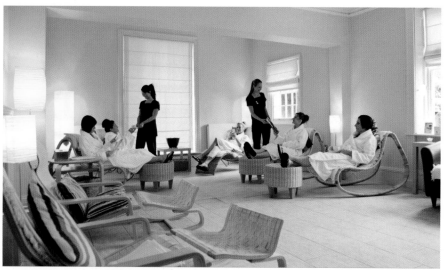
Therapists communicating with clients

COMMUNICATION TECHNIQUES

In the salon, spa or nail studio, the majority of communication with people is face to face. However, there is a growing trend towards the use of technology (eg email, text messaging and social media sites such as facebook and twitter). It is important to be aware of the effect that distance can have on communication.

During conversation only 7% of what we communicate comes from the words we use, 38% comes from the tone of voice we use to say the words and 55% comes from our body language or non-verbal communication. You can therefore see how important it is to pay attention to your tone of voice when communicating over the phone. The tone of your voice will say far more than the words you use.

The way we communicate can be divided into three categories:

- verbal communication
- non-verbal communication
- listening skills.

VERBAL COMMUNICATION

Verbal communication is any communication that is spoken and includes sounds such as laughing or any noises we may make to agree something or confirm a decision (eg 'uh-huh'). When speaking to people you need to be aware of how you are speaking to them. You must make sure you:

- are not aggressive
- speak clearly and calmly
- do not use technical jargon unless it is necessary.

In order to establish and manage a client's expectations, it is necessary to ask them questions. There are two types of questions:

- open questions
- closed questions.

HANDY HINT

When addressing your colleagues and clients you will not speak to them in the same way as your friends. You need to speak to colleagues and clients in a more formal and professional manner.

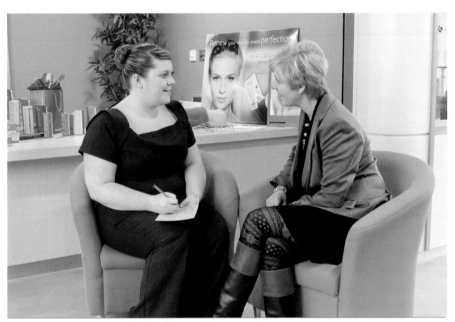

A therapist talking to her client

Open questions

Open questions are used to start a conversation and find out information. They allow you to find out information as they give the client a chance to give you a more detailed response. Open questions begin with 'what?', 'why?', 'when?' and 'how': During a consultation a therapist is likely to ask the following types of open questions:

- What causes your stress?
- Which treatments have you had before?
- How does your skin feel normally?

Closed questions

Closed questions are used to:

- confirm information (eg 'Can I confirm that your appointment is for an Indian head massage?')
- get a short response – 'yes' or 'no' (eg 'Is that pressure firm enough?')
- close a conversation or shorten it if the client is talkative (eg 'Is there anything else I can help you with today?').

 SmartScreen 301 Worksheet 2

NON-VERBAL COMMUNICATION

Non-verbal communication includes:

- body language
- written communication.

Body language

Body language is a large part of non-verbal communication. Without being aware of it, we use our bodies to communicate what we are thinking.

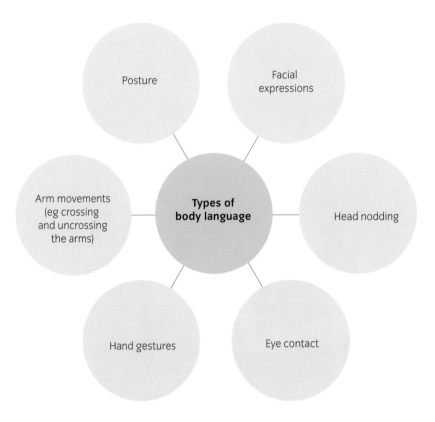

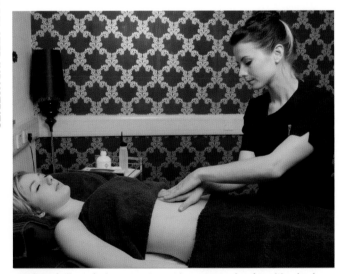

A relaxed client during a treatment is an example of positive body language

Body language can be positive or negative depending on the way in which it is used.

Positive body language

If your client is happy and relaxed, this will show in their body language. Signs to look out for that indicate that your client is enjoying their treatment include:

- relaxed body language – arms uncrossed and sat or laid comfortably
- smiling
- good eye contact with you (if they are not having a relaxing treatment)
- looking sleepy (or actually going to sleep during a relaxing treatment).

Negative body language

Look out for the following negative body language from your client:

- leaning back or away from you
- crossed legs
- crossed arms
- looking away/lack of eye contact.

This may be a warning sign that they are nervous, disinterested or defensive or that they want to leave the salon.

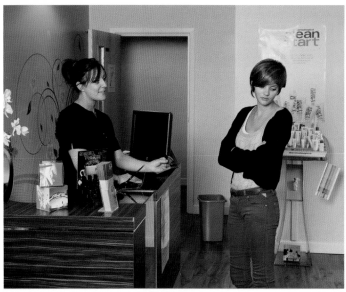

A client showing negative body language

Written communication

Written communication is anything that includes written words.

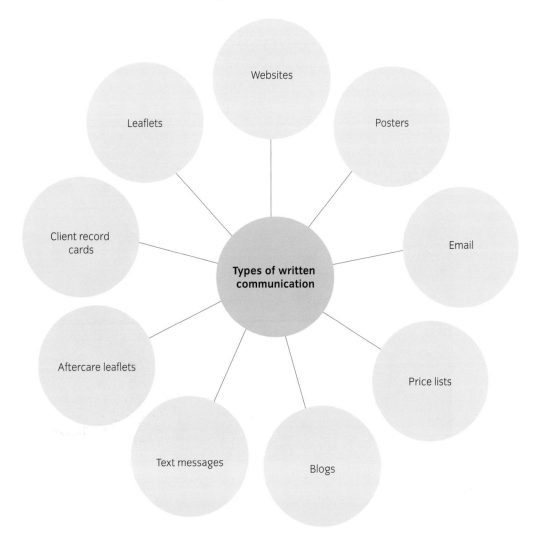

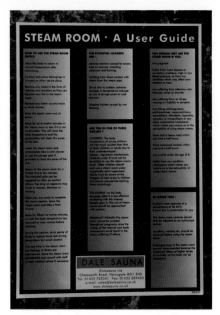

An example of written communication

Concise

Short

Any written information relating to the salon or spa should be clear and **concise**. You should proofread, spell check and check the grammar in any material before it is issued as it is a representation of your salon or spa and it reflects on your professional image.

LISTENING SKILLS

When someone else is talking to you, you should make sure you listen. During a client consultation you should always listen more than you talk. By listening rather than talking, you will gather valuable information. This will assist you when you are deciding which recommendations you are going to make. It also shows the client that you are interested in what they have to say and that it is important.

At the end of the consultation, it is a good idea to repeat back the important points of the conversation to make sure that you have fully understood the information and that you haven't made any assumptions. This technique is known as 'summarising and confirming'.

VISUAL AIDS

Visual aids are a fabulous tool for use when explaining treatments. For example, it is really useful if you have access to before and after photos to show clients the results that a treatment can achieve. If a client has never used a particular product or had a particular treatment before then show them the equipment and products that you are going to use during their treatment and explain the treatment.

INDUSTRY TIP

A good way of encouraging clients to purchase products that you have recommended is to let them try the products. Give them the product and let them try it on their skin.

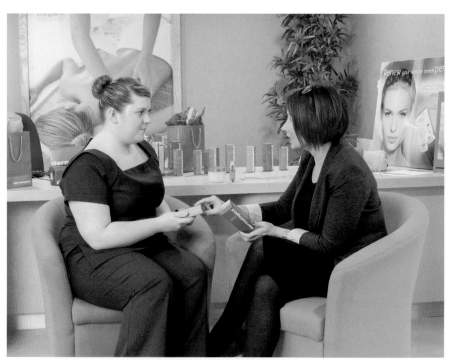

A therapist using product boxes as visual aids with a client

WHY DON'T YOU ...

in pairs, practise a consultation using a visual aid (eg a product) by explaining a piece of equipment. Ask your partner for feedback. Did it help with the consultation? Was it useful to be able to demonstrate/show something? How was it useful? What improvements could you make?

ADAPTING YOUR METHODS OF COMMUNICATION TO SUIT THE CLIENT'S NEEDS

An important part of good communication is being able to adapt your methods of communication to different situations. For example, if a client has a hearing problem, is blind or partially sighted or has a learning disability, you may need to adapt your communication in the following ways.

Communication difficulty	How to adapt your communication
Learning disabilities	■ Speak clearly. ■ Be patient. ■ Avoid technical jargon. ■ Repeat information and check client's understanding.
Deaf or partial hearing	■ Face the client. ■ Use eye contact. ■ Speak normally but clearly. ■ Do *not* shout at the client. ■ If possible, use visual aids (eg pictures of the treatment). ■ Try to discuss the client's needs in a quiet area without other sounds and distractions. ■ Be patient.
Blind or partially sighted	■ Speak normally and clearly. ■ Try to discuss the client's needs in a quiet area without other sounds and distractions. ■ Be patient. ■ Guide your client through the salon – offer your client your shoulder as assistance and walk in front them. Guide them through the salon being sure to mention any steps and potential dangers as you go.

ACTIVITY

Working with a colleague, ask them to close their eyes and place their hands over their ears. Explain a treatment to them. Did they understand you? How did it feel? Did they feel that you fully explained it to them? This exercise should have raised your awareness of what it is like to be someone who is visually impaired or hearing impaired.

PROFESSIONAL BEHAVIOUR WITH COLLEAGUES

It is important to be professional at all times, both in the salon environment and outside of the salon. Working cooperatively with others and respecting colleagues and clients is covered in more detail in Unit 301.

NEGATIVE BEHAVIOUR

Remember that any negative behavior displayed with colleagues will have an impact on everyone around you including clients. Negativity is stressful for everyone and creates a poor working environment. Negative behavior must be addressed and dealt with quickly and effectively.

It is important when wearing your uniform outside of the salon that you remain professional as people might recognise where you work or you might be seen by clients. Within the salon it is important to behave in an appropriate and respectful manner towards your colleagues and clients at all times. The way in which a person behaves reflects the image of the salon.

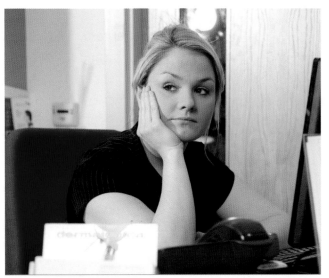

Negative behaviour, such as appearing bored, will leave a poor impression on a client

FOLLOWING SALON REQUIREMENTS

Being professional also includes following safe and hygienic working practices in line with salon requirements and legislation. These are covered in more detail in Unit 301.

PERSONAL SPACE

Personal space refers to the area around us that we consider to be private. If you invade someone's personal space and get too close for comfort they may feel uneasy. Personal space varies from person to person. You will need to enter a client's personal space during some treatments so make sure you are aware of it and how clients may feel.

USING EFFECTIVE CONSULTATION TECHNIQUES TO IDENTIFY TREATMENT OBJECTIVES

The consultation process is an essential part of any beauty or spa treatment. It will allow you to get to know your client and find out their hopes, fears and expectations (ie their objectives for the treatment). Having a knowledge of the client's needs will allow you to select the

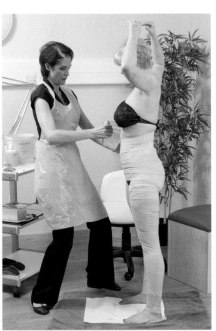

Body wrap treatments require you to enter a client's personal space

most suitable treatment and products and even to start to think about products that will benefit them after the treatment has been completed. During the consultation you should:

- record important or key information
- assess whether the client is suitable for the treatments
- find out and record what the client hopes and needs to achieve from the treatment (ie their expectations)
- decide on which product or treatment will meet the client's needs
- explain the **features**, **actions, benefits** of the treatment and any **special points** in relation to the particular treatment
- provide an opportunity for the client to discuss the treatment and ask questions
- establish a **rapport** with the client and build confidence
- agree on the treatment objectives so the correct products and treatments can be used and any adaptations to the treatment can be made to suit the client's needs
- take details of the client's medical history so you can adapt the treatment if there are any **contra-indications** and provide the most suitable treatment
- take details of any previous treatments so that you can use this information when deciding which procedure to use
- carry out, if needed, an analysis of the client's posture and/or a skin sensitivity or patch test
- add the results of a skin sensitivity test to the consultation form or client's record card
- check for contra-indications.

The very first consultation that you have with a new client will always be more in-depth than later consultations. When the client returns for future treatments, a shorter **review** consultation should still be performed and the treatment plan amended according to the client's needs.

Features
A description (of the treatment)

Actions
What will take place (during the treatment)

Benefits
Effects (that the treatment is likely to have)

Special points
Any particular information to be aware of (about the treatment)

Rapport
A close relationship between two people in which they understand one another's feelings and attitudes

Contra-indication
A reason why a treatment cannot be carried out or needs to be adapted

Review
Assessing or examining something again

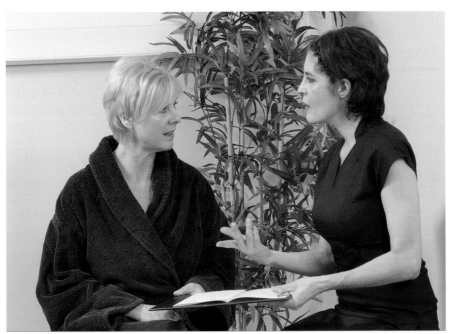

A therapist undergoing a consultation with a client

A consultation should not only be performed at the start of every treatment but also when the client makes their booking. If the receptionist is not a trained therapist they must seek advice from senior therapists or managers about the questions they need to ask and the advice they need to give. When the client books their appointment always ask them if they have had the treatment before. For example, if they have never had a body massage before they may not be aware that they will need to undress or if they have not had a spray tan treatment before they won't know what they need to do to prepare for the treatment. By finding out whether the client has had the treatment, you will be able to provide them with the correct advice so that they come prepared for the treatment.

INDUSTRY TIP

During the consultation process it is essential that you find out about and record details of clients' medical histories in case there are any conditions (contra-indications) that might restrict or prevent the treatment.

SmartScreen 303 Worksheet 5

ACTIVITY

For Level 3 treatments, write a list of questions that the receptionist needs to ask clients when they are booking. Put together an information pack to help any new starters, including descriptions of the treatments, approximate timings and the questions the receptionist needs to ask when taking a booking.

CONTRA-INDICATIONS

A contra-indication is a reason why a treatment cannot be carried out. It might be a contra-indication that prevents the client from being treated at all, or one that might require the treatment to be restricted or modified. Checking for contra-indications must be done prior to any treatment. Ask the client whether they have any contra-indications that might be relevant to the treatment. The client should then sign and date the consultation form to confirm that the information is accurate.

In some cases contra-indications will just restrict treatments. For example, a bruise or an area of open skin will need to be avoided. If you need to adapt your treatment, you should always explain to the client how and why and get their agreement before you start. In some cases, it might be more advisable for the client to rebook the treatment for another time when they can benefit from the full experience.

The following contra-indications will either prevent or restrict treatment so you need to make sure you are familiar with them. For further information on each of the contra-indications listed, refer to pages 32, 46, 52–53, 56, 69–73, 82, 90–91, 99–100, 102, 107–108, 115, 122–124, 128 and 134 in the Anatomy and Physiology chapter.

INDUSTRY TIP

If there is a reason why you cannot carry out a treatment you must explain tactfully to the client why the treatment cannot go ahead.

Contra-indications that prevent treatment

Contra-indication	Action	Contra-indication	Action
Fungal infection	Seek medical advice for all face and body treatments.	Eye infections	Seek medical advice for all face and body treatments.
Bacterial infection		Chemotherapy	
Infestations		Radiotherapy	
Viral infections		Deep vein thrombosis	
Severe eczema		Disorders of the nervous system (eg epilepsy, multiple sclerosis etc)*	
Severe psoriasis			
Severe skin conditions			

* Disorders of the nervous system can prevent or restrict a procedure depending on the treatment that the client is receiving. Please check each unit for further details of nervous system contra-indications.

Contra-indications that restrict treatment

Contra-indication	Action	Contra-indication	Action
Broken bones	Treatments may need to be modified or an alternative treatment offered.	Allergies	Treatments may need to be modified or an alternative treatment offered.
Recent scar tissue		Varicose veins	
Hyperkeratosis		Undiagnosed lumps	
Skin allergies		Recent fractures and sprains	
Cuts and abrasions		Respiratory conditions	
Epilepsy		Circulatory conditions (phlebitis)	
Diabetes		Pregnancy	
Heart disease		Obesity	
High and low blood pressure		Nail conditions	
Skin disorders			
Piercings			

SEEKING MEDICAL ADVICE

If you think that the client should seek medical advice then suggest this. Remember that you are not qualified to make a medical diagnosis and so it is important that the client sees a professional who is medically qualified.

If the client speaks to their medical practitioner and they have agreed that the treatment can go ahead, you should record this. Make notes on the client's record card and get the client to sign to confirm the information and agree to the treatment going ahead.

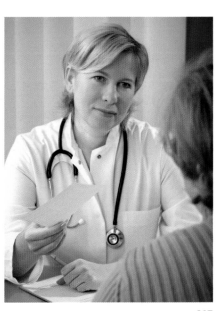

INDUSTRY TIP

Remember, it is important not to discuss information about the client with anyone else in the salon to avoid breaching client confidentiality.

MANAGING CLIENT EXPECTATIONS

In this part of the chapter you will learn about:

- maintaining client confidentiality in line with legislation
- making product and treatment recommendations to meet client requirements
- evaluating client feedback
- identifying methods of improving own working practices
- resolving client complaints.

It is important that you explain what is realistically achievable with a treatment. Be truthful at all times. The client will be more disappointed if you give them an unrealistic expectation than if you are honest and explain that a single treatment will not have the same result as a course of treatments. For example, if a female client wants a bikini ready body after one electrical muscle simulation (body faradic) session it is not going to be possible. You will need to explain to the client how the treatment works and why they will see better results over a course of treatments. If the client will never achieve a bikini ready body, even with a course of treatments, be honest and tactful and suggest other more suitable treatments.

Once you have agreed the treatment objectives with the client and decided what the treatment will include, you should write the information down in the client's treatment plan. You should make a note of any changes to the treatment that need to be made. Ask the client to sign the consultation form. Their signature indicates that they are happy to have the treatment you have recommended as recorded on their record card. Make sure the treatment plan and record card are accurate and filed away securely and in line with the Data Protection Act (see pages 152–153). This will help to maintain client confidentiality.

MAKING PRODUCT AND TREATMENT RECOMMENDATIONS TO MEET CLIENT REQUIREMENTS

When you make product recommendations or sell treatments or products, it is important to:

- know all the treatments the salon provides so you can advise and make recommendations
- have a thorough knowledge of the particular product or treatment you are recommending (ie its features and benefits)
- make sure that the products you are offering the client are appropriate to the treatment that has been performed
- record the information on the client's record card.

For more information on selling products, please see Unit 304.

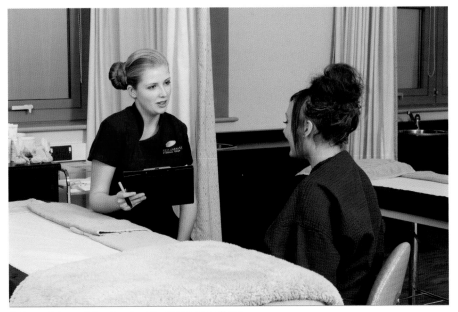

A therapist providing treatment advice to a client

EVALUATING CLIENT FEEDBACK

It is important to gain feedback from the client. Feedback helps you to:

- evaluate the effectiveness of a treatment
- understand how you can improve a treatment
- learn from your experiences.

When you have completed a treatment you should seek confirmation from the client that they are satisfied with the result of the treatment. If the client previously purchased a product, check they were happy with it.

It is essential to gain feedback from the clients as it is one way in which you can improve the service that both you and the salon provide. Do not be nervous about asking clients about their treatment. Ask open questions rather than ones that will just get a one-word answer (eg 'yes'). You want their feedback to be constructive to help you improve. If the client is happy with their service hopefully they will come back and ask for you specifically. Always thank the client for their feedback whether it is negative or positive.

INDUSTRY TIP

If you want honest feedback from a client get a colleague to ask the client for the feedback. Clients might be more likely to give honest feedback to someone else.

INDUSTRY TIP

One way of evaluating your customer care and quality of service is to review how many of your clients come back as repeat business – especially for regular treatments. Repeat business is usually a positive sign. However, there is always room for improvement no matter how good you think you are.

ACTIVITY

Gaining client feedback is one method of finding out how you can improve your skills as a therapist. Can you think of any other ways of finding out how to improve the way you work?

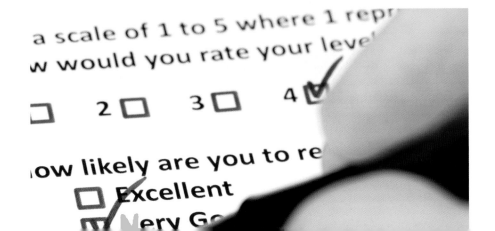

METHODS OF GAINING FEEDBACK

Ideally, you should use a range of methods to gather feedback as different information can be gained from each method:

- verbal questions
- observation – was the client's body language relaxed during the treatment? Did they appear to enjoy their treatment?
- written questionnaires.

RESOLVING CLIENT COMPLAINTS

If a client is unhappy with a product or treatment then it is vital that their complaint is dealt with immediately in a professional manner by:

- listening to their complaint without interrupting them
- identifying exactly what the problem is
- involving the correct people (eg the manager) to deal with the client
- following relevant workplace policies for dealing with complaints
- being patient and understanding
- displaying positive body language – don't become defensive or aggressive towards the client
- offering a complimentary treatment or products (if you are authorised to do so)
- offering to **rectify** the problem immediately
- moving the client to a more private area of the salon if they are becoming loud and aggressive.

The salon should have a procedure for dealing with complaints. Depending on the nature of the complaint you might be able to **resolve** the problem yourself. For example, the receptionist should be able to deal with complaints about bookings or retail products. If you are unable to resolve the problem you might need to refer the complaint to someone else (eg the manager) so that it is dealt with promptly and effectively.

HANDY HINT

It is necessary to distinguish clients who have a genuine complaint from those clients who are complaining because they want money off their treatment or a complimentary treatment. This comes with experience.

Rectify

Put right

Resolve

To find a solution or answer

INDUSTRY TIP

When offering to rectify a problem, check the treatment schedule to make sure there is enough time. If not, book the client in again for a complimentary treatment after checking this with your manager.

INDUSTRY TIP

By offering the client top-quality customer service when dealing with their complaint it will help to keep them as a client. It is in the salon's interest to keep clients as trying to attract new clients costs the salon money (eg marketing and advertising costs).

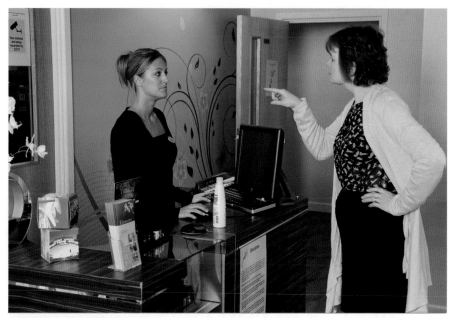

Client complaints should be dealt with calmly and efficiently

TEST YOUR KNOWLEDGE

Use the questions below to test your knowledge of Chapter 303 to see how much information you have retained. These questions will help you revise what you have learnt in this chapter.

Turn to page 499 for the answers.

1 During a conversation, what percentage of what we are communicating comes from the tone we use?
   a 7%
   b 38%
   c 55%
   d 100%

2 Which **one** of the following is a type of electronic communication?
   a A consultation
   b A text message
   c A poster
   d A price list

3 Which **one** of the following types of behaviour should **not** be used when dealing with a problem?
   a A positive attitude
   b Common sense
   c Assertiveness
   d Aggressiveness

4 Which of the following pieces of legislation covers personal information collected in a salon?
   a Health and Safety at Work Act
   b Consumer Protection Act
   c Data Protection Act
   d Sale of Goods Act

5 A client complains that their appointment has been booked for the wrong time. Who should deal with the complaint in the first instance?
   a The receptionist
   b A junior therapist
   c The salon owner
   d The salon manager

6 Which **one** of the following is an example of a closed question?
   a Have you had a massage before?
   b Which treatments have you had before?
   c How often do you have a facial?
   d What are the names of the products you use?

7 Maintaining information in line with the Data Protection Act:
   a helps to prevent the public from seeing how much treatments cost
   b ensures client confidentiality is upheld
   c helps with checking spelling on documents
   d prevents clients reading what you have written about them

8 How long is the cooling-off period if someone buys something from the Internet, TV or from a magazine?
   a 7 days
   b 10 days
   c 15 days
   d 28 days

9 Which **one** of the following is an example of positive body language?
   a Frowning
   b Folded arms
   c Smiling
   d Staring

10 When communicating with a client who is hard of hearing, you need to:
   a face them
   b shout at them
   c write everything down
   d ignore them

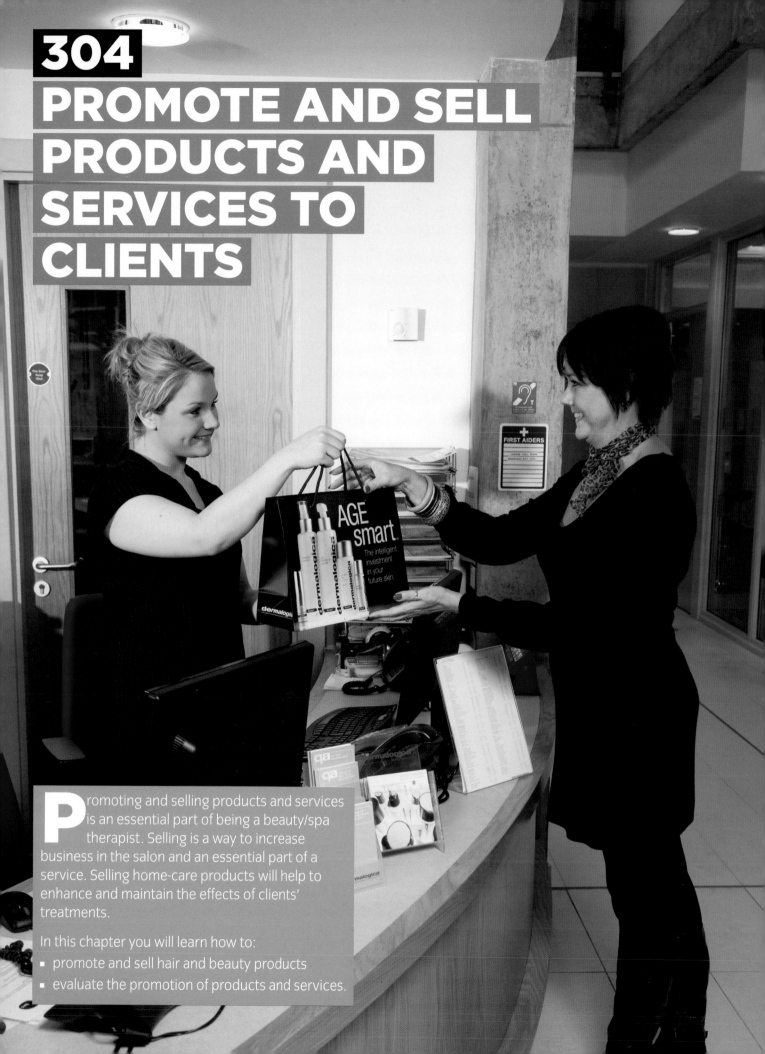

304
PROMOTE AND SELL PRODUCTS AND SERVICES TO CLIENTS

Promoting and selling products and services is an essential part of being a beauty/spa therapist. Selling is a way to increase business in the salon and an essential part of a service. Selling home-care products will help to enhance and maintain the effects of clients' treatments.

In this chapter you will learn how to:

- promote and sell hair and beauty products
- evaluate the promotion of products and services.

WHY PROMOTE AND SELL HAIR AND BEAUTY PRODUCTS?

Many people often buy their beauty products from high street stores rather than buying them from a salon. This means that salons and spas lose valuable retail opportunities to recommend home-care products to the client and sell further treatments and products. These are lost business opportunities for the salon or spa. The therapist may also lose out if their wages include **commission** from product and service treatment sales.

Clients also miss out on an important part of their salon or spa experience. Information and advice on products and treatments could enhance the effects of the treatment and benefit their skin and well-being.

This chapter is about promoting and selling products and giving advice on services and products.

Commission

An amount paid based on sales of products and services

PROMOTE AND SELL HAIR AND BEAUTY PRODUCTS

The keys to successful selling are:

- a good knowledge of products and treatments
- confidence
- professionalism.

In this part of the chapter you will learn about:

- the benefits to the salon of promoting services and products to the client
- effective communication techniques
- the importance of product and service knowledge
- identifying selling opportunities
- interpreting buying signals
- the differences between features and benefits
- the stages of the sales process
- managing clients' expectations
- legislation that affects the selling of services and products.

INDUSTRY TIP

A client's visit to the salon is a special experience for them. Clients need to trust and believe in the therapist's expertise and enjoy their time in the salon. It is therefore important to make sure that you look after your clients in the best possible way.

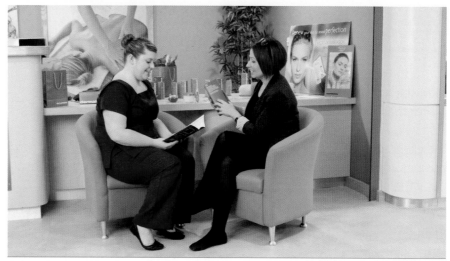

A therapist consulting the price list for a product

BENEFITS TO THE SALON OF PROMOTING SERVICES AND PRODUCTS TO THE CLIENT

Helps to increase the salon's profit and turnover giving the business money to buy new products and equipment

Maintains the clients' interest in your salon's service so they are more likely to return

Encourages clients to try new products and services

Benefits to the salon and therapist of promoting products and services

Provides money for training and updating of staff skills

Helps therapists reach their personal targets

Enhances the reputation of the salon leading to new clients as a result of recommendations

Encourages clients to try new products and services

Improves the professional image of the salon

INDUSTRY TIP

Think of product and service promotion as part of your job and an opportunity to create business. The more your potential clients know about the products and services that you offer in the salon or spa, the more they are likely to try them and to buy!

EFFECTIVE COMMUNICATION TECHNIQUES

The way in which you communicate with clients will impact on your sales technique.

It is important to perform a consultation before a treatment but you can also do a consultation when a client shows interest in just purchasing products. A client consultation is essential to help the stylist or therapist identify:

- any concerns that the client has about their hair, skin or body
- products and services that will benefit the client at home
- opportunities to **upsell** further treatments, rebook and **cross-promote** other services.

A consultation form should always be used to record the information.

Upsell

Persuade a client to buy something additional or a treatment/service of a higher value (eg if a client books an eyebrow treatment and you recommend a facial)

Cross-promote

To recommend another treatment or service from a different professional in your salon (eg if a client books a facial and you recommend a wash and blow-dry)

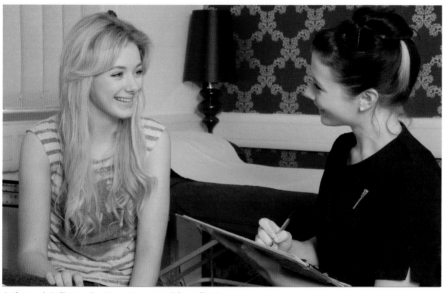

A therapist discussing treatments with a client

VERBAL COMMUNICATION

When communicating with clients, it is important to speak clearly, use simple language and avoid the use of technical jargon so that the client understands what you are saying. Be professional and knowledgeable and use open and closed questions (see page 207). A calm, unhurried manner is necessary when explaining the products and services. Use a positive tone of voice and try to be keen, but not over-enthusiastic, about the products and services you are promoting. If the client is given clear and accurate advice it will allow them to decide whether or not they wish to try or purchase additional items or services.

Open and closed questioning techniques

Questioning techniques should include open and closed questions. Open questions should be used to get information from your client about their requirements. Closed questions have 'yes', 'no' or one-word answers and should be used to confirm decisions.

Examples of open questions include:

- What cleanser do you currently use?
- Why did you book a body massage today?
- What products do you use at home?

Examples of closed questions include:

- Would you like to purchase that cleanser?
- Have you had a body massage before?
- Would you like to book another appointment?
- Would you like a morning or afternoon appointment?

NON-VERBAL COMMUNICATION

Listening skills

Good listening skills are important to fully understand clients' answers to your questions. The clients' answers will contain valuable information that will allow you to select suitable home-care products or treatments for them.

Body language

Your body language should always be open, relaxed and professional.

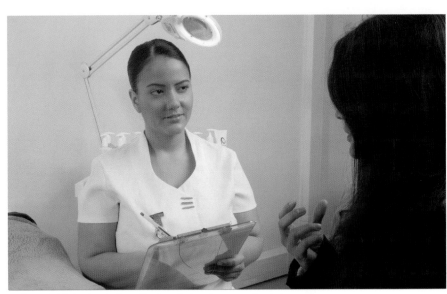

A therapist listening to her client and showing open body language

Position yourself about a metre away from your client when talking to them. This is a comfortable distance for both of you.

Personal appearance

A professional appearance sells! Before you can sell any products or treatments you need to be able to sell yourself. If you look clean and tidy and present yourself and your workplace in a professional way it will give the client the confidence that you are professional and you know your trade.

IMPORTANCE OF PRODUCT AND SERVICE KNOWLEDGE

To be able to promote products and treatments/services, you need to make sure you are familiar with what is available to clients in your salon. You therefore need to know:

- what treatments, services and products are available within your salon – if you are unsure, look at the salon's price list for treatments and products
- how much each product costs

- how much each treatment/service costs and how much a course of treatments costs
- the suitability of the treatment/service for clients
- what the treatment/service involves
- how long the treatment/service takes
- how long products will last (ie their 'shelf life')
- how long a product will last with the correct usage (ie how long a product is likely to last the client if they use it correctly)
- what the features, benefits and results of the products/treatment are.

WHY DON'T YOU...
visit three different types of salons/spas (eg a high street salon, a hotel-based spa and a salon within a department store) or look at their websites. Get a list of their treatments to see what they offer. Have you heard of all the treatments on offer?

KEEPING UP TO DATE WITH INDUSTRY TRENDS

Be knowledgeable about your profession! It is essential to keep up to date with new trends within the industry and products that are new to the market.

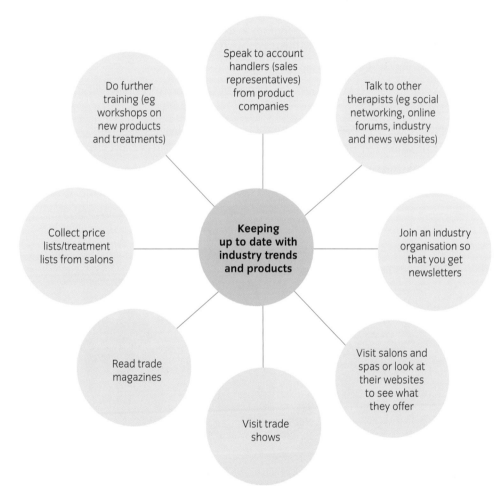

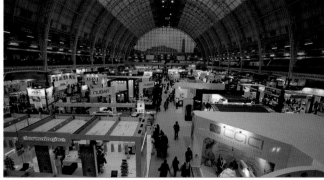

A beauty trade show

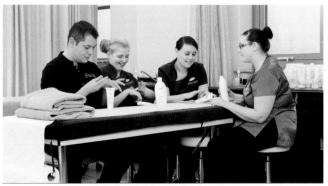

A manager carrying out product training with staff

225

By maintaining and updating your knowledge you are not only arming yourself with the information for selling but you are also continuing your professional development (CPD). The hair and beauty industries are fast paced and ever changing so it is vital to keep up to date with current trends and products. Keeping your knowledge up to date will mean that you can recommend and provide the best possible treatments and products to your clients and provide excellent home-care advice.

KNOWLEDGE OF NEW PRODUCTS AND TREATMENTS/SERVICES

You need to make sure you have a good knowledge of products and treatments/services to give clients confidence when you are selling. You will need to be able to answer the following questions about any new products and treatments/services you are offering or are planning to offer:

Products
- What do they do?
- What is their **unique selling point (USP)**?
- How much do they cost?
- What sizes are available? Are there both retail and professional sizes of the products?
- How exclusive are the products/treatments? Will clients need to come to your salon to purchase them or are they available in high street stores?
- What **point of sale (POS) material** is available to help sell the products?

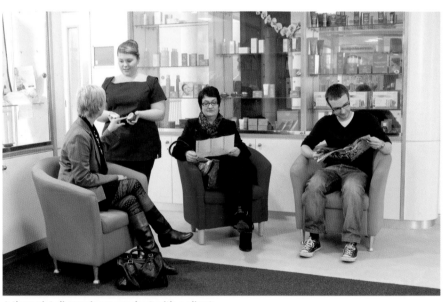

A therapist discussing a product with a client

Treatments/services
- Do clients really want these treatments/services?
- How often does the client need this treatment/service to achieve and maintain results?
- Is this treatment/service just a **fad** or will it be around for a long time?
- Are you able to upsell other products/treatments/services to your client at the time of booking or get them to rebook for further treatments?
- Can you cross-promote other treatments/services to your clients?

Unique selling point (USP)
The one thing that makes a product or treatment different from all others

Point of sale (POS) material
Marketing and advertising materials that are provided to help you sell a product or service

Fad
A passing trend that is fashionable today but gone tomorrow

Equipment

- How expensive is it?
- What maintenance is needed?
- Are the **consumables**/items used within the equipment expensive?
- How many salons in your immediate area have this equipment?
- What are the trade reviews of the equipment like?

Aftercare

- What are the aftercare requirements for the treatment?
- How expensive are the **home-care products** for maintaining the treatment?
- Are there any before and after examples you can use to help sell the treatment/service or products?

Consumables

Items that need to be used with the equipment (eg crystals for microdermabrasion and face pads for microcurrent treatment)

Home-care products

The products recommended and sold to a client to help enhance or maintain the salon treatment they have had

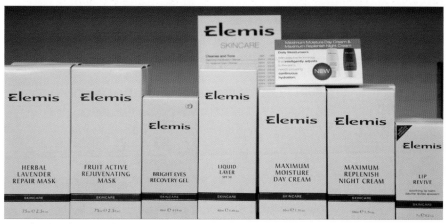

A professional range of skincare products

IDENTIFY SELLING OPPORTUNITIES

Throughout your working day, try to identify opportunities when you can naturally promote additional services or treatments or opportunities for upselling a treatment:

- If a client is booked in for a facial, try to interest them in a luxury facial by explaining what it involves and the benefits. Some clients may not be aware that this service is available.
- If a client comments on a skin condition (eg dry skin), recommend a product or a treatment that will meet their needs or if a client is having a manicure and has dry skin recommend a paraffin wax treatment.

UPSELLING

The key to upselling is to be knowledgeable, confident and assertive. However, remember that there is a difference between being assertive and being aggressive. Avoid using bullying tactics for the **hard sell**; it is intimidating and will lose the salon customers.

When clients visit the salon to buy retail products, try to find additional selling opportunities. For example, a client calls in to the salon to buy her usual cleanser. This provides you with an opportunity to offer her a consultation to see whether:

- the product was correct for her skin type
- she would benefit from additional products, such as a moisturiser
- her skin would benefit from a facial.

Hard sell

High-pressure selling

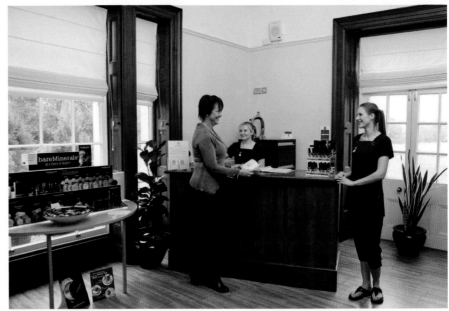
Sales opportunities begin the moment a client walks into the salon or reception area

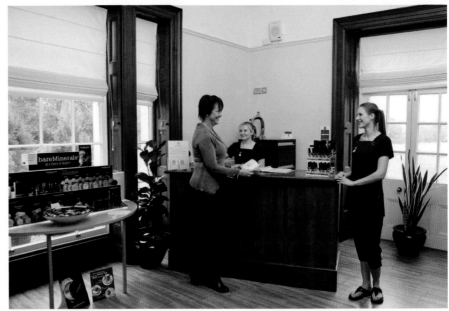

HANDY HINT

Some clients will want to buy products because their friends use them, because celebrities endorse them or because they have used them for years. These products might not be the correct products for them.

INDUSTRY TIP

Don't be negative about products that a client might be using. It is unprofessional and the client may feel that you are challenging their opinions. Listen to the client and reinforce the benefits that your products would deliver.

Sales opportunities start from the moment the client walks in to the salon. The receptionist can also try to upsell additional treatments/services. For example, if the client is booked in for a facial, the receptionist can ask if they would like to have an eyebrow shape as well.

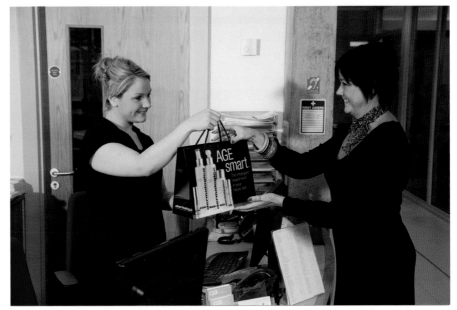
Sale therapist closing the sale of products with a client

INDUSTRY TIP

Look for positive responses from your client. If they seem interested, ask them if they are happy for you to give them product advice for home care.

Opportunities for upselling during a treatment

If the client is booked in for a treatment, explain the products you are using during the treatment and their benefits. This gives you an opportunity to show how they are being used. At the end of the treatment, after you have provided your recommendations, close the sale by asking them which size they would like to buy. If they are interested in booking another treatment/service, ask whether they would like a morning or afternoon appointment.

All companies use opportunities to upsell. Think about some of the places you visit. For example, in fast-food restaurants, they will always ask you if you want to 'go large' when ordering a meal or whether you 'want fries with that' if you just order a burger. They are identifying a sales opportunity and asking every customer. There is quite a high chance that customers will purchase extra items.

It is not difficult to upsell just by asking a question and the majority of the customers do not even realise they have had products promoted to them.

IDENTIFYING AND INTERPRETING BUYING SIGNALS

If clients are looking at retail products or leaflets advertising products in the reception area while they were waiting this could be a **buying signal**. This could provide you with an opportunity to discuss further suitable products. Other examples of buying signals might include:

- a client enquiring about other treatments or products during a treatment
- a client enquiring about the price of a treatment or product.

Buying signal

A visual or verbal indication from a client that they are interested in a treatment or product

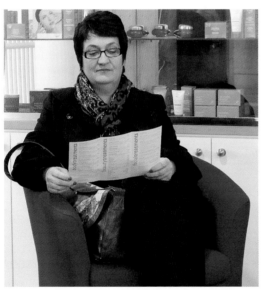

A client reading a treatment list is an opportunity for you to discuss any purchases they would like to make

Use open questions to gain the client's interest. Discuss their interests and/or concerns and then give them solutions by offering them suitable products or treatments.

If they are interested in purchasing the products, demonstrate the products and explain their benefits. The diagram on page 232 shows the stages in identifying a buying signal and turning it into a sale.

FEATURES, ACTIONS, BENEFITS AND SPECIAL SELLING POINTS (FABS)

When you have identified a sales opportunity, knowing the features, actions, benefits and special selling points (FABS) of a product or treatment will really help you to sell it. You will be able to inform the client about what the treatment or product does.

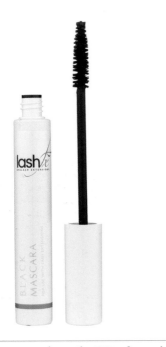

Make sure you know the FABs of a product before you try to sell it to a client

FEATURES

A feature is a description or characteristic of the product or treatment/service; for example, what ingredients a product contains or how much it costs.

ACTIONS

This explains what can be achieved by the treatment/service or by using the product. It explains what the product or treatment/service does and how the client can use it.

BENEFITS

This explains the effects of the product or treatment/service, such as what it does for the client's skin. This is the most important information for a client and so the benefits need to be relevant to them.

SPECIAL SELLING POINTS

This includes any special selling points to be aware of. Special selling points may be, for example, an ingredient found in a product (eg chamomile for soothing) or a particular benefit of a product (eg it smoothes the appearance of fine lines).

THE STAGES OF THE SALES PROCESS

As well as knowing about the features, actions, benefits and special points (FABS) of products and treatments/services, you need to be familiar with the seven steps of the sales process (called the seven 'Ps').

1 PROBE

To probe means to investigate. Probing is done by asking questions. Ask the client about:

- previous treatments/services they have had
- previous products they have used
- the results these treatments/services and products have had.

These questions should be used to begin the consultation looking at the client's home-care routine.

2 PRESCRIBE

Prescribing is using the information to make recommendations. By asking questions during a consultation process, the stylist or therapist is able to use the information to recommend suitable products, services and treatments.

3 PRESENT

Demonstrating (ie presenting) the product to the client is important to allow the client to look at and try the product. For example, try the product out on the client's hands or explain in detail the treatment/service. Explain the features, actions, benefits and special selling points (FABS). Giving them visual aids, such as promotional literature showing before and after pictures and explaining the results. Give the client clear explanations and think about drawing diagrams to help with your explanation. By educating the client about products and treatments

A client sampling a product

they will understand the benefits more easily and will be more likely to follow your advice and buy.

4 PARTICIPATE

If you are selling products, give the products to the client and allow them to use them and smell them. Get the client to compare the results and repeat the features, actions, benefits and special points (FABS).

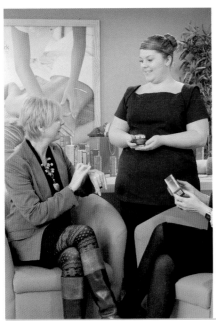 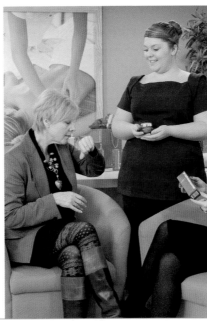

Allow your client to sample and smell the product whilst telling them of its features, actions, benefits and special points

INDUSTRY TIP

It is said that if you repeat something three times it enters the **subconscious** mind. If you can repeat the key features and benefits, it will help them to remain in the client's thoughts.

Subconscious

The part of your mind that you aren't aware of but that influences your feelings and actions

INDUSTRY TIP

At the end of a treatment, go back and talk through the prescription again. Link back to the information that the client gave you during their consultation. In this way, the client will see that you have listened to their concerns and to what they wanted to achieve. This will provide you with an opportunity to make recommendations for the products you have used.

5 PROBLEM SOLVE

Be **proactive** rather than **reactive**. Try to think about any **obstacles** or objections to purchasing a product or additional treatment/service that a client might have and think of some possible answers to them. For example, if a client:

- cannot afford a product, advise them that it is available in a smaller size
- does not have enough cash with them, advise them of other payment methods that are accepted by the salon
- doesn't want to purchase right now, focus on rebooking them for a service or treatment and review the product recommendation at the next visit.

Proactive

Anticipating and controlling a situation rather than reacting to it

Anticipating

Expecting or predicting

Reactive

Acting in response to a situation rather than anticipating it

Obstacle

Something that is in your way and is making it difficult to achieve something

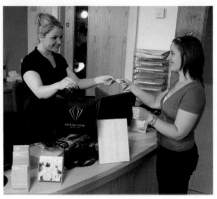

A client purchasing a product

6 PURCHASE

If your client purchases a treatment/service or goods, reward them with a selection of product samples that will work well with their purchases. If they book a course of treatments offer them a discount on home-care products. It is also good to congratulate them on their choices and make them feel positive about their purchases.

7 PROMOTE

Make a record of the client's purchases and schedule them in for a return visit. If they have purchased products, this will give you an opportunity to review how the products are working. You can promote additional products and services at this stage and also advise the client of any special promotions within the salon.

The diagram below shows the stages in identifying a buying signal and completing the sale.

The Seven 'Ps'

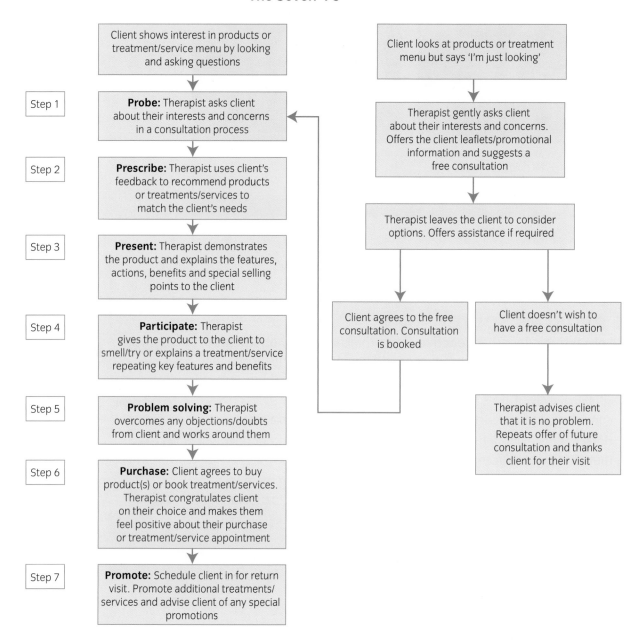

ACTIVITY

Carry out a role play to practise your knowledge of the features, actions, benefits and special points (FABS) of the range of products and treatments/services offered at your college or in your salon. Your friends and colleagues can be your 'clients'. Make notes and recommendations on a consultation form and use diagrams. Use the verbal and non-verbal communication techniques discussed earlier in the chapter to make sure you are asking your client relevant questions. Encourage them to give you clear answers. Recommend home-care products and further treatments from the range you have available at college or from products that you know. The more you practise, the more confident you will be!

HARD SELLING

We have all experienced hard selling. It makes us feel uncomfortable and puts us under pressure. Hard selling is when someone is pushy and does not consider the client's needs; they just want to make the sale or reach their target. We all hate having a wonderful treatment only to be pushed into buying a product before we leave. This is off-putting and might make the client reluctant to return. If the client says 'no' or is not interested, you must accept this and not keep pushing them to buy something.

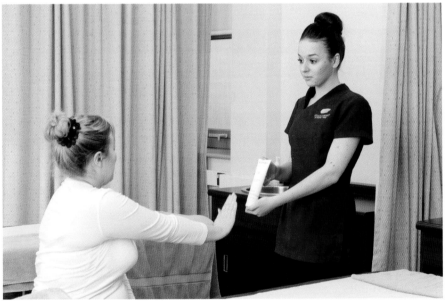

A client refusing a hard sell

MANAGING CLIENTS' EXPECTATIONS

It is important to manage the client's expectations of the treatment/ service or product during the probing stage/consultation stage. This can be done by explaining the results that the client is likely to see after two weeks or a month. Make sure that the client knows how to use the product and that they understand the instructions. Explain that they can only expect to see good results with regular use. Remember, you have to be realistic about the benefits and must *not* promise miracle results after a few days' use. If you do, the client is unlikely to see the results and they will lose faith in the product and you. In future, they may not take your advice or purchase from you.

INDUSTRY TIP

Always deliver excellent service to clients and congratulate them on their choice of products. Clients like reassurance from their therapist and to feel special!

WHY DON'T YOU...
visit some salons or cosmetic counters in stores in your area. Ask the therapist about their treatment and product ranges. Be a customer and see if they promote these to you professionally or if they try the 'hard sell'. Write down the points you liked and the points you didn't like about their sales technique.

LEGISLATION

When promoting and selling products and treatments/services, you must follow the relevant legislation:

- Data Protection Act (see pages 152–153)
- Trade Descriptions Acts (see page 157)
- Sale and Supply of Goods Act (see pages 155–156)
- Consumer Protection Act (see page 154)
- Prices Act (see page 158).

The Prices Act – prices of products and services must be displayed clearly (eg a visible treatment price list or prices clearly marked on products or the shelf that they are displayed on).

The Consumer Safety Act protects customers against any products or treatments that may be dangerous or **defective**.

Defective

Faulty

ACTIVITY

Write down and summarise in your own words two key points for each of the laws stated above. For each law, give an explanation of the consequences for the client if the salon/spa does not obey these laws.

EVALUATE THE PROMOTION OF PRODUCTS AND SERVICES

So far we have covered sales based around clients who are already attending the salon. However you also need to know how to promote your salon so that you attract new clients and build a **client base**. A salon's business is based largely on **repeat custom**.

In this part of the chapter you will learn about:

- the importance of setting and agreeing sales targets
- different methods of evaluating selling techniques
- the importance of reviewing selling techniques and implementing improvements
- evaluating the effectiveness of advertising services and products to a target audience.

Client base

Regular clients who purchase products and services and help keep your business up and running

Repeat custom

Customers who buy products and services again

PROMOTIONAL EVENTS

The aim of product or treatment/service promotions is to boost sales of a particular product, treatment or service. Promotional events are also run to promote a new treatment, service or product and can also be used when opening a new business. Promotional events are often run at quieter times of the year to increase business. Promotional events can include:

- invitation-only evenings – customers are invited to the launch of a new product, treatment or service

- specific promotional evenings or discounted treatments/products aimed at specific customers, such as teenage clients, male clients or mature clients.

Other types of promotional activities include:

- offering discounts when clients purchase so many treatments, services or products in advance
- gift vouchers or discounts for clients who introduce friends and family
- offering free products if clients purchase a less popular service or treatment
- newsletters (via e-mail and text message) to remind clients of special offers
- sending thank-you cards to repeat customers offering a discount
- customer loyalty schemes offering rewards such as a free treatment (eg have five treatments and receive a **complimentary** treatment).

INDUSTRY TIP

Make the free service/treatment one your client has not tried before as this may encourage them to try it again.

Complimentary

Free

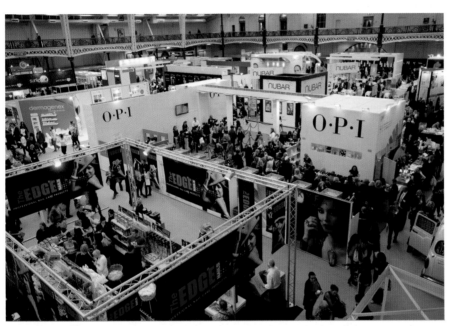

A promotional beauty event

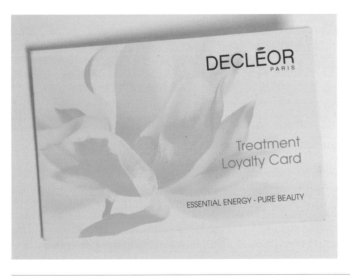

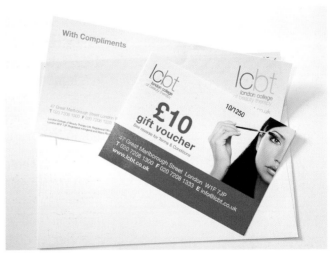

Loyalty cards and gift vouchers can be used by salons and spas

Commission

An amount paid based on sales of products and treatments/services

Productivity

A measure of how efficient a person or business is in producing goods/money

SETTING AND AGREEING SALES TARGETS

Within a salon or spa environment, selling may make up part of your wage. This is called **commission**. **Productivity** and sales targets are often set by managers to encourage staff sales and motivation. They also show the management and employees how much business is being created from product and treatment/service sales.

Targets should be:

- realistic
- recorded
- agreed by staff to help develop their selling skills during the course of their career.

Sales targets show:

- who is selling well – healthy competition is important for both the employees and management and should:
  - motivate individual members of staff to do well by earning commission individually
  - generate more profit for the business
- what is selling well (ie which treatments, services and products are 'best sellers') and which products/treatments/services have done well as a result of a promotion (eg measuring the increase in the number of treatments/services and profit in response to an advert to promote treatments/services/products to teenage clients)
- which products, treatments or services need promoting to ensure all stock and treatments are used effectively.

REVIEWING AND EVALUATING SALES

Different salons and spas have different methods for evaluating sales:

- Computer programmes – some salons will have a computer programme that will show each therapist's productivity and their sales achievements. Users have to log into the system so that it recognises them.
- Paper based-systems – other salons use a paper-based system where therapists write down everything that is sold.

Both of these systems will be reviewed by management to adjust targets if necessary and to give out rewards for achievement.

REVIEWING SELLING TECHNIQUES AND IMPLEMENTING IMPROVEMENTS

It is important for you to review your selling techniques on a regular basis with your manager to make sure that they are effective. Good sales techniques will increase the salon's/spa's business, increase your commission and result in satisfied clients.

Salons may hold sales workshops, either during or after work hours, to train staff in sales techniques and evaluate how they are progressing. These workshops often involve role playing sales situations. The manager and employees visually and verbally demonstrate sales techniques on each other and act out different situations. The group completes an evaluation (written or verbal) of each other's techniques to help improve the team's sales techniques and performance.

WHY DON'T YOU...

in groups within your class, set up a sales workshop. Role play selling situations using the features, actions, benefits and special product details (FABS) and seven steps to selling. Evaluate the group's performance. Ask colleagues to give feedback on your sales technique (ie what went well and what you need to change) and write down how you could improve this in the future.

There are three steps which lead to successful sales:

- Sell yourself – put yourself in your clients' footsteps and think like them.
- Sell by asking not telling – asking questions helps you to find out what the client really wants.
- Sell results – the client buys the benefits of the products, treatment or service so tell them what it does and what results can be achieved.

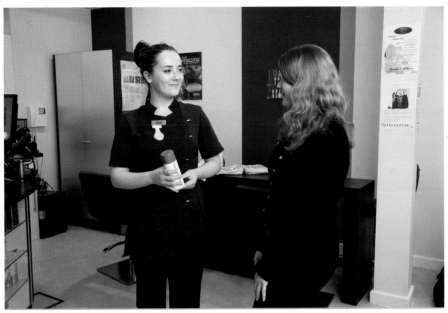
A therapist selling a product to a client

EVALUATING THE EFFECTIVENESS OF ADVERTISING SERVICES AND PRODUCTS TO A TARGET AUDIENCE

It is important for a business to know how successful its advertising and promotions have been in attracting new business. A business needs to decide whether the promotion or advert has been effective so that it can decide whether to use that method of promotion again. The salon therefore needs to evaluate the promotion to see how much new business has been generated as a result of the promotion and whether it was effective. This can be done by:

- client feedback – either verbally or by use of a form or questionnaire
- looking at the type of clients that were attracted (ie did it reach the right target audience – teenagers or mature males for example?).

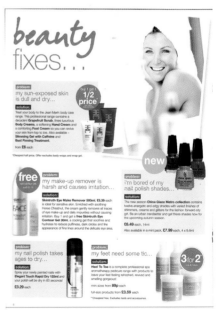
A promotional advert

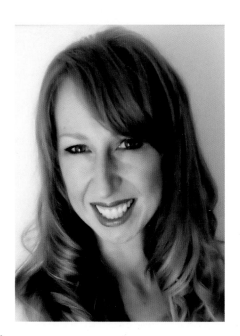

Since the age of 13, I knew I was going to work in the beauty industry. Even at such a young age I had a fascination with health and wellness. I began my training as a beauty therapist in 1991 and completed a two-year beauty therapy qualification. I quickly went on to develop skills in various forms of massage, including clinical aromatherapy, reflexology, sports massage and Thai massage. My interest in the ageing process and my passion for wellness led me to begin practising yoga and to combine this with my therapy skills. I qualified as a yoga teacher in 2007.

The industry is constantly changing with new technologies and therapies being introduced and it is important to keep up with these innovations. To keep up to date with developments, I spent almost 13 years of my career training with product houses such as Elemis, Guinot and Anne Semonin as well as taking night classes and weekend courses in subjects such as glycolic peeling and Hopi ear candling.

During my 20-year career I have worked as a therapist, manager, owner and trainer in a variety of spa environments both in the UK and abroad. As a business owner I gained a variety of skills over and above my beauty therapy training, including marketing, budgeting, and recruitment, as well as both time and people management.

I am presently the Head of Recruitment at Steiner Training, where I manage a number of recruitment staff and I interview hundreds of hairstylists and therapists to work on luxury cruise ships worldwide. My job has enabled me to travel around the globe to some fantastic places and meet lots of interesting people along the way.

The beauty industry offers a variety of opportunities that make it very exciting and also rewarding. There is no other job in the world I would rather do!

TEST YOUR KNOWLEDGE

Use the questions below to test your knowledge of Chapter 304 to see how much information you have retained. These questions will help you revise what you have learnt in this chapter.

Turn to page 499 for the answers.

1 Which **one** of the following Acts states that the price of a product or service must be clearly displayed?
   a Trade Descriptions Act
   b Consumer Protection Act
   c Sale and Supply of Goods Act
   d Prices Act

2 Which **one** of the following Acts states that products must not be falsely described?
   a Supply of Goods and Services Act
   b Trades Description Acts
   c Prices Act
   d Consumer Protection Act

3 Which **one** of the following Acts protects customers against products or treatments that may be dangerous or defective?
   a Supply of Goods and Services Act
   b Trades Description Act
   c Prices Act
   d Consumer Protection Act

4 How do promoting products and services benefit the salon?
   a Makes the staff feel good
   b Fills in time between treatment bookings
   c Increases the salon's profits
   d Keeps the salon owner happy

5 Which one of the following is a benefit of a product?
   a A description of the product
   b The ingredients it contains
   c The container it comes in
   d Personalised to the client

6 Which **one** of the following is a feature of a treatment?
   a A description of the treatment
   b What it does
   c What value it has to the client
   d Why the client should use it

7 Which **one** of the following statements is covered under the Sale and Supply of Goods Act?
   a The service must be carried out with reasonable care and skill
   b Personal information must not be disclosed to a third party
   c Goods must be fit for the purpose for which they are sold
   d Products must not be described misleadingly

8 Hard selling will:
   a Make a client want to buy a product
   b Make a client feel uncomfortable and pressured
   c Help you reach your target
   d Make a client think you are knowledgeable

9 Which **one** of the following should be used to close a sale?
   a Do you want to take anything today?
   b Which one of the products would you like to take with you today?
   c Do you want to buy something next time you are in?
   d The products are expensive so have a think about them

10 Which **one** of the following is a method of verbal communication?
   a Talking
   b Smiling
   c Eye contact
   d Nodding

305/309
PROVIDE BODY MASSAGE AND PROVIDE MASSAGE USING PRE-BLENDED AROMATHERAPY OILS

Massage is a wonderful, versatile treatment when applied professionally and appropriately according to the client's needs. It can be applied in various ways, using a range of techniques to achieve different effects. The origins of massage date back thousands of years and can be found within many longstanding traditions such as Chinese and Ayurvedic medicine. There are illustrations on the walls of ancient buildings of many different cultures depicting massage taking place. It's ingrained in all of us – the power of touch cannot be underestimated and forms the basis of many healing systems.

This chapter also covers massage that includes the use of pre-blended essential oils as part of the treatment. There is not an expectation for you to have extensive knowledge of aromatherapy oils, as you will be using pre-blended oils designed to achieve specific objectives. The aroma and the effect of the essential oil blend as well as the different movements you use add an extra dimension to the treatment.

In this chapter you will learn to:

- prepare for a body massage treatment and be able to prepare for massage using pre-blended aromatherapy oils
- provide a body massage treatment and be able to carry out massage using pre-blended aromatherapy oils.

You should make sure you are familiar with the:

- structure, function, position and action of the muscles of the body
- location, function and structure of the bones of the body
- location, function and structure of the circulatory and lymphatic systems.

PREPARATION FOR BODY MASSAGE

PREPARATION OF THE THERAPIST

As a therapist you will be working in close **proximity** to the client throughout this treatment. It is very important that you are dressed and presented in a professional manner. See Chapter 301, page 168 for more information.

Before you start any treatment you should make sure you are physically prepared and mentally focused. The client is paying for your time and attention and you should avoid any distractions.

HAND EXERCISES

It is important that your hands are warm before you start the massage. This will help to prevent any injury or muscle strain. You can warm your hands up by placing them in warm water for a few minutes. It is also a good idea to exercise your hands to increase their flexibility.

Proximity

Nearness

INDUSTRY TIP

Do chew gum to freshen your breath, but always remember to take it out before starting work with a client – chewing looks unprofessional.

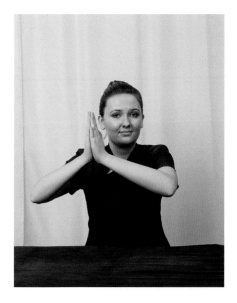

Exercise 1	Exercise 2	Exercise 3	Exercise 4	Exercise 5	Exercise 6	Exercise 7
Make a fist, clenching and then stretching out the fingers.	Run the fingers up and down as if typing or playing the piano to loosen the finger joints.	Thumb circling: rotate one way then the other.	Rotate wrists in a circle, and then rotate in the opposite direction to loosen them up.	Place hands flat together and draw a figure of eight; go clockwise and anticlockwise to loosen up the wrists.	Shake the hands.	Flex one hand and apply pressure to the flexed hand with the other hand to stretch out the wrist.

PREPARATION OF THE TREATMENT AREA

The treatment area should be fully prepared before the client arrives. You should make sure that all work surfaces have been cleaned and are tidy and organised. Clean and disinfect any equipment you will need to use, such as gyratory massage heads, couch and trolley before you begin. Make sure that any equipment or products you may need are ready and easily accessible before you start, so that you do not have to interrupt the flow of your treatment to go and get anything. Check that any equipment you require is plugged in and is in working order.

THE TREATMENT ENVIRONMENT

The client needs to be comfortable during their treatment. The following should all be checked and adjusted if necessary.

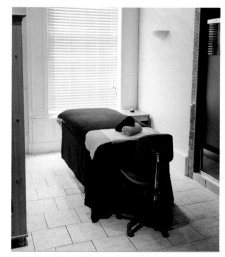

A tidy treatment area

Environmental conditions	Considerations
Lighting	▪ Use subtle lighting. ▪ Make sure to avoid glare in the client's eyes.
Ventilation	▪ Maintain good air circulation. ▪ Avoid draughts.
Sound/music	▪ Choose soft, gentle, relaxing music. ▪ Check that this is OK with the client – some may actually prefer to have their treatment in silence. ▪ Avoid any unnecessary noise during your treatment, or sounds that might disturb the client.
Client privacy	▪ The client will be removing their clothes and parts of their body will be exposed during a massage treatment, so it's important to make sure they have privacy.
Hazards	▪ Check your work area for hazards such as trailing wires. ▪ Reduce any risks to you and your client.
Warmth	▪ You will be exposing parts of the client's body as you carry out the massage routine, so keep the area warm and free from draughts.
Aroma	▪ Make sure the room has a pleasing aroma – avoid the build-up of stale odours, pay attention to personal hygiene and use fragranced products.

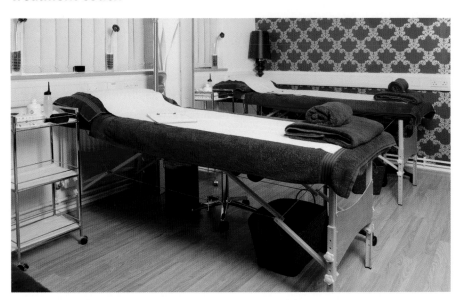

HANDY HINT

Never pour unused products down the sink, especially oils – these will build up on the inside of the pipe and cause bad odours. Eventually the pipe may become blocked. Blot or soak up any products with couch roll or tissue and then place into a refuse bin.

INDUSTRY TIP

As a guideline, to check you are working at the correct height, stand sideways on to the couch and place a clenched fist on the surface. Your knuckles should just touch the couch.

HANDY HINT

Avoid using any more towels than you need to, as these can be bulky and get in the way. A large bath sheet and a small hand towel are often all that you need.

INDUSTRY TIP

Clean up oil from work surfaces such as trollies, as oil residue becomes sticky and is a breeding ground for bacteria.

DISPOSAL OF WASTE

You should have a bin, lined with a new bin liner. To ensure hygiene and avoid cross-infection, dispose of your waste as you work and do not let it collect on a trolley or work surface. Do not let the bin overflow.

EQUIPMENT

Treatment couch

The treatment couch is the main piece of equipment needed to carry out a massage. It should be sturdy, well-cushioned and padded. It is preferable to have a face hole – not all clients like to use this, but it is useful for those who do to stop the neck scrunching up when working on the back. The couch should be adjustable to allow for different therapists to work at it. It should be cleaned regularly with a suitable cleaner for hygiene reasons and to remove any oil residue, and covered with a couch cover.

The couch should be neat, tidy and ready for the client. Towels should be freshly laundered and washed after every client to maintain hygiene standards.

There should be a small pillow or towel for the client to put their head on to support the neck. An additional towel or blanket may be required for warmth but these should be protected from direct contact with the client's skin and covered with couch roll to prevent staining. If the client is very tall you can place a hand towel on the couch and fold it over the client's feet to keep them covered and warm.

Trolley

Position your trolley so it is within easy reach. The trolley should contain all the products that you will require during the massage.

Mechanical equipment

Complete a safety check on any mechanical equipment you plan to use to make sure it is ready, then switch on, ready for use.

- Infra-red – check that the bulb is working and that there is no damage to the lighting case. Make sure that both the bulb and protector are secure.

- Gyratory massage – make sure all the mechanical heads are clean and have been disinfected in hot water and antibacterial soap. They should be allowed to dry and then sprayed with a sanitiser spray such as isopropyl alcohol. Make sure that protective covers are available and on the stand ready for use.

Skincare products

If the client is having their face treated, make sure you remove their make-up before you start your treatment.

Consumables

You will also require some consumables:

- cotton wool to remove cleanser
- tissues
- couch roll to protect towels and maintain hygiene
- spatulas, to decant products hygienically.

<table>
<tr><td>INDUSTRY TIP</td></tr>
</table>

Try to avoid using make-up remover wipes, as these often contain mineral oils which can cause skin congestion. Many clients and therapists use them because they are quick and easy and seem more economical, but in the long term they are not always cost-effective or beneficial to the skin.

THE CONSULTATION

A detailed consultation to establish the client's priorities and needs must take place before every treatment. Further information on the consultation process can be found in Chapter 303.

COMMUNICATION AND BEHAVIOUR

It is important to behave in a professional manner at all times. For more information on appropriate behaviour, communicating with the client and providing a professional consultation, please see Chapter 303.

THE CONSULTATION PROCESS

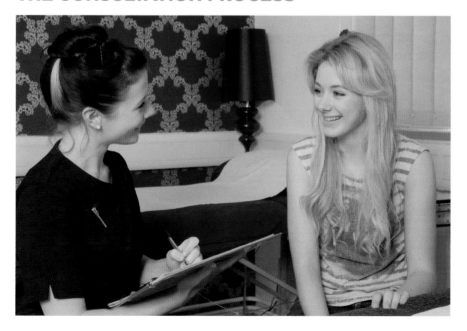

Carry out the massage consultation somewhere quiet and private. Greet your client by name and introduce yourself, then lead your client to the consultation or treatment area. You should sit beside your client so that you do not have any physical barrier, such as the couch, to communication – you should be able to maintain eye contact. You should confirm the treatment the client is booked in for before proceeding any further.

The aim of a consultation is to find out what treatment objectives the client has. It is an opportunity to discuss treatment options or to upgrade the treatment you are giving, if this is possible. To make sure your client leaves satisfied, it is important to listen to the client carefully and match the treatment objectives to their needs. Treatment objectives can be categorised, as shown in the diagram.

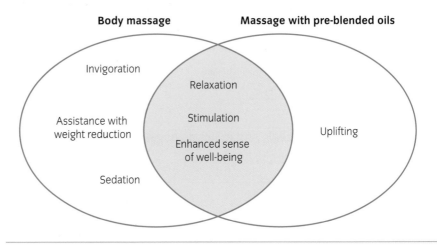

Treatment objectives for each treatment

How these can be achieved will be addressed later in this chapter.

It is vital to agree the treatment objectives with the client during the consultation so you can make the correct choice of oils and massage movements. The client's expectations may not always be realistic or what you are expecting – if so, you need to be tactful and provide the client with a realistic treatment plan. If you feel that the client's expectations are unrealistic you should politely explain this and suggest alterative treatments that can be supported with a home-care routine. Allow the client plenty of time to ask questions.

Remember that as part of a thorough consultation you should include postural analysis and check for contra-indications.

CONTRA-INDICATIONS

A contra-indication is a reason why a treatment cannot be carried out. It may prevent the treatment or restrict it. One of the purposes of the consultation is to check for contra-indications. If there is a reason why you cannot carry out the treatment you should tactfully explain why to the client. If possible, offer the client an alternative treatment. If you think that the client should seek medical advice, suggest this, but remember you are not a medical practitioner and you are not qualified to make any form of diagnosis.

If the client speaks to their medical practitioner and they have agreed that there is no reason why the massage cannot go ahead, you should record this on the client's record card and get the client to sign to agree to the treatment going ahead.

In some cases the contra-indication will just restrict the treatment in some way. An example of this would be a bruise or an open wound that must be avoided. It may be that the treatment will need to be adapted, for example if a large part of a limb is contra-indicated. You should always explain to the client if you are going to have to avoid an area or adapt a treatment – the client must agree to this before you start. It may be advisable for the client to rebook to benefit from the full treatment.

You will need to review the following contra-indications and make sure that you are familiar with each condition before offering a massage treatment.

CONTRA-INDICATIONS TO MASSAGE

The main contra-indications to massage are listed below:

- Contra-indications that prevent a massage treatment – fungal infection, bacterial infection, viral infection, infestation, severe eczema, severe psoriasis, other severe skin conditions, dysfunction of the muscular system, dysfunction of the nervous system, eye infection, deep vein thrombosis, ongoing chemotherapy, ongoing radiotherapy, sunburn.
- Contra-indications that restrict a massage treatment – broken bones, recent fractures and sprains, cuts and abrasions, recent scar tissue, skin disorders, skin allergies, product allergies, epilepsy, diabetes, high/low blood pressure, undiagnosed lumps and swellings.
- Contra-indications that restrict the use of pre-blended oils in a massage treatment – heart disease, hyper-keratosis, respiratory conditions, circulatory conditions, dysfunction of the nervous system, dysfunction of the muscular system, phlebitis, pregnancy.

Thermal and tactile testing

Infra-red uses heat and therefore an important part of the consultation prior to this treatment is to carry out thermal and tactile sensitivity tests:

- Thermal (hot and cold) testing – you will need one hot item and one cold item. You can use special tubes designed for this function, or you can use small bottles to carry out this test. Place the different-temperature items randomly over the treatment area and ask the client to tell you whether they feel hot or cold. If the client cannot feel the difference between hot and cold, they cannot have the treatment, as they will not be able to tell you if something is too hot and burning.
- Tactile (sharp and soft) testing – for this test you need a cotton bud and the pointed end of an orange stick. Press these items randomly over the treatment area, and ask the client to tell you whether what they can feel is sharp or soft.

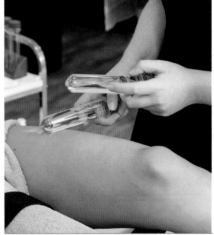

Thermal testing

PRODUCT SENSITIVITY

Pre-blended oils contain ingredients that a client may be sensitive to – for this reason it may be necessary to carry out a test patch (see Chapter 303 for details).

First cleanse the skin with an antibacterial product, then apply a small amount of the product to be tested. If this is a single product, do this in the small dip behind the ear, as this area is hidden. If more products are being tested it may be preferable to use the inside of the forearm. Be careful to remember where you place each product and make sure there is no overlap.

The client should be asked to monitor the area for at least 24 hours or according to the manufacturer's instructions for any redness, irritation, itching or inflammation, any of which would be a contra-indication.

FIGURE AND POSTURAL ANALYSIS

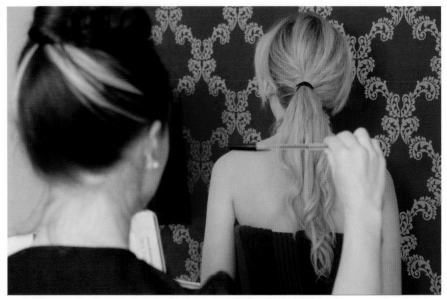

A therapist carrying out a figure and postural analysis

During your visual observations of the client you should consider each of the following general conditions. These will influence your decision about which products and techniques to use. They may also influence the treatment objectives.

AGE

A client's age will affect their skin condition. A young client will generally have good skin tone and elasticity. As skin ages it becomes thinner and less elastic, causing a loss of body contour. If the skin is very thin it should be treated gently to avoid damage. You should avoid movements that drag the skin.

Maintaining muscle tone becomes harder as we age, and muscle tone can become weaker as a result. Poor muscle tone is also associated with a lack of physical activity and is often not related to age. (See the Anatomy and Physiology chapter for more about muscle tone.)

Another factor associated with women as they get older is a loss of bone mass, which can lead to brittle bones. Elderly clients who are thin and frail should always be treated with care. Avoid using tapotement techniques.

SKIN TYPE

General skin types are detailed in the Anatomy and Physiology chapter. You should also be aware of the differences in skin between the different genders (see page 30).

Moist skin

Some clients have naturally moist skin. This is usually due to overactive sweat glands, but can also be caused by anxiety.

Oedematous skin

This is where the skin becomes swollen due to an accumulation of tissue fluid. Some skins are naturally more spongy in texture and this can be quite evident in inactive, overweight clients. If there is very obvious fluid retention, when a finger is pressed into the tissue it will not return to its natural shape quickly. The client should be referred to a GP, as this may be a sign of more a serious condition called oedema.

MALE CLIENTS

Treating a male client will be different from treating a female client. Consider the following:

- Body hair – if the client is very hairy this will influence your choice of massage media and technique, to avoid pulling the hair or generating unnecessary friction.
- Muscle bulk – there is a tendency for male clients to have more muscle definition or bulk, though this does depend on the level of fitness.
- Fat distribution – fat is distributed differently around the body, particularly when there is excess weight.
- Treatment considerations – if a female therapist is massaging a male client, the lower abdomen (below the navel, also called the 'femoral triangle') and inner upper thighs are excluded from treatment. These are **erogenous zones**, and this is done to avoid causing any embarrassment to the client or therapist.

TYPES OF BODY FAT

Body fat is called adipose tissue, and is a type of connective tissue. This tissue is made up of special cells called **adipocytes**. Eighty per cent of adipose fat is subcutaneous and is stored under the skin. Different genders and ethnic groups store fat in different areas. There are three descriptions given to body fat in the context of beauty therapy:

- Soft fat – adipocytes are loosely packed and have some room for movement, making the tissue soft to the touch and easily shifted using a 'wringing' movement.
- Hard fat – this tissue has tightly packed adipocytes with no room for movement, giving a firm, hard surface that is difficult to manipulate.
- Cellulite – fat cells are housed in clusters in free-standing chambers separated by verticals walls of connective tissue. When the fat cells expand the walls collapse under the pressure. This change in structure allows fluid to collect around the cells, resulting in a dimpled appearance of the skin. This condition is common around the thigh and buttock areas but can also be found on the abdomen and upper arms. Loose cellulite is more obvious than compacted cellulite which can be seen by gently squeezing the skin or clenching the muscles in the area.

POSTURAL ASSESSMENT

A postural assessment is used to:

- assess client figure problems and faults
- recognise any problems that may require medical referral
- plan an effective treatment.

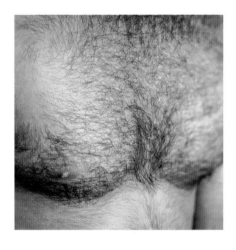

Erogenous zone
Area of the body that has increased sensitivity, eg the inner thighs

Adipocytes
The cells that make up adipose tissue, or body fat

INDUSTRY TIP
Males tend to store excess fat around their middle, whereas women store it on their hips, buttocks and bust.

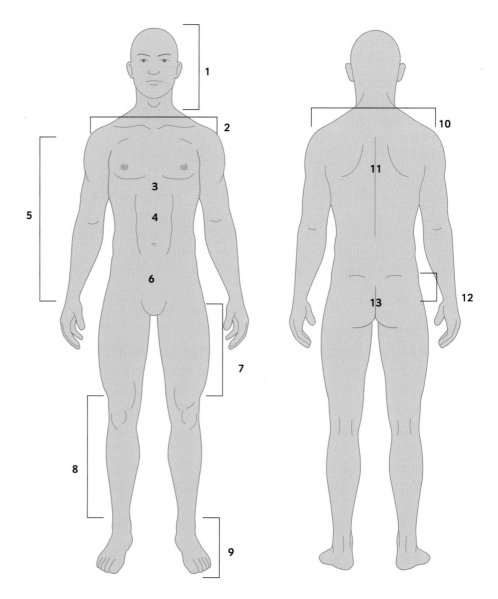

HANDY HINT

When measuring a client's height and weight, always take the measurements on a hard floor – never carpet. The client should remove bulky clothes and shoes first.

Where there are figure faults or other areas of concern the massage can be adapted, for example when working on tight muscles if there is a postural fault, or by choosing an appropriate massage media if the skin is very dry.

The client should be observed dressed and undressed with a minimum amount of clothing (no restrictive underwear) where possible. You should consider their posture and physical requirements and record the following:

- weight
- height
- body frame
- somatype
- posture
- specific body faults.

Postural considerations

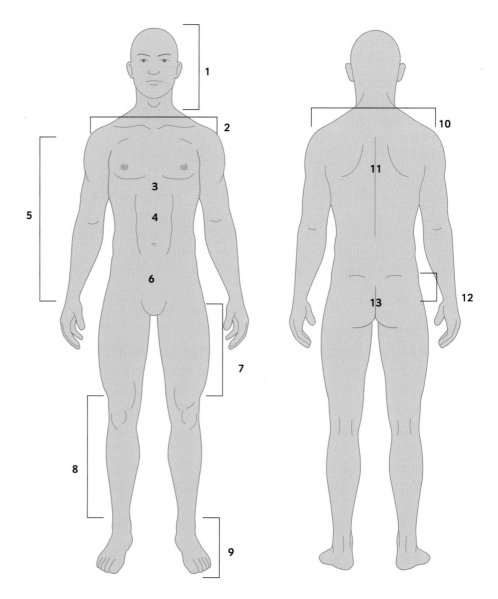

The numbers on each diagram correspond to the following postural considerations on the facing page.

305/309 PROVIDE BODY MASSAGE AND PROVIDE MASSAGE USING PRE-BLENDED AROMATHERAPY OILS

1 Position of head and neck – head should be mid-line, not forward of the shoulders. Ears and eyes should be level.

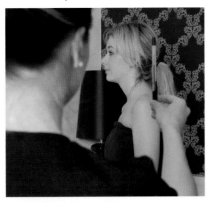

2 Shoulders – do they roll inwards?

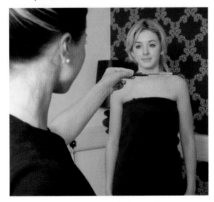

3 Breasts – is there good or poor tone? Is ligament attachment good? Under- or over-developed? Stretch marks?

4 Ribs – the rib cage should be symmetrical, and clavicles should be symmetrical. Is the rib cage very defined or expanded? Pigeon or hollow chest?

5 Arms – solid, muscular, in proportion? Thin or loose crêpey skin? Poor circulation on backs of arms giving rough texture to skin?

6 Abdomen – good or poor muscle tone, giving a flat or protruding stomach? Waist high or low? Any excess fat below waist? Excess skin or stretch marks?

7 Thighs – consider general distribution of fat, including cellulite. Consider proportion – are legs heavy or too thin? Muscular? Stretch marks?

8 Legs – bow legs, hyper-extended knees, knock knees, varicose veins, broken capillaries?

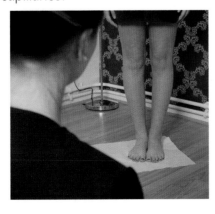

9 Feet – swollen ankles, fallen arches, hallux valgus (bunions), hammer toes, calluses, corns? Note the position of the feet and any abnormalities which may affect posture, such as poor circulation or athlete's foot.

10 Shoulders – note the level of the scapulae. Winged scapula, rounded or very square shoulders, dowager's hump?

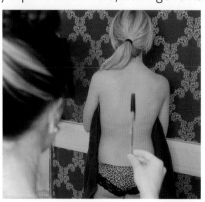

INDUSTRY TIP

People who sit a lot often have more back tension, as this compresses the discs of the spine.

HANDY HINT

To check for a straight spine, ask the client to bend forward and watch how the spine flexes and extends.

11 Back – curvature of spine, kyphosis, lordosis, scoliosis, flat back, round back, excess fat over latissimus dorsi muscle? Note the proportion of the upper back to trunk.

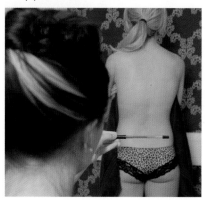

12 Pelvic tilt – dimples on pelvis, if evident, should be level. Does the pelvis tilt forwards or backwards?

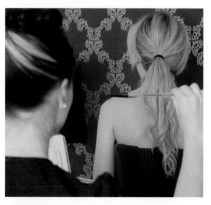

Gluteal folds

The horizontal folds at the base of the buttocks

13 Buttocks – **gluteal folds** should be level. Protruding buttocks may indicate anterior pelvic tilt, excess fat or cellulite. Note the level of gluteal drop – is the gluteal fold in line with the pubis?

THE CITY & GUILDS TEXTBOOK

SOMATYPES

Somatypes are names given to the most common body shapes. Most of us are a combination of more than one.

ACTIVITY

Find three images from magazines to represent each of the different somatypes.

Endomorph	Ectomorph	Mesomorph
▪ Tendency to gain weight. ▪ Hips are wider than the shoulders and shorter limbs. ▪ Heavy build. ▪ Higher percentage of fat to muscle bulk. ▪ Tendency towards padded contours. ▪ Hands may be small and delicate.	▪ Narrow shoulders and hips. ▪ Long, thin trunk. ▪ Long bones, giving long limbs. ▪ Lacks muscle bulk. ▪ Low percentage of fat. ▪ Often underweight with a lack of curves.	▪ Inverted triangular shape – shoulders are wider than the hips. ▪ Boyish physique. ▪ Athletic build; potential for well-toned muscles while active. ▪ Sturdy, straight shoulders. ▪ Low percentage of fat.

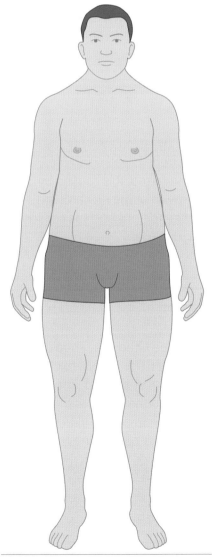

Endomorph

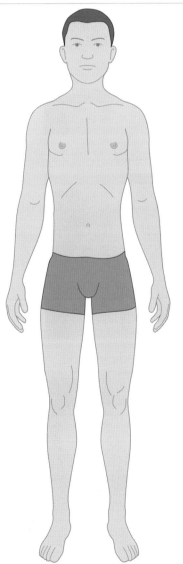

Ectomorph

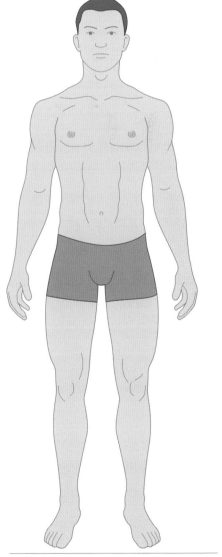

Mesomorph

POSTURAL FAULTS

For more about kyphosis, lordosis and scoliosis, see pages 72–73.

Postural fault	Description and cause
Dowager's hump 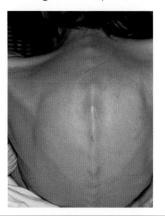	This condition is usually associated with older people. There is advanced kyphosis and rounded shoulders, and as a consequence the head becomes pushed forward. Often caused by fatty deposits which accumulate in the lower cervical and upper thoracic vertebra, creating a pad of adipose tissue which further restricts movement in the area.
Winged scapula 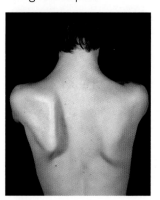	This condition affects the serratus anterior muscles and causes the lower angle of the scapula to stand out prominently, giving a winged appearance.
Pigeon chest 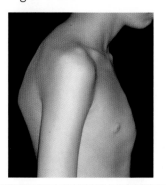	The chest becomes pushed out, as in taking a very deep breath, and the sternum bone raised. It is caused by excessive growth of the rib cartilage, some spinal conditions such as scoliosis or a genetic disorder.
Unbalanced pelvic tilt 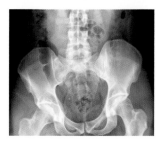	The pelvis can be tilted in a range of directions: forward (anterior), backward (posterior), lateral or rotated. The postural fault and the muscles that are affected will depend on the direction of the tilt. Anterior tilt causes the bottom to stick out, lordosis or flat back. Posterior tilt causes kyphosis and lateral or rotated pelvic scoliosis.

Postural fault	Description and cause
Short limbs 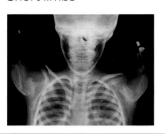	In this condition the limbs are abnormally short and are out of proportion with the rest of the body. It is usually a genetic disorder.
Bow legs 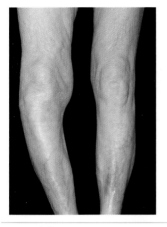	When standing with the feet together, there is a defined arched gap between the legs. It can be caused by nutritional deficiency (lack of vitamin D), leading to rickets.
Knock knees 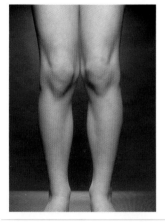	The knees rotate inwards so that they brush together. This condition is caused by slack tendons around the knee joint or an abnormal curvature of the bones of the lower legs.
Flat feet or fallen arches (pes planus) 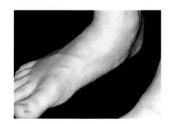	Collapse of one or both of the arches of the feet. This condition can be caused by weak muscles, injury, being overweight or ill-fitting shoes. It may also be hereditary.

PREPARATION OF THE CLIENT

To encourage the client to have confidence in you, always give them clear instructions about what to do, how to prepare and what you are going to do to them. Remember that this massage might be different from other treatments they have had, or it may even be their first massage treatment.

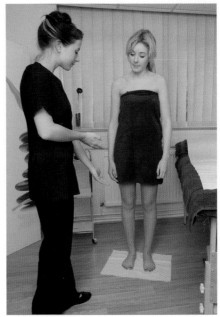

Ask your client to use a foot mat to prevent cross-infection

Ask the client to:

- remove their jewellery, watch, piercings (including from the face and abdomen) and contact lenses; make sure these items are stored safely
- undress down to their briefs (you should leave the client while they do this to protect their modesty)
- get on to the couch once they are ready, and lie on their back, covering their body with a towel (leave this ready for them to use).

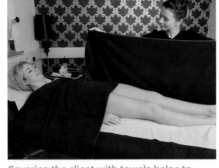

Covering the client with towels helps to maintain client modesty

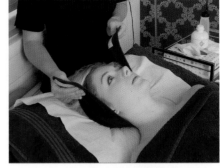

Secure a headband on the client's head to protect the hair from massage products

You should:

- check for contra-indications
- sanitise the client's feet using an antiseptic wipe or spray
- if the face is being included in the treatment, cleanse it to remove any make-up.

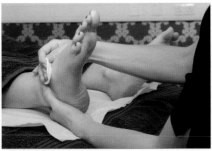

A client's feet being sanitised before treatment

Before the client gets on the couch you may be required to carry out a postural assessment (see pages 249–252).

Once the client is on the couch, you can make them comfortable. Make sure their head is supported on a small pillow, bolster or folded towel if you are starting with the client in a **supine** position. Check that you can still get your hands around the back of their neck and shoulders for when you massage this area so that you don't have to disturb your client later by adjusting the head support. Ask the client if they want their arms tucked under the cover or out.

It is very unnatural to lie completely flat – this puts strain on the natural curves of the body. These should be supported with towels or similar props to help make the client more comfortable. Supports should be placed under the client's knees to support the knee joints and prevent any strain when the client is lying supine. Supports are placed under the ankles when lying **prone**.

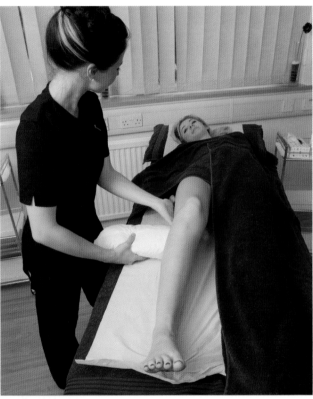

A therapist placing support under the client's knee to make the client more comfortable

Supine

Lying on one's back or spine (think of the 'S' to help you remember)

Prone

Lying on one's front

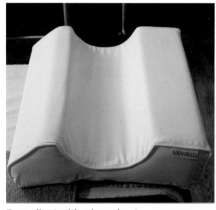

For a client with a large bust, a massage pillow can be used to aid their comfort

PROVIDE A BODY MASSAGE TREATMENT

YOUR POSTURE

Maintaining good posture is essential to enable you to use your body efficiently and to avoid becoming tired or straining ligaments and muscles. During treatment try not to lock any of your joints such as elbows and wrists, and remain relaxed, bending at the knees. Keep your back straight and your shoulders loose. Avoid twisting as much as possible.

INDUSTRY TIP

You can make a support by rolling up a small hand towel. Alternatively many manufacturers have pre-shaped supports which can be purchased.

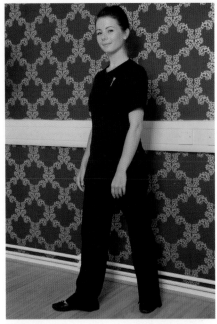
Walk standing

There are two specific stances that are used when providing a massage treatment:

- Walk standing – used when working down the length of the body, for example effleuraging the leg. Stand at the side of the couch with your hip next to the couch, as if about to take a long stride. Weight is transferred from one foot to the other, almost in a rocking motion.

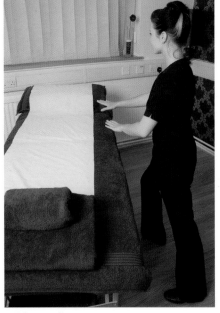
Stride standing

- Stride standing – used when working crossways across the body, for example hacking. Stand facing the couch with feet hip-width apart, and bend at the knees to lower yourself so that your back stays straight.

THE EFFECTS OF MASSAGE THERAPY ON THE BODY

There are two types of effects that can be achieved with any treatment:

- psychological – this is how the treatment makes you feel mentally, eg uplifted
- physiological – this is the effect the treatment has on the body, eg producing an erythema.

PSYCHOLOGICAL EFFECTS

Body massage has many possible effects on the client, including:

- mental relaxation
- feelings of well-being, eg contentment, calm
- uplifting effects
- motivational effects – these can be used as a pleasurable incentive to help the client achieve targets such as weight loss.

THE CITY & GUILDS TEXTBOOK

PHYSIOLOGICAL EFFECTS

Massage affects the systems of the body.

Body system	Effects
Skin	<ul><li>Improves the circulation, bringing oxygen and nutrients to the tissues and improving the general appearance and condition of the skin.</li><li>Sweat and sebaceous glands are stimulated, producing more sebum and making the skin soft and supple.</li><li>Aids **desquamation** as the dead skin cells are rubbed off the surface during massage. This leaves the skin feeling much softer than before.</li><li>Improved circulation gives the skin a healthy glow.</li><li>Oil or cream used nourishes and softens the skin.</li></ul>
Lymphatic	<ul><li>The action on the tissues helps pump the tissue fluid, making it more responsive, especially when directed towards the nearest lymph nodes.</li><li>Stimulates the removal of waste products from the intercellular tissues.</li><li>Excess tissue fluid is directed towards the lymph nodes for filtration.</li></ul>
Muscular	<ul><li>Stimulating the circulation increases uptake of nutrients in the muscle cells and removes waste products, such as lactic acid, from within the muscles.</li><li>The stretching and kneading of the muscle tissue helps to improve elasticity.</li><li>Relieves muscular aches and pains.</li><li>The movement of the muscle fibres during massage helps to keep them more mobile, increasing the circulation and reducing tension.</li></ul>
Skeletal	<ul><li>Increased circulation encourages nutrients into the skeletal system and removes waste products.</li><li>Passive joint movement helps to improve joint mobility.</li></ul>
Respiratory	<ul><li>Circulation to the bronchioles is improved, which brings nutrients to the tissues.</li><li>Mucus may be dislodged.</li><li>Gaseous exchange is improved due to the increased circulation to lung tissue (replenishing oxygen and removing carbon dioxide).</li></ul>
Digestive	<ul><li>Direct massage to the abdominal area increases **peristalsis**, which in turn stimulates digestive enzymes.</li></ul>
Urinary	<ul><li>Aids the removal of waste products and toxins.</li><li>The general increase in cellular activity stimulates urine production to aid removal of waste products.</li></ul>
Endocrine	<ul><li>Release of certain hormones helps maintain homeostasis and a sense of well-being.</li></ul>
Nervous	<ul><li>Stimulates, invigorates or soothes the nerve endings dependent upon the massage technique used.</li><li>**Endorphins** are released, which help to suppress pain.</li></ul>

Desquamation

The removal of dead skin cells from the surface of the skin

Peristalsis

Involuntary muscular movements in the walls of the digestive system that move food through the system

Endorphins

Chemicals released by the pituitary endocrine gland

HANDY HINT

Endorphins transmit electrical signals within the nervous system. When endorphin levels are high we feel less pain and fewer negative effects of stress.

MASSAGE TECHNIQUES

The massage techniques you choose will enable you to achieve your client's treatment objective.

EFFLEURAGE

The word 'effleurage' comes from a French word meaning 'to skim over', and includes stroking movements. During effleurage the whole of your palm and fingers are used. Keep your hands and fingers relaxed so that they can mould to the client's body and maintain maximum contact.

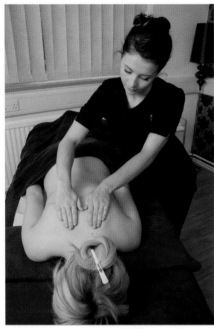

Effleurage movement carried out on the body

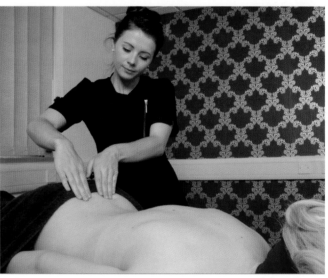

A therapist carrying out effleurage movement

Application of effleurage

- It is used to apply massage mediums to the skin.
- It is used for the first contact and last touch of a massage.
- The movements allow the client to become accustomed to the therapist's touch.
- It links different movements together so that the treatment remains flowing and continuous.
- It assists lymphatic and venous drainage.
- It increases micro-circulation, warms the skin and produces erythema.
- It increases cellular activity and metabolic rate.
- It can be applied in different ways for different effects. If applied slowly and lightly it will induce relaxation; if applied at a brisk pace it will stimulate and uplift.

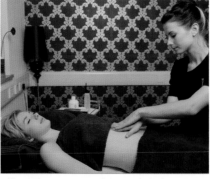

Effleurage movement being carried out on the abdomen

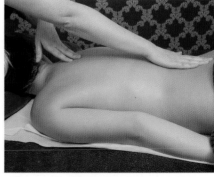

Effleurage movement being carried out on the back

PETRISSAGE

This movement involves lifting and squeezing muscles and tissues, and is often referred to as kneading. Any pressure applied below the heart should always be applied in the direction of the heart. There are several different ways in which petrissage can be applied.

Technique	Parts of the hands and arms used	Method
Kneading	■ Palms of the hand ■ Heels of the hands ■ Forearms ■ Thumbs ■ Fingers	Work in a circular motion. Hands can work singularly or in pairs – the circular direction may be applied in opposite directions for a deeper effect.
Picking up	■ Fingers ■ Thumbs	Pick up tissue with one hand and pass it to the other while gently lifting and squeezing it.
Wringing	■ Palms of the hands ■ Forearms	Use hands in opposite directions, lifting the tissue up, sliding the hands against each other and releasing the tissue again. Use this over larger areas of tissue to prevent discomfort, eg thighs and abdomen.

Technique	Parts of the hands and arms used	Method
Rolling	- Fingertips - Thumbs	Lift the body tissue up with the fingers and then push down towards the fingers using the thumbs.
Ironing (reinforced kneading)	- Palms of the hands - Heels of the hands - Forearms	Place one hand on top of the other and place the palm and fingers on to the body tissue. Apply firm pressure, working in a circular motion.

INDUSTRY TIP

When muscles become overworked they produce too much waste. This causes the muscle fibres to become sticky and immobile and the circulation does not flow easily. We can feel this as an area of hardness or tightness within the muscle as we massage over it. Massage helps to encourage the circulation in this sluggish area, to remove the waste and encourage the muscle fibres to move more freely again.

Application of petrissage

- It can assist lymphatic drainage.
- The squeezing action of the muscles stimulates arteriole circulation, including in the skin, muscles and bones, causing vasodilation and erythema.
- It loosens tight tissue.
- It increases cellular metabolism.
- It stimulates peristalsis when used over the abdominal area.
- Wringing improves muscle elasticity by stretching movements along the length of the muscle tissue, and softens hard subcutaneous fatty tissue.
- Rolling improves skin elasticity, and softens subcutaneous tissue.

FRICTIONS

These are small movements, made either in a circular motion or with a backwards and forwards (transverse) movement, with constant pressure applied. They are often classified as petrissage movements. The palms of the hand or the fingers or thumbs are used to rub the skin and underlying tissue briskly. This action can be done in circles or backwards and forwards in a criss-cross movement.

Application of frictions

- They loosen muscle adhesions.
- They help with rapid increase of the circulation, causing vasodilation and erythema.
- They assist with lymphatic circulation in the area.
- They soften scar tissue by stretching and softening collagen fibres.
- They stimulate nerve endings.

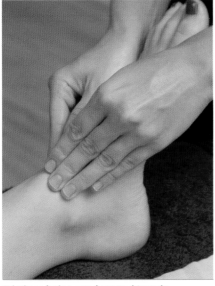

Frictions being used around tarsals

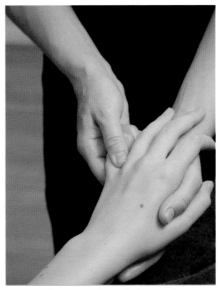

Frictions being used on phalanges

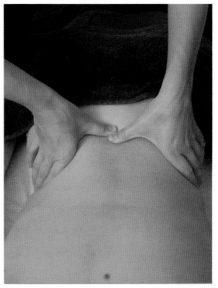

Frictions being used around erector spinae muscles

TAPOTEMENTS

Tapotements are quick, brisk movements that are carried out rhythmically, which is why they are often referred to as percussion movements. They are very beneficial when used appropriately and are no more tiring than other techniques when carried out correctly. Remember that tapotement techniques are not used in pre-blended aromatherapy oil massages.

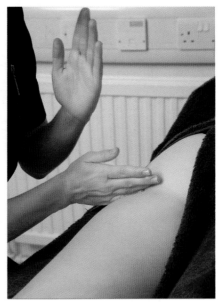

Hacking being used on quadriceps

Technique	Parts of the hands and arms used	Method
Cupping	▪ Cupped hands	With cupped hands and elbows slightly bent, flex and extend the wrist – quickly moving alternate hands up and down on the area. A hollow, clapping noise should be heard as the hands create a vacuum effect between the flesh and the hands. If you hear slapping, review your technique.
Hacking	▪ Ulna border of both hands	Have your fingers held loosely together and relaxed. The little finger and ring finger gently strike the area. Keep your hands working alternately in a brisk rhythm.
Pincement	▪ Fingertips and thumb	Fingertips pick up loose tissue in an alternating action. (This is excellent on areas of poor circulation such as the backs of the arms and the toes.)

Technique	Parts of the hands and arms used	Method
Pounding	▪ Ulna border of loose fists	Think of pounding on a door – hands pound in an alternating action over the area. This movement is only used over areas that are well padded, such as the upper thighs and gluteals.
Beating	▪ Ulna border of loose fists	Keep your thumbs relaxed and tucked into loosely clenched fists, and elbows slightly bent. Alternately press the fists lightly on to the body, developing a brisk, stimulating rhythm. Think of beating batter in a bowl – your hands rotate around each other towards your body, striking the flesh using the ulna border. The circular movement lifts the tissues. This movement is only used over areas that are well padded, such the upper thighs and gluteals.

Application of tapotements

▪ They give a rapid increase in circulation, leading to vasodilation and erythema.
▪ They stimulate nerve endings in the muscles, causing minute muscle contractions as a reflexive response.
▪ They increase cellular metabolism.
▪ They are great over the upper back to help loosen chest mucus.
▪ They can be applied gently towards the end of a treatment to gently wake the client up.

VIBRATIONS

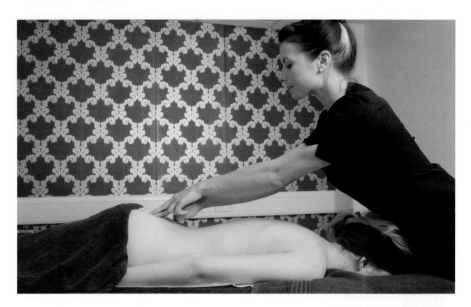

The vibrations technique involves shaking the skin tissue and muscle. It can be applied with the fingers or palms of the hands. Vibrations can be static and applied in one area by trembling the fingertips, forming a vibration on the skin. They can also be applied with the hand moving (which is often easier to do), creating running vibrations over a larger area.

Vibrations are also very effective lymph drainage techniques, but they do need to be light.

Application of vibrations
- They soothe and clear nerve pathways.
- They relax muscle fibres.
- They stimulate lymphatic activity in an area.

PASSIVE JOINT MOVEMENTS

These are used to take a joint such as the ankle or wrist through a range of movements unaided by the client – they just relax. This helps to improve and maintain joint mobility and flexibility. When using this technique the joints should never be forced or overextended.

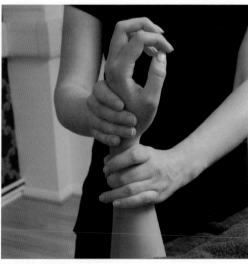

Massage of the metacarpals

LYMPHATIC DRAINAGE – PRE-BLEND MASSAGE TECHNIQUE

These are light movements which work just below the skin to stimulate the drainage of lymph within the body tissues. Lymph, or tissue fluid, vibrates rather than flows like the blood, and moves very slowly – about 1cm per minute. There are two main types of lymphatic drainage movements:

- slow stroking or fanning movements, performed in the direction of the nearest lymph nodes

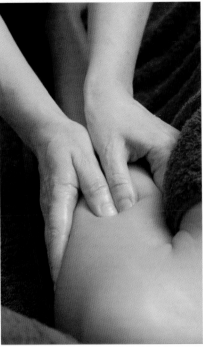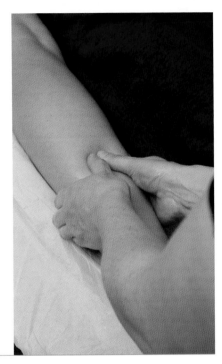

Pressure point movement

- light pumping movements, which squeeze the lymph tissue, creating vacuums which the lymph is sucked into, to drain it.

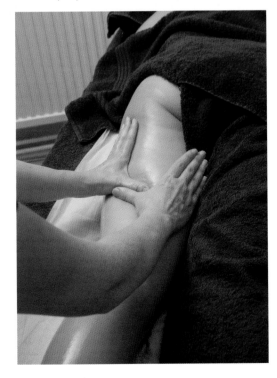

NEUROMUSCULAR PRE-BLEND MASSAGE TECHNIQUE

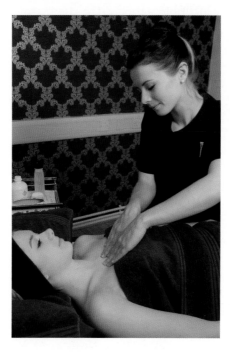 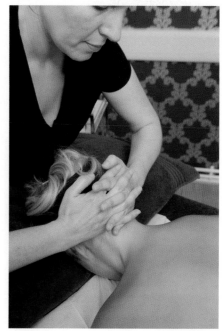

This technique has an effect on both the nerves and muscular tissues. Static pressure is applied to points in a muscle using either the thumbs, knuckles or elbows. These points are usually the tender spots where nodules and areas of dense tissue are found in the muscles. The client takes a deep breath and pressure is then applied as the client breathes out. This pressure is maintained for up to 30 seconds. When the pressure is released, circulation rushes into the area and helps to alleviate the symptoms of muscular aches and pains.

MASSAGE MEDIUMS

There are a variety of massage mediums available to use. When choosing one, consider the following:

- skin type
- skin condition
- client preference
- allergies
- amount of hair in the area
- 'slip' required
- if massage is to be combined with another treatment.

Familiarise yourself with the different skin types and conditions before selecting your massage medium, to ensure you are using the most beneficial product for the client.

MASSAGE OILS

Massage oil is the most popular choice of medium for body massage, as it gives the best slip, allowing the hands to glide easily across the skin's surface.

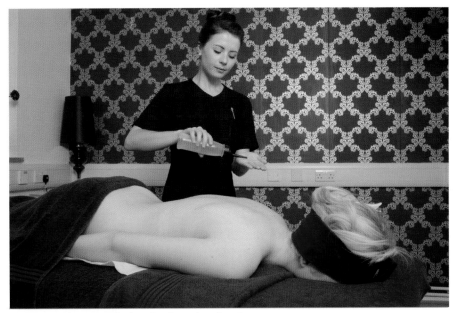

Massage oil being applied to the therapist's hands

The most beneficial oils are vegetable based. The skin readily absorbs natural oils, and they can help to soften and nourish the skin, keeping it supple. Different oils are suitable for different skin types and give different effects.

Mineral oils are the main ingredient in many massage oils and leave the skin feeling soft and supple; however, they have no therapeutic value and can clog the skin. Mineral oils are not absorbed as easily as vegetable oils, because they are made up of large hydrocarbon molecules, by-products of the oil refining process. This kind of oil stays on the surface of the skin for longer and is a popular ingredient in perfumed body lotions and creams.

MASSAGE CREAMS

HANDY HINT

Try to familiarise yourself with different carrier oils and their uses, as this will enhance your treatment results.

INDUSTRY TIP

Avoid buying oils in large quantities, unless you know you are going to use them – oils lose their therapeutic value over time and can go off (go rancid).

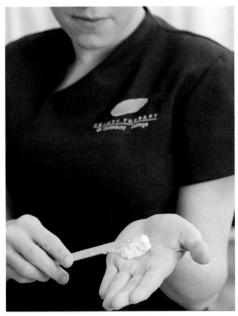

The correct procedure to apply massage cream to a therapist's hands

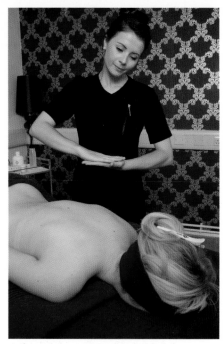

A therapist warming oil in her hands

INDUSTRY TIP

Refresh your product knowledge regularly so that you know what ingredients they all contain.

Massage cream can be very effective on dry skin and is ideal to use on clients who do not like the feel of oil. Creams are easily absorbed into the skin – but it is only necessary to use a small amount as cream spreads widely once warm.

PRE-BLENDED MASSAGE OILS, CREAMS AND BALMS

Many companies produce a range of pre-blended oils to use for massage treatments. Often these are developed for a signature treatment that will follow a set routine.

Pre-blended oils are formulated for specific treatment objectives. Familiarise yourself with the products and their ingredients so that you can be sure they are suitable for use on particular clients.

Pre-blended oils:

- give a sense of well-being
- relax
- stimulate
- uplift.

The benefits of using pre-blended oils are that they are inexpensive, no measuring of essential oils and carrier oils is required, and they are easy to select according to the client's needs. They are often marketed under a brand name, which will give the client confidence in the treatment. The disadvantage of using pre-blends is that the client may not like the smell of the blend most suited to their needs.

POWDERS

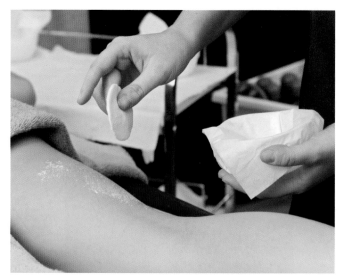

Correct application of a powder media to a client

Choose the finest, unperfumed powders for use with massage. Powder will permit a firmer massage, as it does not provide slip as an oil or cream would. It is rarely used in the industry today, but it is a suitable alternative for use on a client with oily skin or if the client has a perspiration problem. If the skin is dry, powder will dry the skin further, as it will absorb any oil and moisture on the skin's surface.

Powder your hands rather than pouring the product directly on to the client's skin. Keep powder use to a minimum, and avoid shaking it, as it creates a dusty atmosphere and will get in the eyes and nose of the client. Powder has also been found to aggravate respiratory conditions such as asthma.

SAFETY PRECAUTIONS

All products should be used according to health and safety guidelines. There are some further safety considerations when using base or carrier oils and pre-blended oils.

Correct storage

As with all products, correct storage of massage mediums is important. Carrier oils and blended essential oils need to be stored in dark bottles. Check the manufacturer's instructions for correct storage methods.

Toxicity

If a product is toxic, it means it is poisonous. In some cases, it might even be fatal in large quantities (for example, large amounts of essential oils).

Phototoxicity

This means that a product is sensitive to sunlight, and may cause a skin reaction when exposed to ultraviolet rays. If the skin is exposed after having oil applied, the mixture of the essential oil and the ultraviolet rays may result in itching, redness or burning, or an increase in skin pigmentation in the area. The main phototoxic oils are citrus oils.

Irritants

The skin may become irritated when an essential oil is applied to it. The skin cells produce a histamine reaction and the area becomes red, itchy and inflamed. The severity of the irritation will depend on the strength of the blend used.

Over-exposure

Over-exposure to products can cause irritation, sensitivity or result in toxic levels being used.

Disposal of massage mediums

It is a good idea to measure out what you need or to use a container that has a pump dispenser to avoid waste. If there is any product left over after the massage, it should be soaked up with a tissue and placed in a lined bin ready for disposal.

Treatment timings

A full body massage or massage using pre-blended oils will take one hour. If the face and scalp are included it will take 75 minutes. A back treatment on its own will take 30 minutes. If you need to adapt or modify your treatment, it should still last for the expected duration – you will need to extend the treatment in an appropriate area to achieve this.

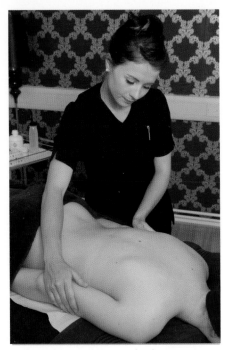
A therapist carrying out a back massage

MASSAGE SEQUENCE

Massages can follow different routines and orders of work. They should be modified to suit each client, and each therapist will perfect their own routines. The exception is when you are performing a signature treatment, where the routine will be set to suit specific products. Each training centre will have a specific routine which will be used for training until you are confident enough to adapt it and work on your own routine.

As a general rule, effleurage is always used first, followed by petrissage. Other techniques may then follow. Frictions are excellent for increasing the circulation quickly. Tapotement is often used last before finishing the treatment area with further effleurage to drain and soothe it.

Select a massage medium suitable for the client's skin type and condition. Apply it to your hands and lower arms up to the elbows. Then apply the medium to the client's skin with light effleurage movements, starting across the décolleté and moving up the neck and face.

ADAPTING MASSAGE TECHNIQUES TO ACHIEVE TREATMENT OBJECTIVES

The massage should be adapted to suit the client's treatment objectives, unless it is a signature treatment following a set routine. The selection and use of techniques will depend on the client's requirements.

The treatment objectives for massage therapy include the following:

- Relaxation – use preheat before treatment to help relaxation (unless using pre-blended oils, when heat should be avoided as it may result in intensified contra-actions). To achieve a relaxation treatment, keep effleurage and petrissage movements slow and light, keep techniques rhythmic and use a relaxation blend. Tapotement should be omitted for pre-blended aromatherapy massage but may be useful towards the end of a body massage to wake the client up.

INDUSTRY TIP

Make sure your hands are warm, as this will be more comfortable for the client. Warm muscles and tendons are more flexible and this will help protect your hands from strain.

INDUSTRY TIP

Warm a small amount of oil in a container – just enough for what you need. Oil should not be kept warm for hygiene reasons, but the application of warm oil is a wonderful experience for the client.

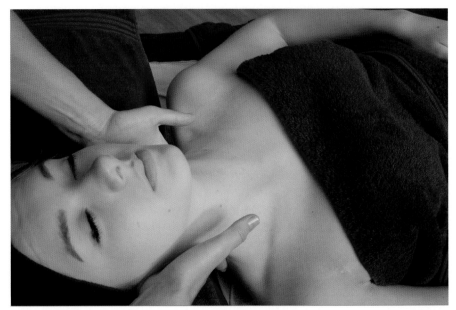
A therapist massaging a client's neck from the front position

- Sense of well-being – the aim of this treatment is to make the client feel happy and content. A pre-blend tailored to this objective could be used.

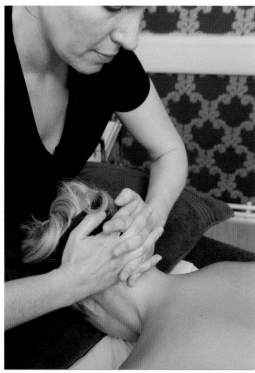

Neuromuscular movement being used

- Stimulation – use brisk, deep techniques and increase petrissage. Frictions are particularly good for stimulation, and incorporate tapotement techniques when carrying out a body massage.

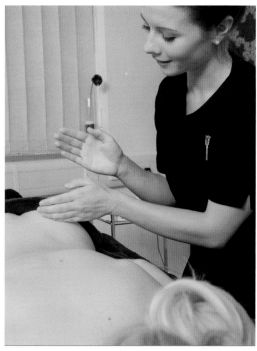

Avoid slow, repetitive effleurage

- Uplifting – use techniques that will not sedate the client – keep up a good pace throughout the treatment and use an uplifting pre-blend such as citrus.

- Sedation – keep techniques light and very slow. Make effleurage slow and long. Using quite repetitive movements, particularly effleurage, as a stroking soothing movement can be quite hypnotic and calming.
- Invigoration – use deep, brisk techniques such as vibrations and tapotement.
- Assistance with weight reduction – work predominantly on the problem areas where fat is stored, such as the buttocks and upper thighs. It is also useful to work over the abdomen. Use slow, deep movements and concentrate on petrissage and tapotement.

To recap on the treatment objectives achievable with the two main types of massage, see page 246.

MASSAGE MODIFICATIONS

When performing a massage treatment the therapist may have to modify (alter) the treatment in order for it to be effective, for example if the client is obese, very muscular or requires a relaxing or stimulating massage.

Obese client
- Deeper movements are necessary.
- The skin may be sensitive.
- Deep petrissage techniques and, when performing a body massage, hacking, cupping, beating and pounding should be used on areas of excess adipose tissue.
- Use a gyratory massage for working on areas of cellulite.

Muscular client
- Use deep, firm effleurage.
- Use slow, deep kneading over tense areas to relax muscles.
- Avoid deep petrissage movements on short contracted muscles, as this may be painful. Use stretching instead.
- Use infra-red to preheat before body massage to warm the muscles.

Elderly client
- Avoid tapotement over bony areas.
- Use gentle pressure throughout as the skeletal system may be more fragile.
- Use infra-red to preheat (body massage only).
- Apply extra frictions around joint areas to stimulate synovial fluid and increase joint mobility.
- Use passive joint movement to increase mobility.
- Use lighter effleurage and stroking, to avoid dragging delicate, thinner skin.

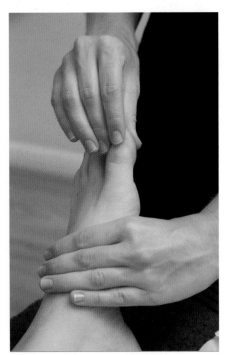

Adapt your treatment depending on your client. Treatment areas like toes on some clients might be fragile

MECHANICAL EQUIPMENT

Mechanical equipment can enhance the effects of the treatment. The two main pieces used are:

- infra-red lamp – this is a portable heat lamp, used to warm the tissues prior to massage
- G5 mechanical massager – this is a mechanical massager with detachable heads which provide different sensations and depths of pressure.

Infra-red is a heat treatment; therefore you need to take the following safety precautions:

- Make sure there are no products on the skin.
- The client's contact lenses should be removed.
- Check for any heat or sun exposure within the last 24 hours.

If carrying out gyratory massage, avoid treatment to the following:

- bony areas
- the abdomen during **menstruation** or pregnancy
- loose, crêpey skin
- excessively hairy areas.

Infra-red lamp

An infra-red lamp provides a deep heat by infra-red rays from the bulb (these rays are part of the electromagnetic spectrum). Infra-red is a heat radiation treatment, and the lamp is also known as a 'non-luminous lamp' as the heat can be felt but the rays cannot be seen.

The rays emitted from the lamp vary in intensity depending on how close the lamp is to the skin and the duration of the treatment. The inverse square law says that the light intensity decreases with the square of the distance from the light source. So the further away the lamp is from the subject, the bigger the area it covers and it can be left on for longer. For example, if the lamp is at a distance of 40cm, it can be left on for five minutes. If the distance of the lamp is doubled to 80cm, the time it can be left on for is is quadrupled to 20 minutes. So if the distance is doubled, the time is multiplied by four. It is much kinder to the skin to have the lamp further away but to leave it on for a longer length of time.

ACTIVITY

Switch on a torch and place it flat against a wall. Move away from the wall and you will notice that as you do so, the light from the torch covers a larger area. This is similar to how the inverse square law works.

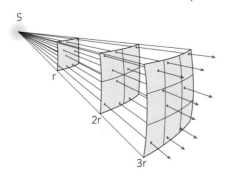

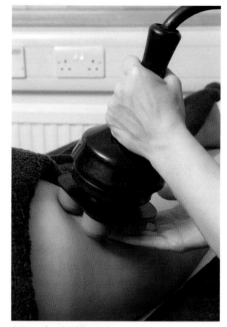

G5 mechanical massage

Menstruation
The proper term for a woman's monthly period

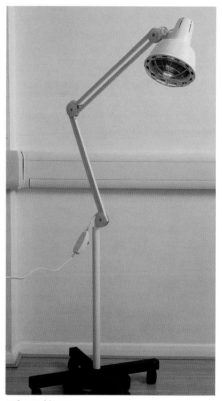

Infra-red lamp

INFRA-RED TREATMENT

Infra-red enhances the treatment by:

- vasodilation – it increases the body temperature slightly
- softening the muscle tissues and relaxing muscles
- stimulating the sebaceous glands and lubricating the skin
- its mild heat having a soothing and calming effect on sensory nerve endings.

APPLICATION OF INFRA-RED TREATMENT

Following consultation and preparation of the client:

1 The most common area treated in this way is the back, so position the client prone, with pillows for support that tilt the body slightly towards the lamp.

2 Ensure the eyes are protected by sun bed goggles, or by draping a towel so that it shields the eyes.

3 Position the lamp so the light rays hit the area at a 90° angle – never put the lamp directly over the client.

4 Follow the manufacturer's instructions on distance and time. Use a tape measure to ensure that the distance is correct. As a guide, lamps are usually left on for 5–20 minutes at a distance of 45–90cm.

5 Observe the skin's reaction throughout, by looking and touching. You should also ask the client how they feel.

6 At the end of the treatment, switch the lamp off and place it in a safe area to cool down. Place a towel on the lamp so that you can move it. This also acts as a warning to others that the lamp may be hot.

7 Continue with further treatment, such as a back massage.

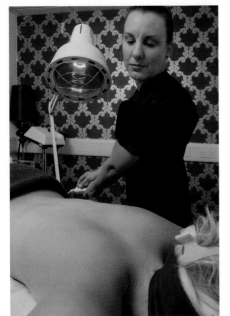

An infra-red lamp being used as part of a massage treatment

GYRATORY (G5) MASSAGE

This kind of massage is performed by a mechanical machine, which works deeper into the muscles. It is ideal for use on bulky areas, such as adipose tissue or defined muscle mass. Gyratory massage can be used in place of manual body massage or alongside it.

The head of the unit, when attached, has a motor that creates a twofold movement – it rotates and moves up and down with a vibrating action. This machine can either be hand held (portable) or floor standing.

Most units have a variable speed selector so that the depth and speed of the vibration can be tailored to the client's needs. There is a range of massage applicator heads that give different effects.

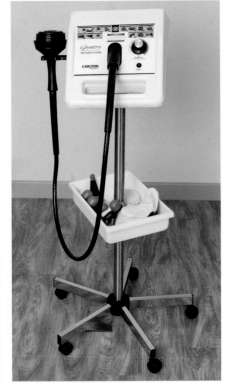

G5 machine

GYRATORY MASSAGE HEADS

G5 head	Uses	Application
Disposable protective cover	▪ Protects sponge covers from cross-contamination – they are not as easily cleaned as rubber heads.	
Soft sponge applicator	▪ Used for effleurage and stroking movements. ▪ It is relaxing and is used to start and complete a treatment. ▪ Excellent for desquamation.	Used in long one-directional stroking movements or circular directional strokes directed towards the head and lymph nodes.
Curved sponge applicator (with protective cover)	▪ Used for effleurage and stroking movements. ▪ It is relaxing and is used to start and complete a treatment. ▪ Excellent for desquamation.	Used on long-line areas, in long one-directional stroking movements directed towards the head and lymph nodes.
Spiky applicator (hedgehog)	▪ Very stimulating. ▪ Produces erythema. ▪ Ideal for desquamation.	Can be used in long sweeping movements or circular directional strokes. Produces a rapid erythema. Do not overuse as it can cause skin irritation.

G5 head	Uses	Application
Multi-pronged applicator	▪ Similar to finger kneading. ▪ Ideal to use for breaking down fatty deposits or for a deeper effect over bulky areas.	Used in circular movements, with pressure towards the heart. The other hand lifts the tissues into the head to create a deep kneading action. Only use on areas where there is sufficient tissue or muscle bulk to avoid bruising.
Multi-ball applicator (egg box)	▪ Good for deep petrissage movements. ▪ Ideal on bulky areas.	Used in circular movements, with pressure towards the heart. The other hand lifts the tissues into the head to create a deep kneading action. Only use on very padded areas such as the thighs and buttocks to avoid tissue damage.
Cone-shaped applicator (round and point)	▪ Good on tension nodules within muscles. ▪ Gives a very deep petrissage over soft tissue.	Used where there are specific areas of tension, such as the back. Continually monitor pressure when using this head, as some tension areas can be very sensitive.

APPLICATION OF GYRATORY MASSAGE

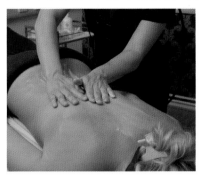

STEP 1 – Apply talc free powder to the treatment area to provide slip and glide for G5 treatment.

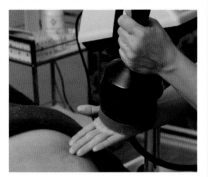

STEP 2 – Introduce G5 to the client slowly by using your hand as a guide. The sponge curved applicator can also be used here.

INDUSTRY TIP

There are variable settings on most gyratory massagers – always read the manufacturer's instructions to ensure you give the client an effective treatment.

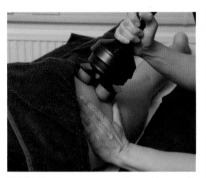

STEP 3 – The egg box applicator is a good choice on areas where spot reduction is required such as the thighs.

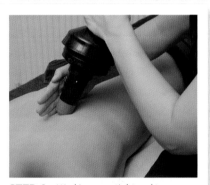

STEP 4 – Working over tight and tense muscles with a cone-shaped applicator can reduce tension.

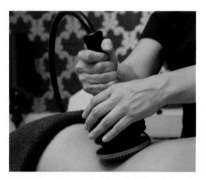

STEP 5 – Use a selection of G5 heads to achieve treatment objectives, building from the sponge head to the hedgehog head.

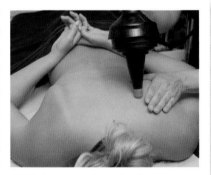

STEP 6 – A cone-shaped applicator (pointer) is an excellent choice when working on nodules around the scapula.

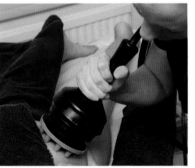

STEP 7 – The multi-pronged applicator is a good choice of head for stubborn fatty deposits around the hips or buttocks.

HANDY HINT

Always protect the client's spine with a guide hand.

The benefits of using a gyratory massage are the same as for normal massage, but more rapid results can be achieved and a deeper massage applied without putting strain on you. Due to the vibrations it is recommended that you do not use the machine for long periods of time to avoid repetitive strain injury (RSI) in the wrists.

G5 can be used as a stand-alone treatment or alongside other electrotherapy treatments. It can be incorporated into a body massage treatment to warm up the muscles first. It is usually concentrated on particular areas of the body, such as the thighs and buttocks, as part of a weight-loss programme. It is also an excellent treatment for the back, to work deep into areas of tension. Another effective treatment is on the backs of the arms, using the sponge and multi-head to improve poor circulation. A treatment is always started and completed using a sponge applicator.

For more information on G5, please consult Chapter 306/307 (on page 330).

HOME-CARE AND AFTERCARE ADVICE

Following the treatment you should give the client suitable aftercare advice. This will help to maximise the benefits of the massage. The clients should be advised to do the following for 12–24 hours after the treatment:

- Relax and avoid any strenuous activity – this will give the body time to heal and cleanse.
- Avoid physical exercise.
- Ensure that food intake following the treatment is light – avoid spicy foods and heavy meals as these may cause discomfort.
- Avoid alcohol, which will put toxins back into the body.
- Increase water intake, to keep the body hydrated and flush waste products out of the body.
- Avoid stimulants such as caffeine in coffee, tea, fizzy drinks and energy drinks.
- Avoid ultraviolet light and sunbathing – the skin will be more sensitive and pre-blended aromatherapy oils may be phototoxic.
- Drive with extra care if calming or relaxing pre-blends have been used – keep the windows slightly open to ensure client remains alert.
- Leave oils on the skin and hair to allow them to penetrate – if pre-blended oils have been used the essences need time to change chemically for a longer-lasting effect; oils on the hair will leave it glossy and hydrated.

There is also longer-term advice to consider:

- Suggest that the client follows a home skincare routine to maintain treatment results and objectives.
- Encourage the clients to use any pre-blended oils you have used at home – and there may also be supporting products such as bath or body products, candles or prepared blends that can be used in a burner.

AFTERCARE ADVICE SUMMARY

- Recommend products for your client to use that they will benefit from.
- Suggest further treatments to maximise results and reduce the effects of stress. Let the client know how often they should return for repeat treatments.
- Where appropriate, discuss lifestyle changes the client could make to improve their physical well-being. Be tactful and only discuss issues that the client has raised. Suggestions might include:
  - ways to increase physical activity
  - healthy eating advice

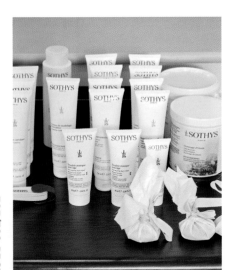

Suggesting products for a long-term skincare routine as part of the aftercare advice

INDUSTRY TIP

For safety and insurance reasons you must never recommend the use of individual aromatherapy oils unless you have been trained as an aromatherapist.

- tips on finding time to relax and destress
- help with reducing or giving up smoking
- reducing caffeine and alcohol intake
- drinking more water.
- It may be appropriate to recommend other treatments from a counsellor, lifestyle coach or aromatherapist to your client. Again, be tactful and only discuss issues that the client has raised.
- Advise on postural awareness according to the client's needs.
- Advise the client what to do if they have a reaction or contra-action.

ACTIVITY

Think of some lifestyle changes that you might discuss with a client. Make a list of the benefits to the client from following the advice you give.

CONTRA-ACTIONS

Sometimes a contra-action is referred to as a 'healing reaction'. They are less likely to happen with a body massage when using a carrier oil, but may occur if pre-blended oils have been used, as the essential oils they contain can have a more dynamic effect on the systems of the body.

SEVERE ERYTHEMA/SKIN IRRITATION

This might be due to over-stimulation of the skin or to excessive heat being applied (infra-red or overuse of gyratory massage). It could also be a sign that the skin is reactive to a product. Stop and review what you are doing. If you are applying massage, are you using appropriate techniques? Cool compresses (or cold stones if you have them) should be applied to the skin to reduce the circulation.

ALLERGIC REACTION TO A PRODUCT

The skin will feel hot and the client will feel irritation, tingling or itching. Remove the product completely with lukewarm water. Apply a cool compress and discontinue treatment. Refer the client to a medical practitioner if the irritation does not subside. Sometimes the reaction can be delayed and it may reoccur once the client has returned home. In this case, advise the client to bathe the skin with lukewarm water and apply a cool compress. They should seek medical advice immediately if the symptoms worsen.

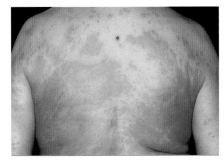

A client after an allergic reaction to a product

LETHARGY

Following a good relaxation treatment it is not unusual to feel very sleepy and relaxed. Sometimes this can go on for longer than desired and this is a sign that the body needs to rest and heal. The client should be advised to follow their body signals and rest and relax for as long as possible. An early night is always a good remedy.

HEADACHE

During a massage treatment the body begins to get rid of waste products from cellular activity. These flood into the circulatory system and to the liver and kidneys to be filtered out and removed. If the waste products build up to a higher level than can be eliminated quickly the client may experience a headache. Advise the client to sip water to keep the body hydrated, and to rest until the headache goes away.

NAUSEA

During massage the circulation is redirected to the area being treated. If a client has had a meal before their treatment, the blood will be directed away from the digestive system, and this will cause the client to feel nauseous. Ideally the client should not have a massage for at least an hour after eating. If the client has eaten recently, always avoid massaging the abdomen. Sometimes the experience of the body re-establishing **homeostasis** can make the client feel nauseous. Advise the client to sip water and rest until the feeling subsides.

Over-application of infra-red to the back of the neck and the vibrations from the gyratory massage on the back can also make some clients feel nauseous – if this occurs, stop the treatment.

HEIGHTENED EMOTIONS

When the body is in a relaxed state it 'lets go'. Emotions that have been held in are suddenly released and a client may get very emotional – probably tearful and weepy. The best remedy is to have a box of tissues handy and listen to the client if they want to talk. Offer the client reassurance that the feeling will pass. Avoid hugging the client or becoming emotional yourself, as this will not help. Sit with the client and place a hand on the forearm or shoulder. Offer them a drink to sip and take them somewhere quiet to rest if possible until they are feeling calmer. On rare occasions the client may become very chatty and hyper, sometimes laughing out of character. Again, allow the client to chat and rest somewhere quiet until they feel more balanced.

FREQUENT URINATION

During a massage treatment the body begins to get rid of waste products from cellular activity. This is transported by the circulatory system to the liver and kidneys. The body needs plenty of fluids (water) to help eliminate the waste products from the kidneys, which will result in more frequent urination.

BRUISING

Bruising should not occur during treatment. However, it may occur if gyratory massage is used for too long, too deeply or over bony areas. If there is bruising you should review your technique, as this is a sign of poor practice and a heavy-handed technique.

It is possible that the client may have a blood condition that makes them more susceptible to bruising – if so, this needs to be considered and discussed with the client beforehand.

BURNS

Burns should never occur. They can happen if you:

- fail to check and monitor infra-red equipment
- use infra-red equipment for too long, too close to the body.

Homeostasis
The body's balanced state

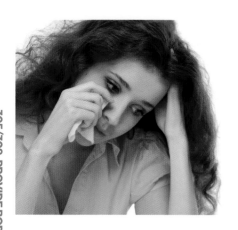

HANDY HINT

For skin irritation or an allergy it is often advisable to suggest a client speaks to a pharmacist rather than a GP. This will be quicker and the pharmacist will usually have something that can be purchased over the counter without the need for a prescription.

If a burn does occur, apply cool water to the area for at least 20 minutes and seek further treatment from a first aider.

MUSCLE ACHES

It is important to use effleurage and other techniques which help to stretch out the muscles at the end of a massage or mechanical treatment. This is to prevent a rapid increase in circulation to an area, which is then suddenly stopped. This will prevent the drainage of waste products from the area, leaving the muscles feeling tight again rather than helping to remove any tension. Over-treating an area can also cause this.

ADDITIONAL CONTRA-ACTIONS RELATED TO PRE-BLENDED OILS

The following may occur as a response to the use of essential oils, although most are rare:

- heightened emotions
- insomnia (if stimulating blends are used late in the day)
- hallucinations (reactions to certain oils, eg clary sage when combined with alcohol)
- respiratory reactions (an oil blend may have a strong or sharp aroma that catches the client's breath)
- increased secretions, as a result of systems of the body working more efficiently.

Any of these contra-actions is a usually sign that the body is attempting to balance itself, but may also be a more serious adverse reaction to an essential oil.

CLIENT FEEDBACK

It is important to gain feedback from the client. If you carried out an effective consultation and met your client's objectives, your feedback should be positive. When you have completed the treatment you should seek confirmation from the client that they are satisfied with the results, and make a note of this on the client record card.

INDUSTRY TIP

If you want objective feedback, get someone else to carry out a questionnaire. Clients are more likely to complete one if they feel it is being organised by someone impartial.

Use the questions below to test your knowledge of Chapter 305/309 to see how much information you have retained. These questions will help you revise what you have learnt in this chapter.

Turn to page 499 for the answers.

1 Which **one** of the following is an effleurage technique?
   a Pounding
   b Hacking
   c Stroking
   d Beating

2 Which **one** of the following methods is used to apply powder to the client?
   a Decanting it directly on to the client
   b Shaking it on to the client's skin from the container
   c Placing it in a bowl and dusting it on to the client with cotton wool
   d Applying it to the therapist's hands, then the client

3 When is a healing reaction most likely to occur?
   a During treatment
   b Immediately following treatment
   c Up to three days following treatment
   d Up to a week following treatment

4 Which **one** of the following is an absolute contra-indication to infra-red?
   a Wearing contact lenses
   b Having sunburn
   c Low blood pressure
   d Menstruation

5 Which **one** of the following is the **best** way to clean gyratory massage heads?
   a Hot soapy water and a brush
   b Antibacterial soap and an alcohol spray once dry
   c Disinfectant spray, then rinse in hot water
   d Wiping with a cleansing wipe and place in a UV cabinet

6 Which **one** of the following is a contra-indication to a body massage treatment?
   a Eczema
   b Psoriasis
   c Broken skin
   d Urticaria

7 Which **one** of the following is the law that relates to the use of infra-red?
   a Inverse triangle law
   b Inverse square law
   c Inverse circle law
   d Inverse star law

8 Which **one** of the following is an effect of an infra-red treatment?
   a Increased pigmentation
   b Vasoconstriction
   c Healing abrasions
   d Vasodilation

9 Which **one** of the following gyratory massage applicators is most suitable for a soothing treatment?
   a Spiky applicator
   b Sponge applicator
   c Cone-shaped applicator
   d Multi-ball applicator

10 Which **one** of the following mediums is used for gyratory massage?
   a Powder
   b Cream
   c Oil
   d Gel

306/307
PROVIDE FACIAL AND BODY ELECTROTHERAPY TREATMENTS

As the term suggests, electrotherapy treatments use an electrical current. Electrotherapy treatments:

- improve the skin's condition
- improve muscle tone
- aid lymphatic drainage.

Often a client will need a course of treatments to be able to see the results. It is not always possible to see a result after only one treatment.

In this chapter you will learn how to:

- prepare for facial and body treatments using electrotherapy
- provide facial and body treatments using electrotherapy.

PROVIDE FACIAL AND BODY ELECTROTHERAPY TREATMENTS

Within this chapter, you will cover the following facial and body electrotherapy treatments:

- high frequency
- galvanic
- electrical muscle stimulation (EMS) (also known as faradic)
- vacuum suction (also known as lymphatic drainage)
- microcurrent
- G5 (body only).

It is essential that you understand fully:

- the effects and benefits of these treatments
- how the equipment works
- some basic electrical terminology
- the correct products to use with the equipment
- the length and frequency of the treatment
- any noises or sensations associated with the treatment (so that you can explain them fully to the client).

> **HANDY HINT**
>
> Anatomy and physiology go hand in hand with these units as it is vital to know the structure and functions of the face and body in order to provide an effective treatment. Refer back to the Anatomy and Physiology chapter to refresh your knowledge.

PREPARE FOR FACIAL AND BODY ELECTROTHERAPY TREATMENTS

In this part of the chapter you will learn about:

- consultation
- contra-indications to electrotherapy treatments
- selecting equipment and products for electrotherapy treatments
- preparation of a client for a facial electrotherapy treatment
- preparation of a client for a body electrotherapy treatment.

> **HANDY HINT**
>
> You must look professional and act and behave in a professional manner at all times:
>
> - a clean, ironed uniform
> - clean shoes with enclosed toes
> - hair tied back off your face
> - minimal jewellery
> - professional make-up.

> **HANDY HINT**
>
> The client's treatment may take more than an hour so you need to make sure that they are comfortable throughout if you want them to return.

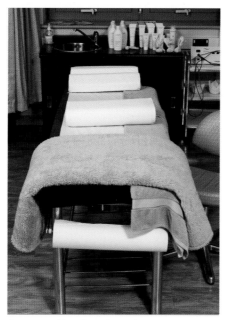

A prepared treatment couch

PREPARING YOURSELF, YOUR WORK AREA AND YOUR CLIENT

You should be fully prepared prior to a client arriving for their treatment. You need to make sure that:

- all the equipment and products are to hand and that once the treatment begins you will not need to leave your client unattended
- the trolley and couch are clean and prepared
- the treatment environment (ie lighting, sound, heating and ventilation) is suitable and makes the treatment experience pleasant for the client. This may vary from client to client so check that they are comfortable before you begin
- you are fully prepared to meet, greet and treat your client.

CONSULTATION

Consultation is a vital process during which you should assess the client's needs and objectives and their suitability for the treatment. More detailed information on the consultation process and communication techniques can be found in Chapter 303, Client care and communication in beauty-related industries (pages 212–215).

During the consultation you will need to:

- discuss what the client hopes to achieve from the treatment
- give the client a full explanation of the treatment (ie what is going to happen – sensations, sounds)
- explain realistic achievements associated with the treatment
- record details of their medical history and previous treatments (to make sure you are using the correct procedure for them)
- perform a figure diagnosis including checking the client's body type and condition (for details on body types and conditions, please consult pages 248–255 in Chapter 305/309).

Allow the client plenty of time to ask questions as they may be nervous or they may not have had an electrotherapy treatment before.

CONTRA-INDICATIONS TO ELECTROTHERAPY TREATMENTS

In addition to the general contra-indications listed in Chapter 303 (page 215), there are a number of contra-indications that are specific to facial and body electrotherapy treatments:

Contra-indication	Treatment	Restricts/ prevents treatment	Reason
Pacemaker	All facial and body electrotherapy treatments.	Prevents treatment	▪ Could affect the rhythm of the heart.
Metal plates or pins Piercings Excessive metal in a particular area (eg dental fillings, bridge work)	All facial and body electrotherapy treatments.	Restricts treatment	▪ Might increase electrical current through the body and therefore make the treatment uncomfortable.
Sunburn	Any electrotherapy treatment of the sunburnt areas.	Restricts	▪ Erythema could develop.
Nervous clients	All facial and body electrotherapy treatments.	Restricts	▪ Treatment will not be enjoyable for client.
Acne rosacea	All facial electrotherapy treatments.	Restricts	▪ Treatment will be painful. ▪ High risk of cross-infection.
Migraines	All facial electrotherapy treatments.	Restricts	▪ May cause a migraine.
Recent botox injections	Facial microcurrent treatments.	Prevents	▪ Risk of interference with botox treatment.
Collagen/dermal fillers	Facial microcurrent treatments.	Prevents	▪ Risk of interference with collagen/dermal filler treatment. Could displace collagen or fillers and have a negative effect on the cosmetic procedures.
Recent breast implants	Breast-lift microcurrent treatments.	Prevents	▪ Risk of interference with implants. Could dislodge or affect the implants.
Muscular injuries	Body electrotherapy treatments.	Restricts	▪ Might make the condition worse.
Intrauterine device (IUD)	Body electrotherapy treatments.	Restricts	▪ If IUD is copper avoid working over the abdominal area (ie over the uterus).
Very bony areas	Body electrotherapy treatments.	Restricts	▪ Might be painful for client if treatment is applied over bony areas, which have little tissue.

Contra-indication	Treatment	Restricts/prevents treatment	Reason
Obesity	Body electrical muscle stimulation (EMS) (or faradic) treatments.	Restricts	■ Adipose tissue is an insulator. ■ The muscles might not contract resulting in an ineffective treatment.
Loose crêpe-like skin	Vacuum suction treatments.	Restricts	■ Suction will cause capillary and tissue damage.
Excessive body hair	Vacuum suction treatments.	Restricts	■ Suction will drag on the hair. ■ Will be uncomfortable for the client.
Recent stretch marks	Vacuum suction treatments.	Restricts	■ The skin tissue is already delicate. ■ Vacuum suction could cause further trauma.

Once you have completed the consultation with your client and have decided on the programme or treatment that meets their objectives, you can begin treatment.

> **HANDY HINT**
>
> If a client has booked a course of treatments with the aim of 'losing inches', record the size of the area at the start of the course and at the end of the course of treatments.

> **HANDY HINT**
>
> The best results are achieved when clients:
> ■ have a course of treatments
> ■ follow a healthy eating plan.
>
> Nutrition has an effect on the skin.

 SmartScreen 306 Worksheet 3

SELECTING EQUIPMENT AND PRODUCTS FOR ELECTROTHERAPY TREATMENTS

To achieve the best results, clients will need a course or series of treatments. Throughout the course of treatments you might need to change the equipment you are using to meet the client's needs. You might also need to use more than one piece of equipment to achieve the treatment objectives. It is therefore important that you understand which pieces of equipment work well together and the course of treatments that will suit your clients.

To select the correct piece of equipment you also need to understand:

■ how the equipment works
■ the electrical current it uses
■ what it is used for
■ specific contra-indications and contra-actions
■ how application to the face and body differs
■ how to prepare for the treatment (yourself, your client and your work area)
■ how to carry out a consultation to:
  ■ find out about a client's needs/objectives
  ■ agree a treatment plan
  ■ carry out a skin analysis and figure diagnosis.

> **HANDY HINT**
>
> If you need to, refer back to your Level 2 beauty therapy book to remind yourself of the products, tools and equipment for carrying out a facial.

> **INDUSTRY TIP**
>
> In addition to the electrotherapy equipment you will need:
> ■ any accessories that are to be used alongside the machine
> ■ products, tools and equipment for carrying out a facial.

Flammable

Easily set alight

PREPARATION OF A CLIENT FOR A FACIAL ELECTROTHERAPY TREATMENT

The actual techniques you use during the treatments will obviously vary. However the preparation for the client will be similar. The following steps outline the preparation of the client for facial electrotherapy treatments.

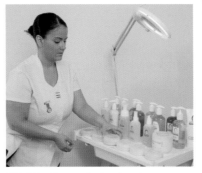

STEP 1 – Prepare the treatment room including the equipment.

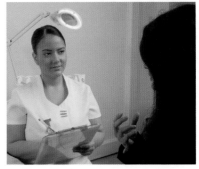

STEP 2 – Perform a consultation and tactile and thermal sensitivity tests on the area to be treated. Ask the client to remove *all* jewellery from the area to be treated. If it cannot be removed, cover it with insulating tape.

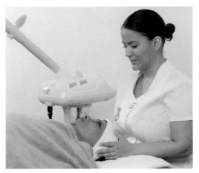

STEP 3 – Cover the client with towels/blankets and protect the client's hair with a net or towel.

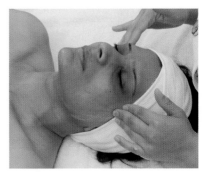

STEP 4 – Cleanse, tone and exfoliate the skin. Make sure the toner doesn't contain any alcohol, as alcohol is **flammable**.

PREPARATION OF A CLIENT FOR A BODY ELECTROTHERAPY TREATMENT

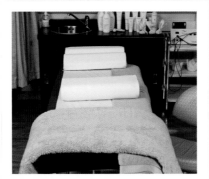

STEP 1 – Prepare the treatment room including the equipment.

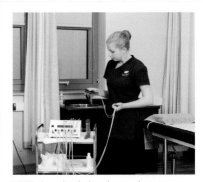

STEP 2 – Check that the machine is working properly.

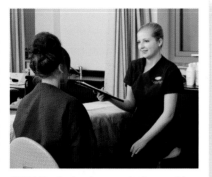

STEP 3 – During the consultation, explain the treatment procedure to the client and give them the opportunity to ask questions.

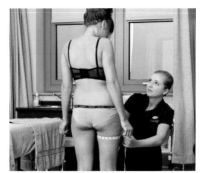

STEP 4 – Carry out a body analysis including: body measurements (ie height and weight), a muscle tone test and a cellulite test. The results must be recorded on the client's record card.

HANDY HINT

Ask the client to remove *all* jewellery prior to treatment and insulate any cuts or blemishes with petroleum jelly.

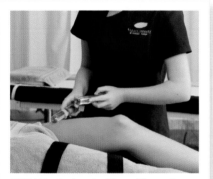

STEP 5 – Perform tactile and thermal sensitivity tests on the area to be treated.

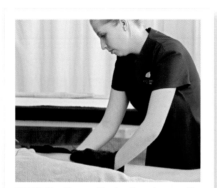

STEP 6 – Cleanse the treatment area with a body cleanser and exfoliate as appropriate or wipe over the area with a sanitiser, such as witch hazel.

HANDY HINT

Make sure that the client's body is warm. Ideally the client will have had a sauna or been in a steam room for the best results; however an infrared lamp can be used instead.

CARRY OUT FACIAL AND BODY ELECTROTHERAPY TREATMENTS

In this part of the chapter you will learn about:

- high frequency treatment
- galvanic treatment
- electrical muscle stimulation (EMS)
- vacuum suction
- microcurrent treatment
- mechanical massage
- general contra-actions to electrotherapy treatments
- general home-care and aftercare advice for facial and body electrotherapy treatments.

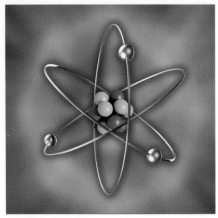
A model of an atom

Atom
The smallest part of a chemical element that can exist

Nucleus
The centre of the atom

Neutrons
Uncharged particles

Protons
Positively charged particles

Electrons
Negatively charged particles

Anion
A negatively charged atom which has more electrons than protons

Cation
A positively charged atom which has more protons that electrons

Ion
An atom that has lost or gained some electrons

Electrical current
A flow of electrical charge

Volts
The force needed to push the energy around an **electrical circuit**

Electrical circuit
A pathway through which electrical current flows from its source through a **conductor** and back to its source

Conductor
A material that is a good transmitter of electricity (eg most metals)

ELECTRICITY

Electricity is a form of energy that is made from electrons which are part of an **atom**. Everything on the planet is made from atoms. Each atom is made up of:

- a **nucleus**
- **neutrons**
- **protons**
- **electrons**.

- If an atom contains the same number of protons and electrons it has no charge because it is balanced.
- If the atom has more electrons than protons it is negatively charged (–ve) (technically known as an **anion**)
- If it has more protons than electrons it is positively charged (+ve) (technically known as a **cation**).

When the balance between the protons and electrons is upset, an atom may gain or lose an electron (an **ion**). The loss of an electron from an atom is what creates an **electrical current**.

ELECTRICAL CURRENTS

The electrical current for electrotherapy equipment can come from two sources:

- Mains electrical supply: equipment is plugged into a wall socket. This type of current is called alternating current (or ac current) and is at 240 **volts**.
- Battery power: equipment runs on a battery that produces electricity from a chemical reaction. This type of current is called direct current (or dc current).

Alternating current (ac)

An alternating current changes direction – it flows one way and then in the opposite direction. It continually repeats this forwards and backwards cycle. This cycle happens many times per second and is measured in hertz (Hz). This is the frequency of the current. UK mains' electrical supply is 50Hz, which means the direction of the current changes 50 times every second. The pressure needed to make the current work is measured in volts (V). UK mains electrical supply is 240V.

When you apply an electrical pulse (during electrotherapy treatments) you can vary the width of the pulse, the depth of the pulse and the frequency (rate of pulses) to have different effects.

1 For example the current may flow at 2 milliamps (mA) in one direction and then 2mA in the opposite direction – this would look like a square wave (Figure 1).

1 Square wave

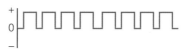

2 If the current starts at 0mA and builds up to 2mA, then returns to 0mA before changing direction, it will look like a wave (Figure 2.)

2 Wave flow (sine)

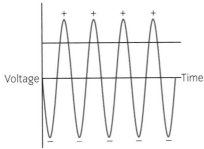

WHY DON'T YOU...
look at a battery. There will be a +ve symbol on one end and a –ve symbol at the other. The battery has an electrolyte solution inside it which helps the current flow from +ve to –ve.

Direct current (dc)

Direct current flows from positive (+ve) to negative (–ve). Electrodes are needed to complete this circuit from positive to negative. An electrode is a device that **conducts** electricity (a conductor) and helps current to flow from positive to negative. Positively charged electrodes are called anodes and negatively charged electrodes are called cathodes. Both of these electrodes are needed to make the circuit complete so that it works. The current passes through an **electrolyte** solution to get from positive to negative.

Conducts
Transmits energy (ie electricity)

Electrolyte
A substance that conducts electricity

Currents used within electrotherapy treatments

A direct current is used in galvanic treatments and a modified direct current used in EMS and microcurrent treatments.

Treatment	Current	Wave form
Galvanic	Direct current – constant direct flow.	**Galvanic wave**
EMS (faradic)	Modified direct current – alters depending upon the machine programme selected for the treatment.	**Faradic wave 1** Brief burst of current, ie pulse (lasting 1 millisecond). Interval when no current flows (lasting 9 milliseconds). Time in milliseconds: 5 10 15 20 25 30 35 40. **Faradic wave 2** Current. Surge eg 2 seconds. Rest period eg 1 second. Time. **Faradic wave 3** Current. Rest period. Time.

Treatment	Current	Wave form
Microcurrent	Modified direct current: ■ alters depending upon the machine programme selected ■ current usually builds up like a wave.	**Microcurrent wave 1** A basic interrupted direct current shows as a square wave **Microcurrent wave 2** Gradual attack **Wave flow (sine)** Voltage / Time **Microcurrent wave 3** The waveform can either attack or decay more gradually

INDUSTRY TIP

Indirect high frequency is mainly used on the face and neck.

Electrode

A device that conducts electricity (a conductor) and helps current to flow from positive to negative

Saturator

A device which is normally made from glass; this is used on the skin to conduct the electrical current to the client

ACTIVITY

The frequency of client visits to undergo treatment can vary from salon to salon and from treatment to treatment. Find out how may treatments your salon suggests for each one.

HIGH FREQUENCY

High frequency can be used on the face or the body (usually the back) to improve the skin's condition.

There are two kinds of high-frequency treatment:

■ Direct high frequency – a glass **electrode** is applied directly to the skin in the treatment area.
■ Indirect high frequency – the client holds the electrode/**saturator**. The current passes through the client's body and into the therapist's hands as the therapist is carrying out the massage.

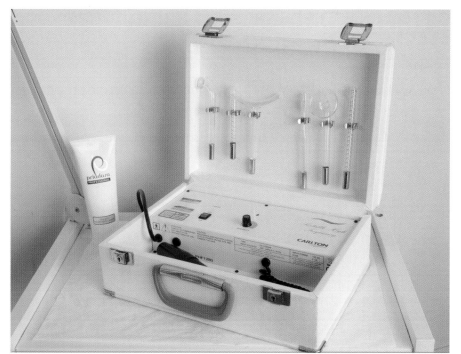
High-frequency machine

How does it work?

The high-frequency machine uses an **oscillating** alternating current. The **frequency** of the machine (ie the number of times per second that the current changes direction) is very fast – up to 250,000Hz. As the pulses of current are very quick, rather than causing the muscles to contract, the high-frequency machine creates a gentle heat which increases circulation and warms and relaxes the treatment area. This high-frequency current also causes a buzzing noise.

Tools and equipment used in high frequency
Electrodes

There is a selection of glass electrodes that can be used for high-frequency treatments. They vary in size and shape and are selected according to the area of the face or body that is being treated.

Inside the glass electrode is a gas. The current passing through the electrode causes the gas to **ionise**. The type of gas will determine the colour that the electrode glows.

Gas	Colour that the electrode glows
Argon	Violet
Mercury vapour	Blue
Neon	Orange

Oscillating

Quick moving

Frequency

The number of times per second that the current changes direction. It is measured in hertz (Hz) (eg 250,000Hz means that it changes direction 250,000 times per second)

Ionise

To convert into ions by removing one or more electrons

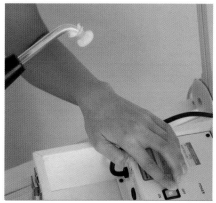
Testing a high-frequency machine

HANDY HINT

Being made from glass, the electrodes are very delicate and need to be treated with care. If you drop them they will smash and break.

INDUSTRY TIP

Be sure to make your client aware of the noise of the machine prior to treatment.

DIFFERENT TYPES OF HIGH-FREQUENCY ELECTRODES

Electrode	Use
Mushroom electrode	▪ Available in a variety of sizes – the smaller the electrode the more stimulating the effect. ▪ Can be used on the face or the body.
Horseshoe electrode	▪ Curved. ▪ Used over contours of the body and neck.
Roller electrode	▪ Used on large flat areas (eg the back).
Fulgurator	▪ Used for a technique called '**sparking**', which is used on papules and pustules.
Glass saturator Metal saturator	▪ Either a metal bar or a glass tube containing a metal spiral. ▪ Used for indirect high frequency.
Rake saturator	▪ Used in hair. ▪ Stimulates circulation and encourages hair growth.

Sparking

The electrode can be used to create a spark by lifting the apparatus away from the skin; this creates a break in electrical flow. Then, by adding the electrode back to the skin's surface this reconnects the current. This process should be used wth caution as it can damage the skin.

> **INDUSTRY TIP**
>
> Remember to use caution when 'sparking'. You may cause tissue damage if you spark for too long or lift the electrode too far from the skin.

Products used in high frequency

Product	Use
Powder (talc free)	▪ Applied to the body during direct high frequency. ▪ Also applied to the hand the client is going to hold the saturator with. ▪ Absorbs any moisture.
Oxygenating cream	▪ Recommended by some manufacturers when using direct high frequency. ▪ Has a soft creamy feel. ▪ Should be used with face gauze to stop the electrode sliding over the area too quickly.
Gauze	▪ Used alongside oxygenating cream. ▪ A piece of gauze is applied to the face. ▪ May be necessary to cut a hole in the gauze for the eyes, mouth and nose. ▪ Gauze face masks with eye and mouth holes already cut out are available from some suppliers.

INDUSTRY TIP

Place the electrodes into a tray lined with tissue if the machine you are using does not have a storage section.

INDUSTRY TIP

It is important to use a talc-free power. Talc is a known carcinogenic which means that it can cause cancer.

Effects and benefits of high frequency

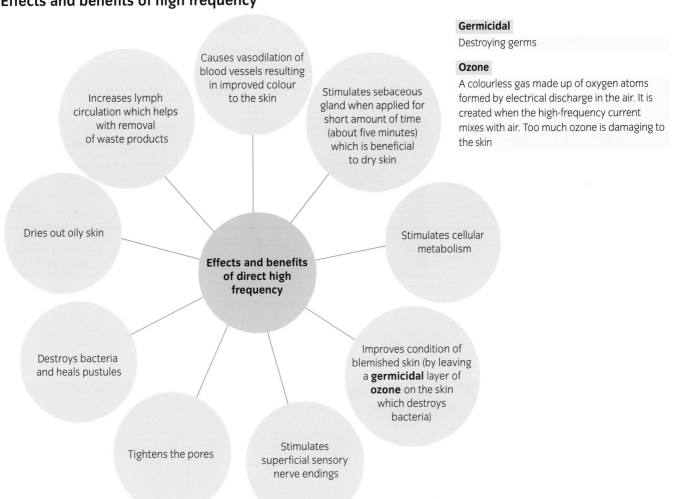

Germicidal

Destroying germs

Ozone

A colourless gas made up of oxygen atoms formed by electrical discharge in the air. It is created when the high-frequency current mixes with air. Too much ozone is damaging to the skin

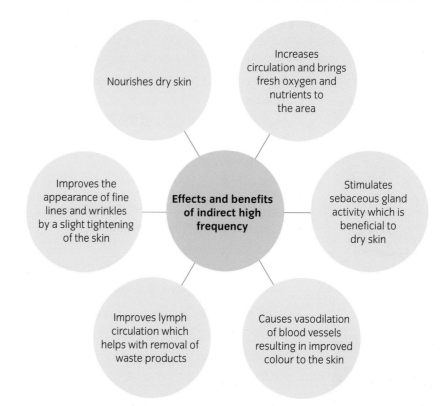

Effects and benefits of indirect high frequency

- Nourishes dry skin
- Increases circulation and brings fresh oxygen and nutrients to the area
- Improves the appearance of fine lines and wrinkles by a slight tightening of the skin
- Stimulates sebaceous gland activity which is beneficial to dry skin
- Improves lymph circulation which helps with removal of waste products
- Causes vasodilation of blood vessels resulting in improved colour to the skin

Contra-indications to high frequency

Please refer to general contra-indications to electrotherapy treatments on pages 288–289.

Application of direct high frequency to the face

Carry out steps 1–4 from facial electrotherapy preparation (see page 290).

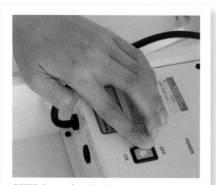

STEP 1 – Explain the buzzing noise to the client before you begin the treatment.

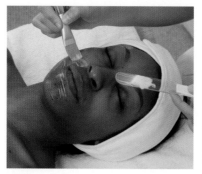

STEP 2 – Apply oxygenating cream and gauze or powder to the treatment area.

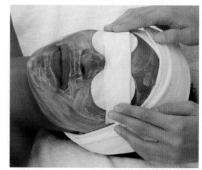

STEP 3 – Secure an eye pad on the client.

HANDY HINT

Double-check that the machine's dials are all at zero before you turn the machine on.

HANDY HINT

Remember tissue damage can be caused if sparking is done for too long or if the electrode is lifted too far from the skin.

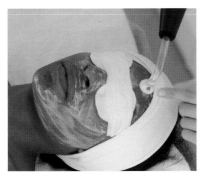

STEP 4 – Starting with the mushroom electrode, place the electrode in contact with the client's skin before switching on the current. Turn up the intensity according to manufacturer's instructions.

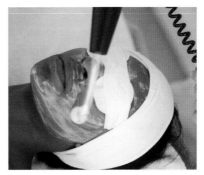

STEP 5 – In a small circling motion, work the electrode across the treatment area. Spark if necessary.

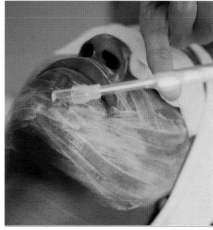

Sparking occurs when the electrode is lifted from the skin

HANDY HINT

Sparking happens when the electrode is lifted about five millimetres from the skin. The current leaps to connect with the skin causing a spark.

HANDY HINT

Switch the intensity back to zero before removing the electrode from the skin.

Application of direct high frequency to the body

Carry out steps 1–6 from body electrotherapy preparation (see pages 290–291).

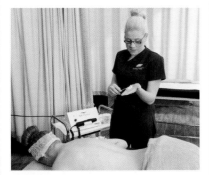

STEP 1 – Apply an appropriate medium to your hand using cut-out method.

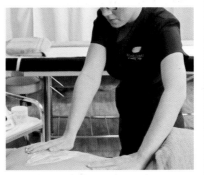

STEP 2 – Apply the product to the treatment area, spreading it out evenly.

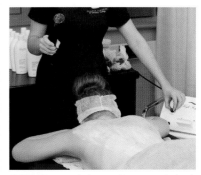

STEP 3 – Switch the machine on and check the intensity dial.

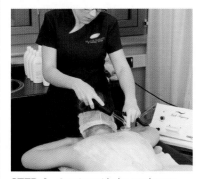

STEP 4 – Starting with the mushroom electrode, place the electrode in contact with client's skin before switching on the current. Keep contact with the electrode to avoid sparking.

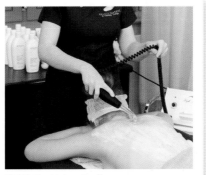

STEP 5 – Using circular movements, carry out the procedure to the treatment area.

INDUSTRY TIP

For the cut-out method a therapist removes cream from the pot with a spatula and applies it to their own hand and they then dispose of the spatula. This method prevents cross-contamination.

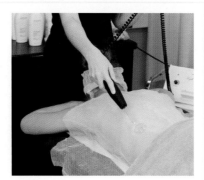

STEP 6 – Gauze can be used on the treatment area.

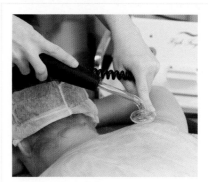

STEP 7 – Once the treatment procedure has been completed, remove the electrode from the treatment area, remembering to keep contact to avoid sparking.

Application of indirect high frequency to the face

Carry out steps 1–4 from facial electrotherapy preparation (see page 290).

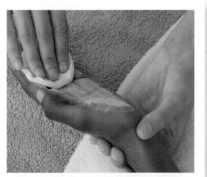

STEP 1 – Apply powder to the client's hands and double-check that any jewellery has been removed. Place a sanitised saturator into the client's hand, ensuring they have a firm grip on it.

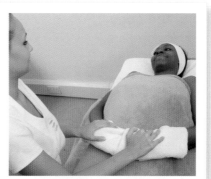

STEP 2 – A hand towel can be used to secure the electrode in the client's hand.

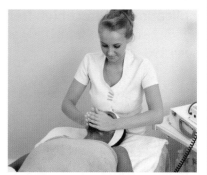

STEP 3 – Apply a medium (eg massage cream) to the treatment area.

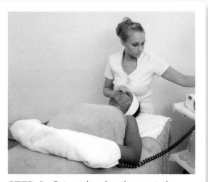

STEP 4 – Put one hand on the area to be treated and make small circular movements. Switch the machine on and turn up the intensity. The client will feel warmth in the area. Check the intensity is suitable for them and place both hands on the area to be treated.

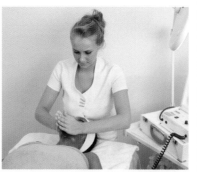

STEP 5 – Massage the area to be treated, avoiding tapotement, as lifting away from the client's skin may cause sparking. Do not lose contact with the skin.

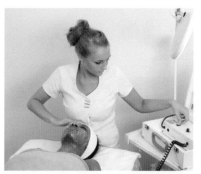

STEP 6 – Remove one hand and turn the intensity back to zero. Continue to massage for a few minutes to allow the current to disperse before removing the hands completely from the skin.

SmartScreen 306 Worksheet 2

ACTIVITY

Carry out some research into the use of direct high frequency alongside galvanism. How many skincare companies use both direct high frequency and galvanism together as one of their signature treatments? You could visit a trade show to try to find out this information as well as seeing it in action!

INDUSTRY TIP

Facial direct high frequency is a highly effective treatment when used in conjunction with facial galvanism. Together they contribute to improved skin condition.

HANDY HINT

Do not perform tapotement movements as part of the massage as they will break contact with the skin and cause irritation.

HANDY HINT

Observe the client's skin reaction throughout the treatment. Application time is 8–12 minutes in line with the manufacturer's instructions.

Application of indirect high frequency to the body

Carry out steps 1–6 from body electrotherapy preparation (see pages 290–291) and steps 1–3 from direct high frequency to the body (see page 299).

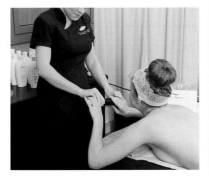

STEP 1 – Place the indifferent electrode into client's hand and protect with a towel.

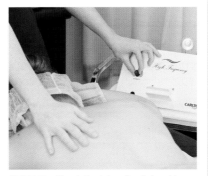

STEP 2 – Check the intensity dial and keep one hand in contact with the client's skin.

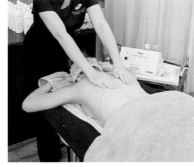

STEP 3 – Carry out the massage procedure across the client's back. Remember not to lose contact.

Contra-actions to high frequency

Refer to pages 330–331 for general contra-actions to electrotherapy treatments.

Home-care and aftercare advice for high frequency

Refer to page 331 for general home-care and aftercare advice for electrotherapy treatments.

HANDY HINT

Losing contact with the client can cause discomfort to them through sparking.

GALVANIC

Galvanic treatment improves the skin in two ways:

- desincrustation: removal of surface blockages and thorough cleansing of the skin – it literally means to remove a crust that covers an object
- iontophoresis: the introduction of water-soluble substances into the skin – this technique is used to push products into the skin.

On the face, it helps improve the skin's texture through desquamation, it cleanses the skin and helps to introduce beneficial ingredients into the skin to improve the skin's condition.

HANDY HINT

Facial galvanic treatment and direct high frequency treatment should be used together to help deep cleanse problematic skin.

On the body, it improves the appearance of cellulite, increases lymphatic flow and can help as part of a weight-loss programme.

How does it work?

A galvanic current is a low-voltage, direct current that flows in one direction. It works on the basic laws of **polarity** (ie like poles repel each other but opposite poles attract each other:

- +ve attracts −ve
- +ve repels +ve
- −ve repels −ve.

Polarity

The galvanic machine has a polarity switch for selecting and changing polarity. The machine also has sockets for connecting electrodes. An **anode** (an electrode with positive polarity) and a **cathode** (an electrode with negative polarity) are needed for the system to work because opposite poles attract. Products containing positively or negatively charged ions are used during galvanic treatments.

Example of how a galvanic facial treatment works:

1 A gel containing anions (negatively charged ions) is applied to the skin.
2 The client holds an **indifferent electrode** (a metal bar electrode) in their hand which has a positive polarity (ie an anode).
3 The roller electrodes (the **active** electrode) that are negatively charged (ie a cathode) are applied to the face.
4 This creates a circuit (from positive to negative) allowing the current to flow.
5 As the polarity of the roller electrodes is the same as the polarity of the gel, they are repelled and the ions in the product are attracted through the skin to the positive electrode in the client's hand.

> **INDUSTRY TIP**
>
> The polarity of the products and the machine setting will have an effect on the treatment. It is important to remember that like poles repel so:
>
> - negative (−ve) to negative and positive (+ve) to positive would push away from each other
> - positive to negative and negative to positive would be attracted to each other as opposites attract.

Effects of the electrodes used in galvanic treatment

Anode (+ve polarity)	Cathode (−ve polarity)
Acid reaction (hydrochloric acid)	Alkaline reaction (sodium hydroxide)
Vasoconstriction	Vasodilation
Pores are tightened	Pores are relaxed
Decreases erythema	Sebum is softened and broken down (**saponification**)
Soothes nerve endings	Stimulates nerve endings
Decreases lymph	Increases lymph
Skin tightening	Skin softening

Polarity
Like poles repel each other but opposite poles attract each other

Anode
A negative electrode

Cathode
A positive electrode

Indifferent electrode
The electrode held by the client that completes the circuit

Active electrode
The electrode that comes into contact with the client's skin

> **HANDY HINT**
>
> The active electrode (eg rollers) must be the same polarity as the galvanic solution/gel so that products are pushed into the skin.

> **HANDY HINT**
>
> The active ingredients in galvanic solutions are marked with a plus (+) or a minus (−) to show whether they are positive or negative. Always check that the correct polarity of cosmetic products are used to make sure that an effective treatment is achieved.

Saponification
The breaking down of fat by an alkali to form soap

Equipment used in galvanic treatment

Equipment	Use
Galvanic body unit	• For galvanic body treatments.
Indifferent metal bar electrode	• Held by the client. • Wrapped in a sponge envelope. • Completes the electrical circuit.
Indifferent metal plate electrode	• Placed under the client's shoulder. • Wrapped in a sponge envelope. • Completes the circuit.
Ball electrode	• Ideal for treating the sides of the nose, the chin and around the eyes.
Roller electrode	• Two rollers are used on the face and neck area in a slow rhythmic rolling motion.
Tweezer electrode	• Lint soaked in desincrustation fluid is wrapped around the points. • Used to target problematic areas.

HANDY HINT

A therapist would choose whether to use the bar or plate electrode but they would not use both at the same time.

Equipment	Use
Carbon electrodes	■ Used for galvanic body treatments.
Metal plate electrode and sponge envelopes	■ Used for galvanic body treatments. ■ Body pads are covered with damp sponge envelopes.
Metal free elastic straps	■ Used to secure carbon electrodes or plate electrodes to the body during galvanic body treatments.

Carbon pads

With body galvanic treatments the electrodes are in the form of carbon pads which are applied to the skin. A positive electrode (pad) will be positioned opposite a negative electrode (eg a positive electrode on the biceps and a negative electrode on the triceps). The electrodes will have different leads depending on whether they are positive or negative:

■ black lead and –ve symbol = negative electrode
■ red lead and +ve symbol = positive electrode.

INDUSTRY TIP
Check that the sponge envelopes do not have any splits or breaks in them and that they are not creased when on the body as this can cause a build-up of current.

INDUSTRY TIP
The red electrode is the indifferent electrode and the black electrode is the active electrode.

Different padding sequences

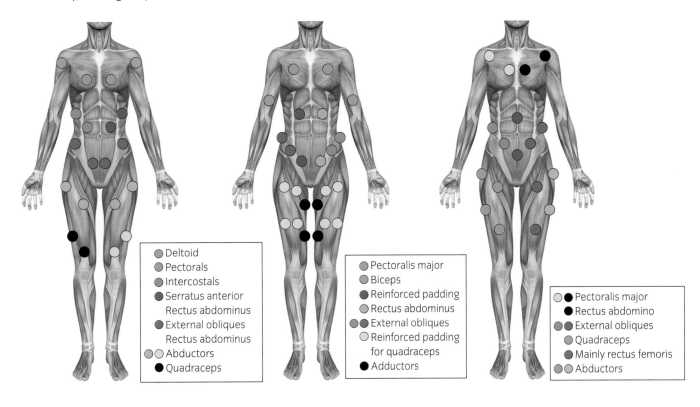

- ○ Deltoid
- ○ Pectorals
- ○ Intercostals
- ● Serratus anterior
  Rectus abdominus
- ● External obliques
  Rectus abdominus
- ○○ Abductors
- ● Quadraceps

- ○ Pectoralis major
- ○ Biceps
- ● Reinforced padding
- ○ Rectus abdominus
- ○● External obliques
- ○ Reinforced padding
  for quadraceps
- ● Adductors

- ○● Pectoralis major
- ● Rectus abdomino
- ●○ External obliques
- ○ Quadraceps
- ● Mainly rectus femoris
- ○○ Abductors

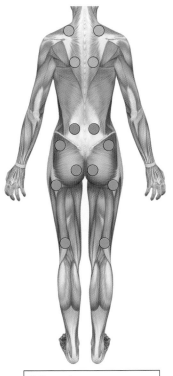
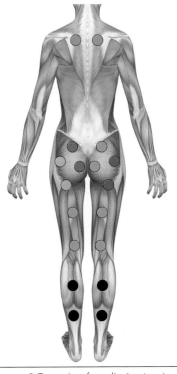
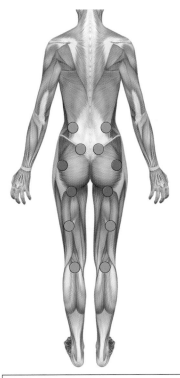

- ○ Trapezius
- ○ Latissimus dorsi
  (also for lower back pain)
- ○ Gluteals
- ○ Outside thighs

- ○ Trapezius: for relieving tension
- ●●●○ Reinforced layout for buttocks
- ○ Hamstrings
- ● Gastrocnemius

- ○ Latissimus dorsi
- ● Gluteus maximus
- ○ Hamstrings: mainly biceps femoris

HANDY HINT

Your tutor will have shown you different pad-up techniques. You may
need to adapt the sequence depending on the client's needs.

Products used in galvanic treatment

Products	Use/benefits
Cleansers and toners	▪ For preparing the skin for treatment.
Galvanic products: ▪ active solutions (eg gels, creams and serums) ▪ saline solution.	▪ Chosen for specific treatment requirements such as toning, firming, anti-cellulite. ▪ Saline solution used for galvanic body treatments; this acts as a conductor for electrical current on the skin.
Masks	▪ Enhances the treatment, has properties such as anti-ageing, firming and nourishing.
Moisturisers, eye gels and lip balms	▪ Protect and nourish the skin, eyes and lips.
Disinfectant	▪ For disinfecting the equipment before and after use.

Effects and benefits of galvanic

Diuretic

A drug or substance that tends to increase the amount of urine flushed from the body

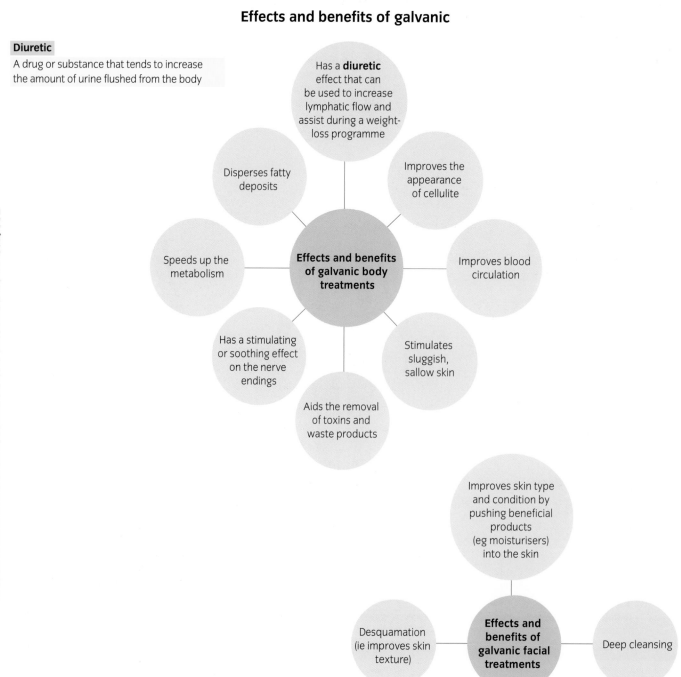

Precautions

It is important to perform all the following safety checks before carrying out galvanic treatments to avoid the risk of galvanic burns:

- Make sure all jewellery (both client's and therapist's) is removed.
- Cover cuts/blemishes with petroleum jelly.
- Do not exceed 2–3mA on the galvanic unit (as per manufacturer's instructions).
- Make sure that the sponge pockets are not spilt or ripped.
- Make sure that wires are not split or damaged.
- Check that the machine has been PAT tested and that it is still valid.
- Make sure that the client does not have any contra-indications that prevent treatment.

 SmartScreen 307 Worksheet 1

 SmartScreen 306 Worksheet 3

Contra-indications to galvanic treatment

In addition to the general contra-indications listed in Chapter 303 on page 215, it is important that you are aware of these contra-indications to treatment:

- pregnancy (and post-pregnancy until the postnatal check or GP's advice)
- metal plates and pins
- pacemaker
- epilepsy
- diabetes
- cuts or abrasions in the treatment area
- varicose veins
- kidney disorders due to the diuretic effect of the treatment.

Application of galvanic to the face – desincrustation

The cathode is the active electrode.

Carry out steps 1–4 from facial electrotherapy preparation (see page 290).

HANDY HINT

Apply petroleum jelly to any broken areas of skin to insulate.

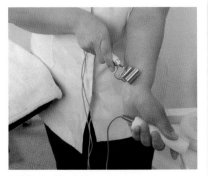

STEP 1 – Check the equipment prior to use.

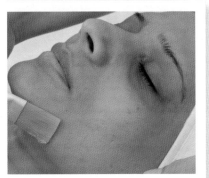

STEP 2 – Apply the negatively charged desincrustation product (eg cream, gel, ampoule) to the client's skin.

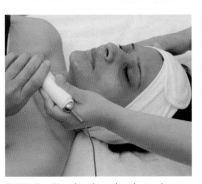

STEP 3 – Give the client the electrode to hold or place one under their shoulder making sure it is not touching any metal (such as a bra strap) and that the electrode is covered with either dampened lint or a sponge pocket.

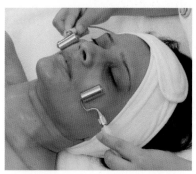

STEP 4 – In small circling motions, work the electrode across the treatment area for between three and five minutes for general cleansing and eight to ten minutes for oily areas.

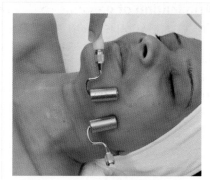

STEP 5 – Carry out the roller sequence starting on the jaw line.

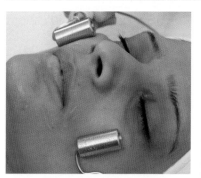

STEP 6 – Use the rollers on the cheek area.

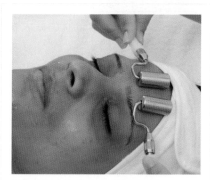

STEP 7 – Use the rollers across the forehead.

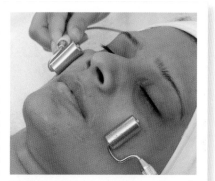

STEP 8 – Iontophoresis can be performed at this point. If you aren't applying iontophoresis then reverse the polarity for two to three minutes to tighten the pores and restore the pH balance of the skin, before applying a mask.

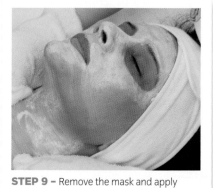

STEP 9 – Remove the mask and apply toner and moisturiser.

Application of galvanic to the face – iontophoresis

The anode (+ve) is the active electrode).

Carry out steps 1–4 from facial electrotherapy preparation (see page 290) and give the indifferent electrode to the client as per the instructions above.

(see page 290)

HANDY HINT

Select the correct polarity (if the solution is +ve, the polarity should be +ve and vice versa).

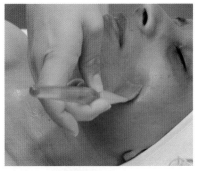

STEP 1 – Apply iontophoresis products to the face and throat area using a mask brush.

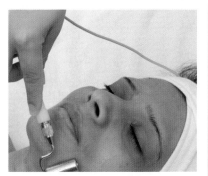

STEP 2 – Pick up one of the rollers and start on the neck. Slowly turn up the intensity and wait for 30 seconds to allow any resistance to be broken down. Then turn up the intensity again until the client feels a tingling sensation. As with desincrustation it should not exceed 1.5mA.

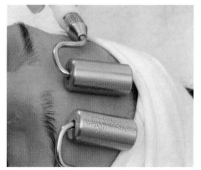

STEP 3 – Pick up the other roller so that two rollers are used in sequence. Start at the neck and work in a sequence up the face to the forehead. Make sure that the two rollers do not clash. Work in a slow, smooth rhythmic manner for five to seven minutes.

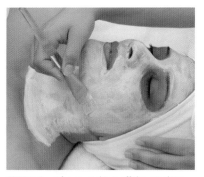

STEP 4 – After switching off the machine and removing the indifferent electrode from the client's hand, remove the iontophoresis product from the skin unless the instructions recommend you apply a mask over them.

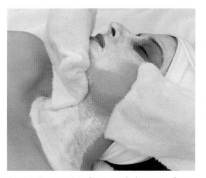

STEP 5 – Apply a face mask, leave on for the recommended time and remove with warm water or a hot towel.

INDUSTRY TIP

An alternative method of application is using electrodes. Refer to the manufacturer's instructions as to how to use these.

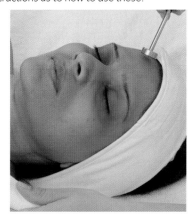

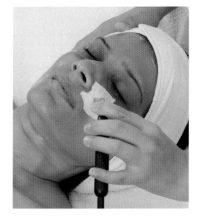

HANDY HINT

Reduce the current slowly. Once the current has reached zero, keep the rollers moving for a moment or two to allow any leftover current to disperse.

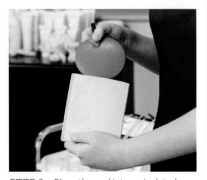

Application of galvanic to the body

The purpose of galvanic body treatments is to introduce active substances into the tissues to increase fluid loss and mobilise fatty tissue.

Carry out steps 1–6 from body electrotherapy preparation (see pages 290–291).

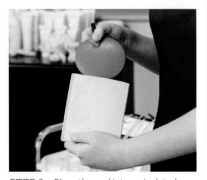

STEP 1 – Place the pad into an isolated protector pad or pocket.

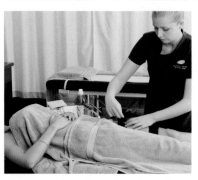

STEP 2 – Secure elastic straps in position on the treatment area.

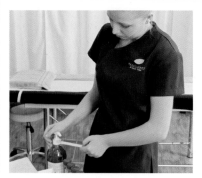

STEP 3 – Dispense the active product for use on the treatment area.

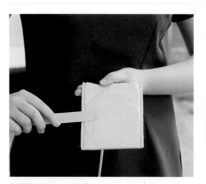

STEP 4 – Apply the active product onto the insulated pad. This can also be applied straight to the treatment area.

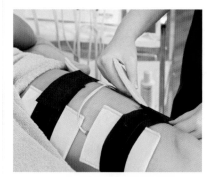

STEP 5 – Place the pads in the correct position for the treatment objective.

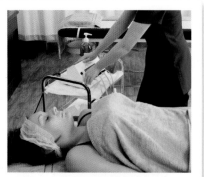

STEP 6 – Make sure that all dials are at zero and that the polarity is on negative. Turn on the machine slowly and check that the client feels a tingling or prickling sensation.

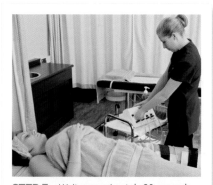

STEP 7 – Wait approximately 30 seconds and increase intensity. Always check the client's response and the treatment area for any erythema (in line with the manufacturer's instructions).

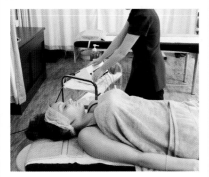

STEP 8 – Reduce the intensity and reverse the polarity for the last three to five minutes. In line with the manufacturer's instructions, switch the intensity back up as this helps to neutralise any irritation caused by chemical formation on the skin.

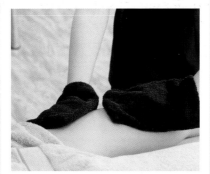

STEP 9 – Remove the pads from the client and clean the area.

HANDY HINT

At the end of the treatment, turn the dials to zero and make sure there is no current (mA) registering. Switch off the machine at the mains.

HANDY HINT

You must increase the current slowly because of the skin's initial resistance.

Contra-actions to galvanic

You need to be aware of general contra-actions such as product allergies. However there are also some contra-actions that are specific to galvanic treatments.

Contra-action	Description	Action to be taken
Sensitisation due to intensity of the treatment or products	▪ Severe erythema.	▪ Apply a cool compress. ▪ If it happens during treatment, reverse the polarity for two to three minutes, then apply a cooling soothing gel.
Galvanic burn	▪ Usually the result of poor practice (eg not applying enough product or over-treating the area). ▪ A chemical burn results from a concentration of alkali on the skin. ▪ Skin is dark, split and surrounded by an inflamed red ring.	▪ Flush the area with lots of cool water. ▪ Apply a dry sterile dressing. ▪ Advise client to seek medical advice immediately.
Metallic taste	▪ If the client has fillings or bridgework they may taste metal in their mouth.	▪ Use rubber gum shields to help prevent this.

Home-care and aftercare advice for galvanic

Please see page 331 for general advice for home-care and aftercare advice for electrotherapy treatments.

ELECTRICAL MUSCLE STIMULATION (EMS) (OR FARADIC)

The first EMS device was patented in 1948 by Dr Sebastian Hawkins (an osteopath and chiropractor).

How does it work?

EMS causes stimulation of the muscles to help tone and strengthen them.

- An alternating low frequency, interrupted and surged direct current of electricity is used.
- A carbon block (facial) or carbon pads (body) are positioned on the **motor point** of a muscle and the current surges causing the muscle to contract the current then stops allowing the muscle to relax.
- If a contraction is not achieved it may be due to incorrect positioning or due to layers of adipose tissue hiding the movement.

Equipment used in EMS

An EMS unit can be purchased as a single facial or body unit or as a combined facial and body unit.

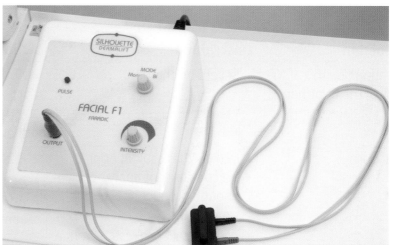

Facial faradic machine

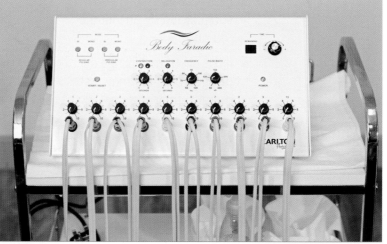

Body faradic machine

Motor point

The part of a muscle that is stimulated and where a visible contraction can be caused with a minimal amount of stimulation

Voluntary muscle contraction

Muscle contraction that you consciously control

An EMS unit produces a low-frequency direct current of between 10 and 120Hz. The EMS unit has a number of controls and settings that the therapist needs to familiarise themself with.

Control/setting	Description
On/off switch	■ Usually has a light to show that the unit is switched on. ■ If using a body unit there might be a master switch to switch all of the attached pads on or off at once.
Timer	■ Some units have preset times or the programme time can be selected manually and displayed during the treatment.
Frequency control	■ Controls the number of pulses per second. ■ Determines the depth of stimulation.

Pulse sequence button	Description
Monophasic pulse sequence	■ Current flows in one direction. ■ Helps to lift muscles. ■ The current travels in one direction only from negative to positive. The polarity of the pads remains constant throughout, meaning that there is more strength under the negative pad, which should be placed on the weaker muscle. ■ A monophasic pulse sequence is always used during a facial EMS treatment because it flows in one direction only. Only an upward movement of the muscle should be stimulated as the aim of the treatment is to lift and tone muscles.
Biphasic pulse sequence	■ The polarity of the pads change so that the current always travels from − to +, but as the pad polarity changes the current runs in one direction and then the other direction of each pulse. ■ Helps with strengthening and toning of the muscle. ■ This is best used in longitudinal padding.

Pulse control	Description
Stimulation	■ The amount of time the pulse of the current will flow for to stimulate the muscle before a rest. ■ Usually set between half a second and two and a half seconds.
Relaxation	■ The length of the rest period when the current does not flow. ■ Usually a few seconds to a minute so that the muscle does not become too relaxed before stimulation occurs again.
Mode control	■ Either constant or variable. ■ Controls the sequence of the contractions.
Constant mode	■ The length of the stimulation period and rest periods remains the same during the treatment.
Variable mode	■ Varies the length of the stimulation and rest periods during the treatment. ■ Ideal for nervous clients as they do not know when to expect the next stimulation so are not able to tense the muscle in anticipation. ■ Only used on the body.
Pulse width	■ Increasing pulse width is similar to increasing the intensity. ■ If the pulse width is increased there will be greater stimulation.

Control/setting	Description
Modulated pulse	■ Gentle stimulation. ■ Builds up to its preset intensity gradually. ■ Causes a more gentle contraction to be produced.

Pulse control	Description
Unmodulated pulse	■ Intense stimulation throughout the whole stimulation period. ■ Ideal for deeper muscles or if there is a large amount of adipose tissue present.
Intensity control	■ Controls the strength of the current. ■ If the dial is turned up, the intensity increases.
Master output control	■ Can be used to turn up all the current settings at the same time. ■ Only used once the client has become used to the contractions.

Electrodes	Description
Block	■ Used on the face. ■ A carbon block with both negative and positive polarity. ■ Attached to the EMS unit with a cable. ■ Positioned on the facial muscles to stimulate contractions.
Pads	■ Used on the body. ■ Contain carbon. ■ Placed on the **origin** and **insertion** of the muscle to achieve a contraction. ■ The black pad (or one with a black lead) is placed on the insertion of the muscle. ■ The red lead/pad is placed onto the origin of the muscle. ■ The black pad has a negative charge which gives a stronger muscle contraction if using the monophasic mode.

Origin

The point where a muscle begins

Insertion

The other end of a muscle that moves when the muscle contracts

 SmartScreen 306 Worksheet 5

Padding

There are three types of padding used for positioning the electrodes on the body for an EMS treatment:

■ Longitudinal padding – padding that extends from the top of a muscle to the bottom of a muscle, near the origin and insertion of a muscle. Pads are placed on the upper and lower motor points of long muscles such as the rectus abdominus, rectus femoris and trapezius.

■ Duplicate/dual padding – a pair of pads is placed on the motor points of muscles with similar actions that are adjacent to one another (eg the external obliques and the rectus abdominus).

■ Split padding – a pair of pads is split and the electrode is placed on the motor point of the same muscle group on opposite sides of the body (eg right and left pectorals, right and left gluteus maximus).

Other equipment used in EMS

Equipment	Description
Steamer or infra-red lamp	■ The muscles should be pre-heated using a steamer or infrared lamp prior to treatment to get the maximum benefit. ■ Relaxes the muscles ready for **passive exercise** and reduces the risk of injury.
Non-metallic elastic straps	■ Used to secure the pads to the body during a body faradic treatment.

Passive exercise
Exercise without physically moving the muscles

Products used in EMS

Product	Description
Cleanser	■ Used to wipe over the area prior to treatment. ■ Should be oil free so there is no barrier that would prevent good muscle contraction. ■ Witch hazel or an antiseptic wipe can also be used.
Saline solution	■ An electrolyte which is a good conductor of current. ■ Can be used with both facial and body EMS treatments. ■ To make a 1% saline solution, dissolve one teaspoon of salt in a pint of hot water.
Exfoliator	■ Exfoliation prior to treatment may be needed. ■ Prepares the skin by removing any barriers to treatment.
Cellulite gel	■ Applied over areas of cellulite at the end of the treatment. ■ Can be recommended to the client for home care.
Antiseptic	■ For wiping over the electrodes after treatment once they have been washed.

Effects and benefits of EMS for the face

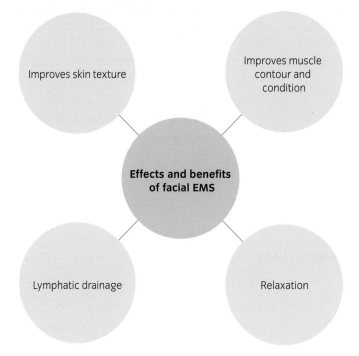

Improves skin texture

Improves muscle contour and condition

Effects and benefits of facial EMS

Lymphatic drainage

Relaxation

Effects and benefits of EMS for the body

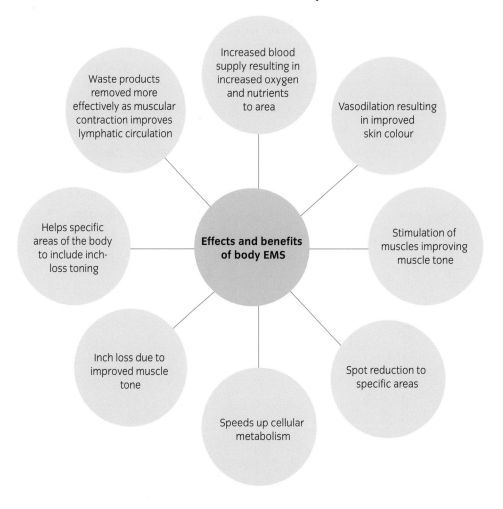

Waste products removed more effectively as muscular contraction improves lymphatic circulation

Increased blood supply resulting in increased oxygen and nutrients to area

Vasodilation resulting in improved skin colour

Helps specific areas of the body to include inch-loss toning

Effects and benefits of body EMS

Stimulation of muscles improving muscle tone

Inch loss due to improved muscle tone

Spot reduction to specific areas

Speeds up cellular metabolism

Contra-indications to EMS

Please refer to pages 288–289 for general contra-indications to electrotherapy treatments.

Application of EMS to the face

Carry out steps 1–4 from facial electrotherapy preparation (see page 290). Remember to test that the equipment is working before you start.

(see page 290)

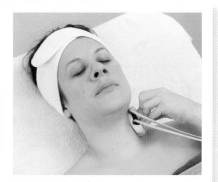

STEP 1 – Soak a piece of gauze in saline solution and place it around the block electrode.

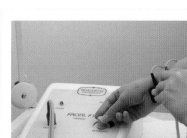

STEP 2 – Test the machine in front of the client so they can see it before they experience it.

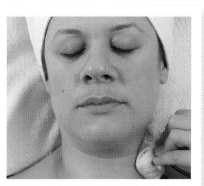

STEP 3 – Place the electrode in contact with the client's skin before switching on the current. Turn up the intensity until a muscle contraction can be seen.

STEP 4 – When a contraction has been observed, work the muscle six to eight times before switching the intensity back to zero and repositioning the electrode on the next muscle. This should take approximately 10–15 minutes to complete the full face.

Ampoule

An ampoule is a vial which contains a fluid/serum that has properties to help the area such as anti-ageing, toning, nourishing

The following is a sequence that can be used for your facial faradic routine, however your tutor may have taught you a different sequence.

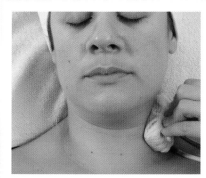

STEP 5 – Neck (sternocleidomastoid).

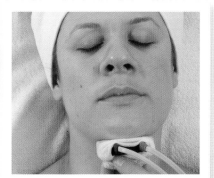

STEP 6 – Chin (digastric).

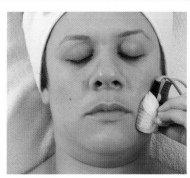

STEP 7 – Cheek (masseter).

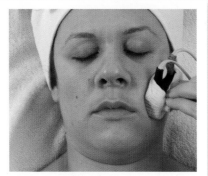

STEP 8 – Upper cheek (risorius).

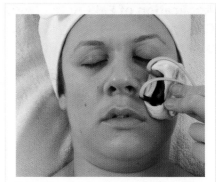

STEP 9 – Cheekbone (zygomaticus).

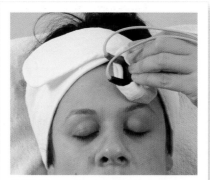

STEP 11 – Forehead (frontalis).

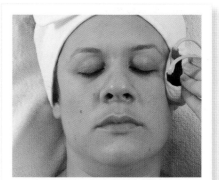

STEP 10 – Eye (orbicularis oculi).

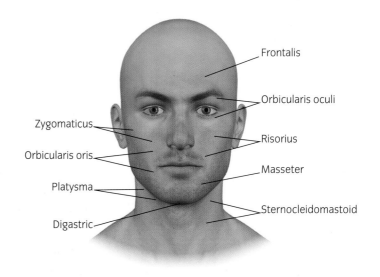

The areas of the face and neck for treatment with EMS

HANDY HINT

If necessary, at this point a facial massage towards the lymph nodes can be performed for five minutes to remove the lymph waste that has been released during the muscle stimulation.

Application of EMS to the body

Carry out steps 1–6 from body electrotherapy preparation (see pages 290–291).

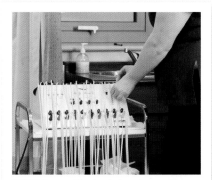

STEP 1 – Double-check that the machine dials are all set to zero.

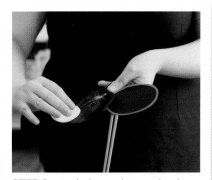

STEP 2 – Apply the conductor gel to the area. Alternatively, saline solution can be applied to the electrodes or pad instead.

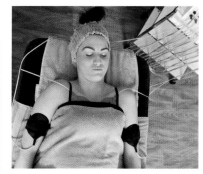

STEP 3 – Position the pads on the treatment area identified in the consultation and objectives.

Steps 4 to 8 are examples of a pad layout. Please refer to the training manual or manufacturer's instructions for alternative pad-up techniques.

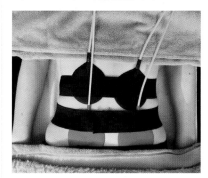

STEP 4 – Abdomen.

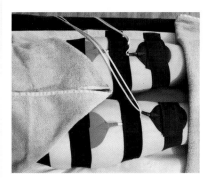

STEP 5 – Upper front thigh.

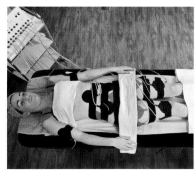

STEP 6 – Full front body.

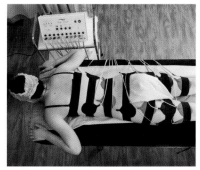

STEP 7 – Full back body.

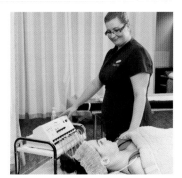

STEP 8 – Explain the sensation to client and what they can expect during the treatment when you turn up the machine.

> **HANDY HINT**
>
> Not all units will switch themselves off automatically. If the unit you are using does not have an automatic switch-off function, ensure it is timed accurately so that you don't under-exercise or over-exercise the muscles.

> **HANDY HINT**
>
> Once the treatment is finished, remeasure the client and inform them of their inch-loss results, and then allow the client time to dress in privacy. During the measuring tactfully recommend to them a course of treatments alongside a healthy eating plan to gain the most beneficial results.

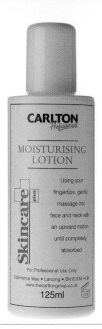

A moisturiser for use after an electrical treatment

Body brushing

Can loosen and remove any dry skin from the area and increase blood flow. It is a great way to look after your body at home and can be carried out before getting into the shower or bath

 SmartScreen 306 Worksheet 6

Mechanical method

Doesn't involve passing an electrical current through the body

Ventouse

Glass cup used in vacuum suction

With EMS for the body, always remember to:

- Select the programme appropriate to the client's needs.
- Cover the client with a blanket to keep them warm.
- Turn up the intensity until a contraction can be seen. Do this until all the muscles are contracting.
- After ten minutes, turn up the intensity control again to achieve a stronger contraction – depending on the client and how well the muscles contract.

Contra-actions to EMS

Please refer to pages 330–331 for general contra-actions to electrotherapy treatments.

Home-care and aftercare advice for EMS

As with all treatments, advise the client to follow a healthy lifestyle (ie reduce or quit smoking, limit alcohol and caffeine intake and take regular exercise). Specific home-care advice related to EMS treatments might include:

- use of an anti-cellulite body product
- **body brushing**
- drinking plenty of water
- following a course of treatments – 10–15 treatments, with two to three treatments in the first week and then an average of two treatments per week
- further monthly treatments once the initial course of treatments has been completed.

VACUUM SUCTION

Vacuum suction is a **mechanical method** of lymphatic drainage treatment.

How does it work?

It is performed using a **ventouse** which is applied to the skin with a straight and light gliding manner towards the lymph nodes. This encourages drainage of lymph fluid from within the lymph spaces. Although the unit operates by using an electrical current, no current passes through the body or face.

Equipment used in vacuum suction

Equipment	Use
Vacuum suction unit	▪ Creates a vacuum that causes skin tissue to be sucked into a ventouse. ▪ Simple to use. ▪ Has an on/off switch and intensity control for the amount of vacuum needed.
Facial cup	▪ For lymph drainage on the face. ▪ Also for deep cleansing.
Body cups	▪ For stimulation of the circulation. ▪ Also for lymphatic drainage of the body.
Comedone ventouse	▪ For extraction of comedones.
Flat-head ventouse	▪ Desquamation along fine facial lines. ▪ For lymphatic drainage without over-stimulating the skin.
Pore blockage ventouse	▪ For comedone or pore blockages when there is a group present.

Effects and benefits of vacuum suction

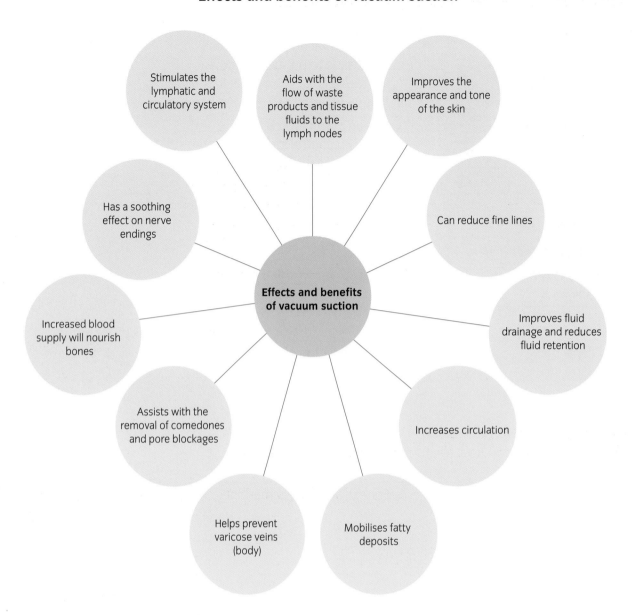

Effects and benefits of vacuum suction

- Stimulates the lymphatic and circulatory system
- Aids with the flow of waste products and tissue fluids to the lymph nodes
- Improves the appearance and tone of the skin
- Can reduce fine lines
- Improves fluid drainage and reduces fluid retention
- Increases circulation
- Mobilises fatty deposits
- Helps prevent varicose veins (body)
- Assists with the removal of comedones and pore blockages
- Increased blood supply will nourish bones
- Has a soothing effect on nerve endings

Contra-indications to vacuum suction
Please refer to pages 288–289 for general contra-indications to electrotherapy treatments.

Application of vacuum suction to the face
Before performing vacuum suction, you need to know where the lymph nodes are positioned.

LYMPH NODES OF THE FACE AND NECK

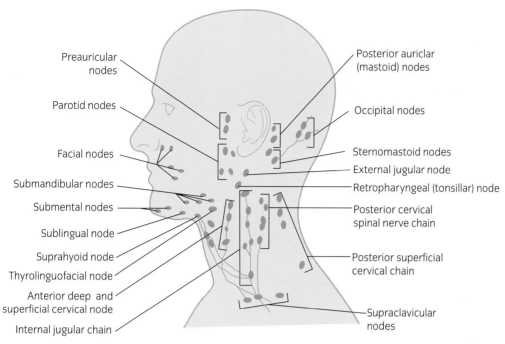

Preauricular nodes

Parotid nodes

Facial nodes

Submandibular nodes

Submental nodes

Sublingual node

Suprahyoid node

Thyrolinguofacial node

Anterior deep and superficial cervical node

Internal jugular chain

Posterior auriclar (mastoid) nodes

Occipital nodes

Sternomastoid nodes

External jugular node

Retropharyngeal (tonsillar) node

Posterior cervical spinal nerve chain

Posterior superficial cervical chain

Supraclavicular nodes

SmartScreen 306 Worksheet 10

SmartScreen 307 Worksheet 2

Facial vacuum suction procedure

Carry out steps 1–4 from facial electrotherapy preparation (see page 290).

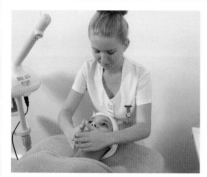

STEP 1 – Prepare the client's skin for treatment with either massage oil or cream.

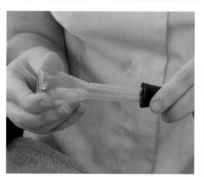

STEP 2 – Select the correct cup for facial use.

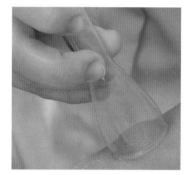

STEP 3 – Test the vaccum suction machine on yourself.

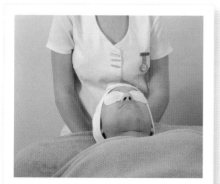

STEP 4 – Explain to the client the sensation that they will experience.

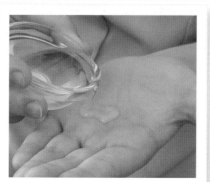

STEP 5 – Apply the medium for the vacuum suction procedure.

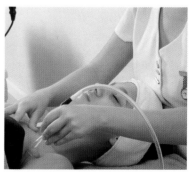

STEP 6 – Start at the decolletage area and draw to the lymph node.

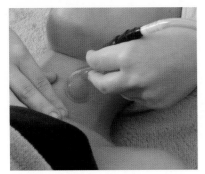

STEP 7 – Carry out the neck routine.

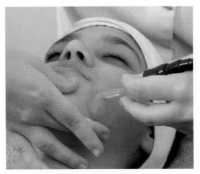

STEP 8 – Draw across the jaw line.

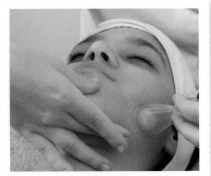

STEP 9 – Work across the cheek area.

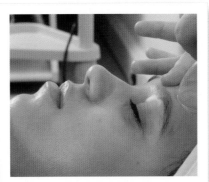

STEP 10 – Work across the forehead, remembering to reduce the vacuum when working on this area.

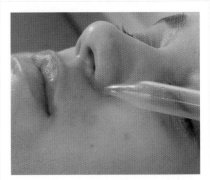

STEP 11 – If you are working on a congested area, use the correct ventouse.

Application of vacuum suction to the body

Carry out steps 1–6 from body electrotherapy preparation (see pages 290–291).

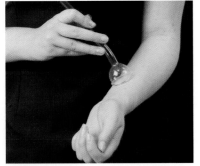

STEP 1 – Select the correct cup size for the treatment area and test this on yourself.

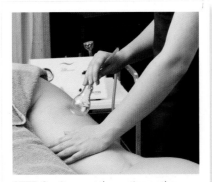

STEP 2 – Carry out the routine on the treatment area identified during the consultation. Always work towards the nearest lymph node.

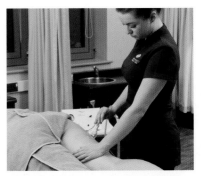

STEP 3 – Work across the treatment area taking care not to overlap drainage too much which can cause excessive erythema.

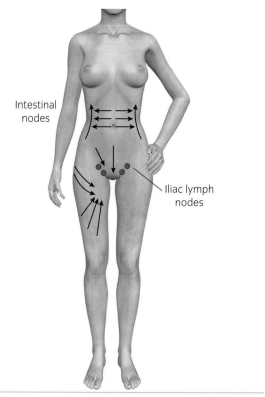

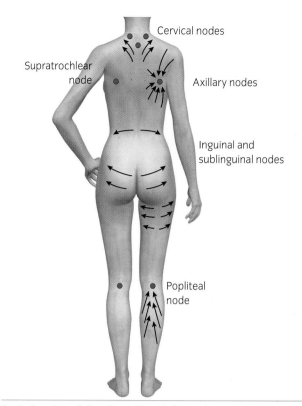

Anterior view of direction of lymph flow using vacuum suction

Posterior view of direction of lymph flow using vacuum suction

Contra-actions to vacuum suction

Please refer to pages 330–331 for general contra-actions to electrotherapy treatments.

Home-care and aftercare advice for vacuum suction

Please refer to page 331 for general home-care and aftercare advice for electrotherapy treatments.

> **HANDY HINT**
>
> For body cups that don't have an air hole, place a fingertip under the edge of the cup to break the seal.
>
> *Never* pull a cup off the skin without releasing the vacuum suction first as this can cause capillary and tissue damage.

ACTIVITY

Using a blank outline of the human body, draw circles on the face and body to show the location of the lymph nodes. Then try to label them or name them.

MICROCURRENT

Microcurrent is often referred to as a non-surgical lift, as it helps to lift and firm body and facial contours. Microcurrent was originally used for the medical treatment of Bell's palsy, strokes, facial paralysis, pain control and scar healing, before becoming a beauty/spa treatment.

> **HANDY HINT**
>
> Ageing limits the effectiveness of treatments. An ageing skin and body are usually less responsive to treatments than a younger skin and body. Therefore, a more mature client may need more treatments to see effective results.

How does it work?

It works by stimulating the muscles. However it doesn't create the same level of muscle contraction as EMS. This is because microcurrent stimulates the Golgi tendon organ (GTO) within the muscle rather than the motor point of the muscle.

The client feels very little sensation during a microcurrent treatment. The treatment uses a modified direct current with a frequency that is very similar to the body's own bioelectrical impulses. It therefore works in **synchronisation** with the body. Microcurrent is measured in **microamps**.

Synchronisation

Operation at the same time

Microamp

One millionth of an amp (symbol is μA)

325

Equipment used in microcurrent

Microcurrent machines have advanced greatly over the years and the following types of machines are available:

Type of microcurrent machine	Use
Combination systems 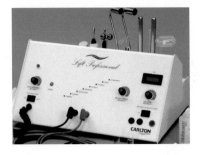	▪ Pads are applied to specific points. ▪ Probes are also used to stretch and re-educate the muscles.
Probe system 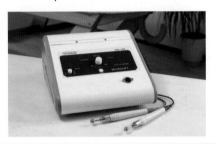	▪ Microcurrent is applied through probes for the face and gloves for the body. This equipment will vary between manufacturers.
Twin system 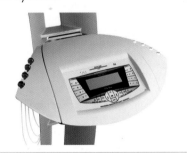	▪ Can be used either with probes or pads.

The majority of programmes on the microcurrent machines are preset. Therefore all the therapist needs to do is apply the pads to the treatment area as recommended by the manufacturer, select the programme and press go.

Products used in microcurrent

In addition to sanitising products and exfoliators, you will need positively (+ve) ionised gels which contain ingredients such as collagen and act as a conductor to the current. Some equipment manufacturers will have their own ranges of products that they recommend for use alongside their machines.

Tools used in microcurrent

▪ Cotton buds cut to 1.5cm may be needed for facial probes.
▪ Adhesive tabs to fix pads in place throughout the treatment.

Microcurrent also has positive and negative polarity, which is selected automatically on preset programmes and is easily recognised with probes as they have two leads, one of which plugs into the negative outlet and the other into the positive outlet.

HANDY HINT

Gloves are not always used in the probe system. Some units have them and some don't. If the system doesn't have gloves, probes would be used on the body instead.

INDUSTRY TIP

If you are using the probe method it might not be as simple as just applying the pads, selecting the programme and pressing go. There are different techniques to follow relating to each individual machine so you need to refer to the manufacturer's instructions.

HANDY HINT

Try to use paper cotton buds rather than plastic ones as facial probes, as paper is a better conductor than plastic.

Effects and benefits of microcurrent

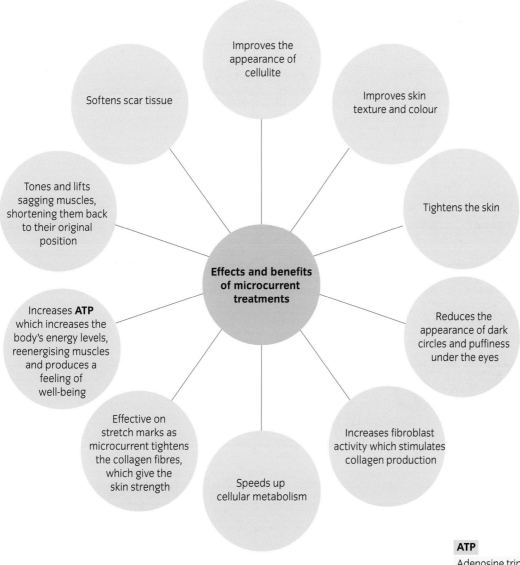

Improves the appearance of cellulite

Improves skin texture and colour

Softens scar tissue

Tightens the skin

Tones and lifts sagging muscles, shortening them back to their original position

Effects and benefits of microcurrent treatments

Increases **ATP** which increases the body's energy levels, reenergising muscles and produces a feeling of well-being

Reduces the appearance of dark circles and puffiness under the eyes

Effective on stretch marks as microcurrent tightens the collagen fibres, which give the skin strength

Increases fibroblast activity which stimulates collagen production

Speeds up cellular metabolism

ATP

Adenosine triphosphate – a chemical substance found in all living tissue that provides energy for muscle contraction

INDUSTRY TIP

Increased fibroblast activity stimulates collagen product. This then rehydrates the skin and encourages moisture retention. Fine lines are plumped out and the appearance of wrinkles is reduced.

Contra-indications to microcurrent

There are three specific contra-indications to facial microcurrent treatment. These are:

- botox
- collagen
- fillers.

Stages of a microcurrent treatment

There are generally four sequential stages to a microcurrent treatment:

1 increasing the circulation to the epidermis
2 drainage and relaxation; this aids the lymphatic system by removing toxins
3 muscle toning, lifting slack tissue and improving the pores
4 firming of muscles, reducing scar tissue, increasing circulation, second detoxification, improving skin texture, stimulating collagen production.

Application of microcurrent to the face

Carry out steps 1–4 from facial electrotherapy preparation (see page 290).

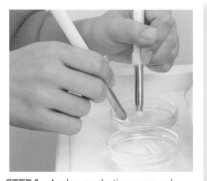

STEP 1 – Apply a conductive cream, gel, serum or ampoule to the client's face and neck in line with the manufacturer's instructions. If you are using probes for the facial treatment, these can be positioned on dry skin prior to applying the conductive skin because they don't need to be stuck to the skin. Follow the manufacturer's instructions.

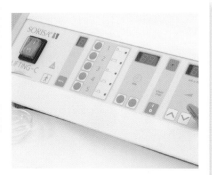

STEP 2 – Double-check that the machine dials are all set to zero. If you are using probes on the face, place a cotton bud soaked in the conducting cream, gel or serum (often collagen gel) into the metal area on the probe. Select the required programme and then apply the pads or probes following the manufacturer's suggested sequence.

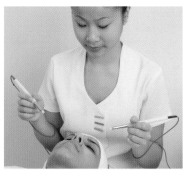

STEP 3 – Explain the sensation to the client.

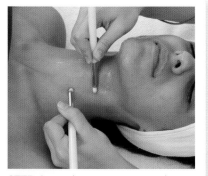

STEP 4 – Work in sequence across the face, starting with the neck.

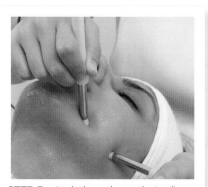

STEP 5 – Apply the probes to the jaw line.

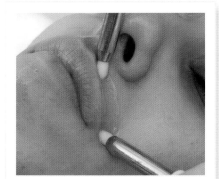

STEP 6 – Apply the probes to the upper lip.

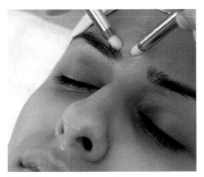

STEP 7 – Apply the probes to the brow line.

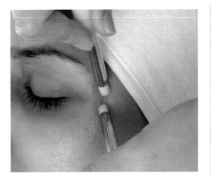

STEP 8 – Apply the probes to the eye area.

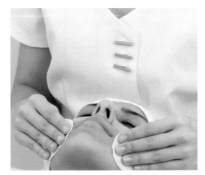

STEP 9 – Remove products and apply toner and moisturiser.

Application of microcurrent to the body

Carry out steps 1–6 from body electrotherapy preparation (see pages 290–291).

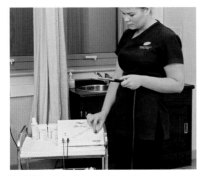

STEP 1 – Select the treatment programme on the microcurrent unit.

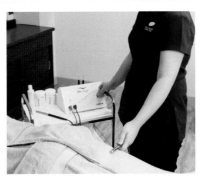

STEP 2 – Test the current on the client.

HANDY HINT

A mask may be applied followed by toner and moisturiser and any specialist products such as eye gel or lip balm.

HANDY HINT

Perform facial massage towards the lymph nodes for five minutes to remove the lymph waste which has been released during the muscle stimulation.

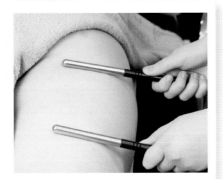

STEP 3 – Follow the manufacturer's recommended sequence either using gloves or probes.

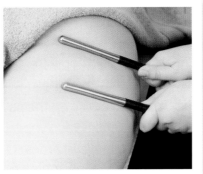

STEP 3 – The lifting sequence used in larger areas to maximum effect.

HANDY HINT

At the end of the programme, massage the remainder of the product into the client's skin or use specialised post-treatment products (eg cellulite gel).

INDUSTRY TIP

- For a bottom lift, before treatment measure from the lowest point of the bottom to the back of the knee when the client is standing up.
- For a breast lift start at the nipple and measure around the back of the neck finishing at the other nipple.
- Repeat these measurements after the treatment to show the client the amount of lift achieved.

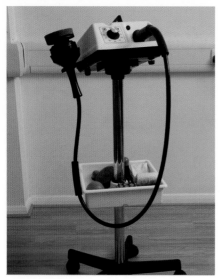

A salon G5 unit

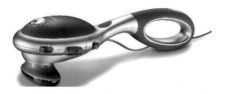

A handheld G5 unit with an infrared feature included

 SmartScreen 307 Worksheet 11

Contra-actions to microcurrent

Please see below for general contra-actions to electrotherapy treatments.

Home-care and aftercare advice for microcurrent

Please refer to page 331 for general home-care and aftercare advice.

OTHER ELECTRICAL TREATMENTS

Mechanical massage

Mechanical massage is a massage that produces a deeper effect than manual massage. It is often used on muscles and fatty tissue to soften and disperse them and is good for exfoliation, improving the skin condition, increasing blood and lymph flow and is also good for spot reduction. There are two types of mechanical massagers (often known as G5 which is also covered in the massage chapter, see pages 276–280:

- a larger salon unit
- a hand-held mobile unit.

GENERAL CONTRA-ACTIONS TO ELECTROTHERAPY TREATMENTS

A contra-action is an undesirable effect which happens during or as the result of a treatment. It is essential that the therapist knows how to deal with a contra-action and that they can also advise the client on how to deal with one if it occurs once they have left the salon/spa. The most common contra-indications following a facial or body electrotherapy treatment are:

Contra-action	Cause	Action to be taken
Excessive erythema (all electrical treatments)	Over-stimulation of the circulatory system.	■ Usually settles and disappears after a few hours. ■ Apply a cool compress to reduce any further heat in the area. ■ If it is still red and uncomfortable after 24 hours, the client should notify the salon and contact their doctor in case there is another cause.
Allergic reaction/ irritation (all electrical treatments)	Reaction to a product that has been applied to the skin.	■ Excessive erythema and inflammation. ■ Might be accompanied by itchiness. ■ Remove all products from the skin immediately using cool water and apply a cool compress to reduce any heat in the area. ■ If the reaction is severe and has not disappeared after 24 hours, the client should contact their doctor and notify the salon of the results.

Contra-action	Cause	Action to be taken
Muscle fatigue (spasms or cramps) (faradic or microcurrent)	■ A lack of oxygen to the muscle and a build-up of waste products (eg lactic acid). ■ Over-working the muscle.	■ Stop treatment and massage affected area to remove waste products and introduce fresh oxygen and nutrients to the area.
Galvanic burns (galvanic treatment)	Over-intensity used	■ Stop treatment and apply a cold compress to the affected area.

GENERAL HOME-CARE AND AFTERCARE ADVICE FOR FACIAL AND BODY ELECTROTHERAPY TREATMENTS

Following a facial or body electrotherapy treatment, you should give your client suitable aftercare advice to follow. This advice will help the client maximise the benefits of the treatment.

■ Provide recommendations for the correct skincare routine (eg products that will enhance their treatment).

■ If a body treatment, promote the use of a body brush to the client and explain how to use it.

■ Encourage the client to:
  ■ drink plenty of water and reduce caffeine intake
  ■ quit smoking
  ■ follow a healthy eating plan
  ■ take regular exercise

■ Encourage the client to book a course of treatments:
  ■ muscle toning treatments (EMS and microcurrent): ten treatments with one to two a week and then monthly to maintain the effect
  ■ vacuum suction, high frequency and galvanic: up to twice a month.

■ Explain how to deal with a contra-action if one occurs.

INDUSTRY TIP

If the client has a contra-action, write this up on their record card so the products/ treatment can be avoided or altered in the future.

SmartScreen 307 Worksheet 9

HANDY HINT

Body brushing is a great piece of aftercare to provide. Suggest to the client that they brush the body in circular motions towards the heart to stimulate circulation, remove waste and encourage desquamation.

HANDY HINT

It is good to be tidy in your salon! After the client has left, clean and sanitise the machine in line with the manufacturer's instructions and store away correctly. With the vacuum suction machine, wash the ventouses in hot soapy water, using an antibacterial soap, and leave them to dry before putting them away.

Use the questions below to test your knowledge of Chapter 306/307 to see how much information you have retained. These questions will help you revise what you have learnt in this chapter.

Turn to page 499 for the answers.

1 What does iontophoresis mean?
  a To degrease the skin
  b To push water-soluble products into the skin
  c To remove the stratum corneum
  d To perspire

2 What is the maximum percentage that the ventouse can be filled to during vacuum suction?
  a 15%
  b 18%
  c 20%
  s 23%

3 Petroleum jelly is used in electrical treatments to:
  a Cover minor breaks in the skin
  b Act as a medium for roller electrodes
  c Cover the indifferent electrode
  d Change the polarity

4 Where is the corrugator muscle situated?
  a At the back of the head
  b In between the eyes
  c Around the lips
  d Under the chin

5 During a galvanic treatment, which of the following effects are created at the positive electrode (anode)?
  a Vasodilation, skin tightening, soothing of nerve endings
  b Vasodilation, stimulation of the nerve endings, saponification
  c Vasoconstriction, skin tightening and soothing of nerve endings
  d Vasoconstriction, stimulation and soothing of the nerve endings

6 What is the sensation created by a microcurrent treatment?
  a Sharp shooting pains
  b Sweeping and gliding
  c Tingling
  d Little to no sensation

7 Where are the quadriceps muscles located?
  a Abdomen
  b Chest
  c Legs
  d Arms

8 Longitudinal, duplicate and splits are all types of pads used in:
  a Microcurrent treatment
  b Vacuum suction treatment
  c EMS treatment
  d Galvanic treatment

9 What is the maximum time limit for a first body galvanic treatment?
  a 20 minutes
  b 15 minutes
  c 10 minutes
  d 5 minutes

10 What colour is a high-frequency glass saturator containing mercury vapour?
  a Orange
  b Green
  c Violet
  d Blue

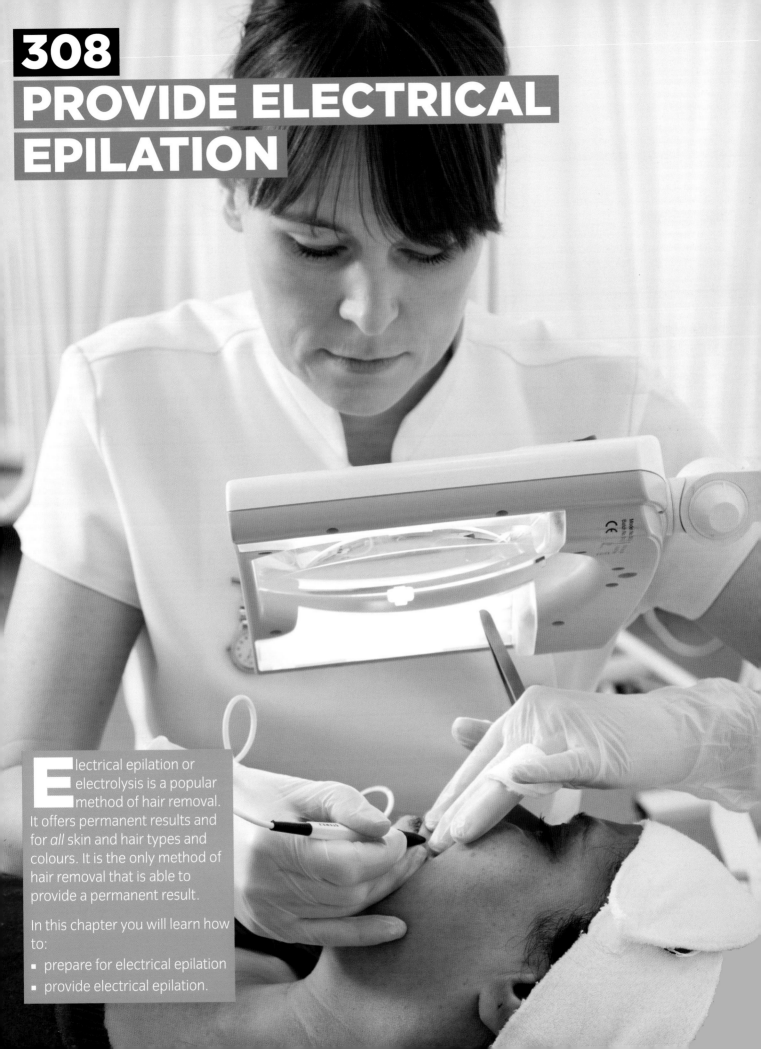

308
PROVIDE ELECTRICAL EPILATION

Electrical epilation or electrolysis is a popular method of hair removal. It offers permanent results and for *all* skin and hair types and colours. It is the only method of hair removal that is able to provide a permanent result.

In this chapter you will learn how to:

- prepare for electrical epilation
- provide electrical epilation.

WHAT IS ELECTRICAL EPILATION?

According to the *Oxford English Dictionary* electrolysis is:

- 'the chemical decomposition produced by passing an electric current through a liquid or solution containing ions'
- 'the removal of hair roots or small blemishes on the skin by the application of heat using an electric current'.

Electrical epilation involves the insertion of a very fine needle or probe down the hair follicle into the dermal papilla. An **electrical current** from an epilation machine travels down to the needle tip where the current destroys the **dermal papilla**.

Each hair needs to be treated repeatedly because each hair has its own blood supply and individual growth cycle. By repeatedly treating the blood supply to each hair its source of nourishment is reduced and the hair becomes weaker, finer and often lighter. Eventually it will stop regrowing.

Successful, effective and safe electrical epilation relies on the therapist's skill. You need to learn and practise:

- probing accuracy
- controlling and using the correct levels of current
- your chosen method of electrical epilation
- electrical epilation techniques
- releasing hairs without traction.

There are three different methods of electrical epilation:

- galvanic
- short-wave diathermy (or thermolysis)
- the blend method.

ADVANTAGES AND DISADVANTAGES OF ELECTRICAL EPILATION

Advantages	Disadvantages
Provides permanent hair removal.	Client can feel discomfort when the electrical current is applied.
Is successful on *all* types and colours of skin and hair.	Works best on small areas such as the upper lip and face.
Results in a natural look – fine downy hair can be left and only the darker unwanted, and more noticeable hairs, treated.	Results take time as each hair has to be treated individually a number of times.
Can improve clients' self-esteem and self-confidence.	

Electrical current

A flow of electrical charge. Electricity is a form of energy that is made from electrons which are part of an atom. If an atom loses or gains an electron it creates an electrical current. Please see pages 292–294 in Chapter 306/307 for further information on electrical currents

Dermal papilla

This is located inside the hair bulb. Blood vessels in the dermal papilla provide nutrients and oxygen to the epidermis. The size of the dermal papilla varies with the size, shape and growth cycle of the hair

HANDY HINT

You should refresh your knowledge of hair growth for this chapter. Please refer to pages 46–53 in the Anatomy and Physiology chapter.

LEGAL HEALTH AND SAFETY CONSIDERATIONS FOR CARRYING OUT ELECTRICAL EPILATION TREATMENTS

Any business and therapist(s) carrying out electrical epilation must register with the local authority. It will issue a certificate documenting that the business and therapist(s) have been inspected and approved to carry out this type of treatment. This is a requirement of The Local Government (Miscellaneous Provisions) Act and covers all skin piercing treatments (ie electrical epilation, ear piercing and tattooing).

The premises will be inspected by an inspector who will check to make sure that:

- the equipment is safe and relevant for use
- the equipment has been **PAT** tested
- needles and other contaminated or hazardous waste are disposed of safely and correctly
- all needles are sterile, used only once and in date
- appropriate sterilisation and sanitisation products and methods are being used for equipment and the working environment
- all products are stored correctly and safely according to the manufacturers' recommendations
- there is a washable floor surface
- there are hand washing facilities.

An environmental health officer (EHO) from the local authority will issue a certificate of authorisation if they are satisfied high standards are being maintained. By displaying this in the reception area, clients will see that the premises have been checked and approved by the local authority. The local authority will carry out further visits to ensure standards are being maintained at all times. If a salon falls below the required standards it will be issued with an improvement notice. This will state what improvements need to be made and give a timescale in which to make the improvements. If the improvements are not made, then the salon may be prosecuted and may even end up closing down.

In extreme circumstances an inspector may close the premises immediately. This is done only if they feel that there are high levels of danger and that the business needs to close to rectify them.

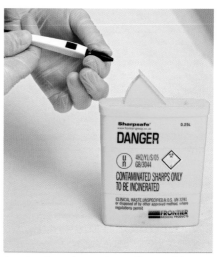

As a legal requirement, needles used in epilation must never be used more than once and should be disposed of safely

PAT testing

Portable appliance testing. Portable electrical equipment needs to inspected and tested annually for electrical safety

ACTIVITY

Contact your local authority and ask for a copy of the laws relating to skin piercing and any other specific local regulations that might apply.

INDUSTRY TIP

The three most important aspects to becoming skilled at electrical epilation are practice, practice and practice. It is a difficult skill to learn but just like riding a bike it becomes easier with practice.

In this part of the chapter you will learn about:

- preparing yourself, the client and the work area
- consultation
- skin and hair types
- contra-indications to electrical epilation treatments
- selecting products, tools and equipment for an electrical epilation treatment

PREPARATION OF THE THERAPIST

You should ensure the highest levels of hygiene, safety and professionalism when carrying out electrical epilation treatments. High standards of appearance, behaviour and attitude, and excellent communication skills are required. You need to be highly skilled and want to constantly improve your skills as electrical epilation demands greater levels of skill than many other beauty therapy techniques. It can certainly carry the most risk if not performed correctly.

You should be well presented, with:

- a clean, ironed uniform
- a tidy personal appearance, hair tied back, no false nails, no jewellery, clean fresh breath
- good personal hygiene
- enclosed flat or low-heeled shoes (for safety reasons).

PREPARATION OF THE CLIENT

Unwanted hair growth can be a cause of embarrassment to the client and can affect their whole mental and physical well-being. To protect their privacy, it is vital to carry out a detailed consultation in a quiet private location. The client will then feel able to discuss fully and openly their requirements, concerns about the treatment and their hopes and expectations. They will also feel more comfortable about showing you the area of unwanted hair growth. The more relaxed and comfortable the client is made to feel the more at ease they will be.

PREPARATION OF THE WORK AREA

The treatment room needs to be a welcoming and comfortable environment. You need to take into consideration general aspects of comfort (such as temperature, lighting, ventilation) for both you and the client. In addition, there are some special considerations for electrical epilation treatments that you must think about to make sure that treatments are performed effectively and safely.

LIGHTING

Clear and bright lighting is needed for an electrical epilation treatment as the therapist needs excellent visibility when probing the follicle.

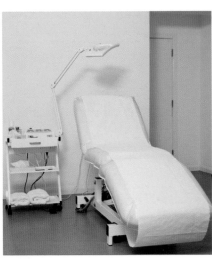

A clean and tidy work area

MUSIC

Electrolysis is not a particularly relaxing treatment; therefore relaxing music that you normally play in the salon may be played at a slightly higher level – but not too loudly. (Note: a licence is needed to play music: see page 160.)

CONSULTATION

Consultation is a vital process during which you should assess the client's needs and objectives and their suitability for the treatment. More detailed information on the consultation process and communication techniques can be found in Chapter 303 (pages 212–215 and 206–211).

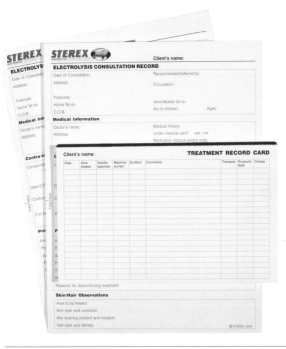

An electrolysis consultation form

- Greet the client in a warm, friendly, professional and polite manner.
- Ask the client how they wish to be referred to (ie by first name or by using their title and surname).
- Explain that all the information you are recording is strictly confidential, and will be stored in line with the Data Protection Act (see pages 152–153 in the Legislation chapter).
- Complete the client's record card with:
    - their doctor's name, address and contact details
    - a full medical history to make sure that no contra-indications will prevent you from carrying out the treatment
    - a history of the client's hair growth – eg how long the unwanted hair has been present and whether it has changed in colour or texture
    - details of any previous hair removal methods as this may mean that the treatment is contra-indicated.

HANDY HINT

It is important to ask the client how they wish to be referred to because:
- it is professional to do so
- some **transgender** clients can have strong preferences regarding gender identity.

Transgender

A transgender person is someone who feels that their gender is different from the one they were given at birth. Many transgender people know from a very early age that they do not identify with their biological gender. Some come to this conclusion much later in life; see the industry study at the end of this chapter

HANDY HINT

If they are a first-time client remember to take down their name, address and contact numbers and ask them for a date of birth rather than age.

INDUSTRY TIP

You should check thoroughly the client's medical history to see if they have any disorders of the endocrine system such as polycystic ovary syndrome. Hormone imbalances have an effect on hair growth.

LASER

Light Amplification Stimulated Emission of Radiation

IPL

Intense pulsed light

- Explain the hair growth cycle (ie anagen, catagen and telogen) to the client (see pages 50–51 of the Anatomy and Physiology chapter). By explaining the hair growth cycle, you can stress that you will be able to treat all visible hairs above the skin but there may be hairs lying dormant under the skin which may take weeks to reach the surface.

- Discuss the treatment options available and explain what electrical epilation involves. Explain the sensation that the client can expect to experience.

- Stress the importance of a course of regular treatments. Explain the duration and costs of the treatment.

- Ask the client's permission to take a photograph of the treatment area so that they can see before and after pictures and so that you can attach this to their record card.

- Give the client the record card/treatment plan to read and ask them to sign and date it.

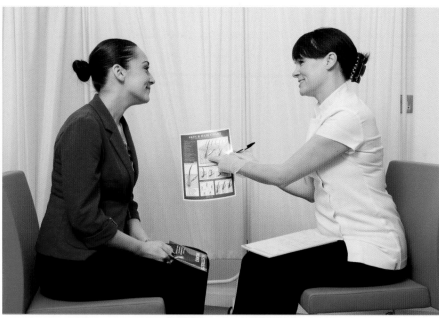

Therapist carrying out a consultation with an epilation client

SKIN AND HAIR TYPES

As part of the consultation, it is important to carry out a detailed analysis of the client's skin type and hair as these will have an impact on the electrical epilation treatment.

Skin types and conditions

The table below shows how different skin types can affect electrical epilation treatments.

WHY DON'T YOU...
design your own skin and hair chart as a visual aid to help you explain the hair growth cycle to your clients.

Insulator
Something that does not allow electrical current to pass through

Skin type/condition	Effect on electrical epilation treatments
Oily or combination skin	■ Usually has a higher level of moisture in the lower skin tissues so treatment can be very effective. ■ Has good elasticity so the hair follicles are open which makes probing easier. ■ Can be thick and coarse with pustules and papules and a disturbed pH balance so care must be taken to prevent cross-infection. ■ Sebum on the skin will act as an **insulator** to the current.
Dry or dehydrated skin	■ The epidermis may be dry or dehydrated due to the lack of sebum or moisture. ■ Found in any age group but particularly in post-menopausal women. ■ Due to build-up of skin cells within the follicle blocking the pore, needle insertion may be more difficult. ■ A lack of suppleness in the skin and hair follicles may also make needle insertion more difficult. ■ There is little sebum present on the skin so there is no insulation against current. ■ Care must be taken not to burn the client. ■ Due to the lack of moisture, higher levels of current are required to produce the best possible effect. ■ Use gold needles to make insertion easier and because they are unlikely to cause an allergic reaction. ■ Requires space to be left in between needle insertions.
Sensitive skin	■ Finely textured. ■ Reacts very quickly to the current with pronounced erythema. ■ Often found in the fine 'English rose' type skin. ■ Thin and fragile skin with dry patches but can also apply to both oily and dry skin types. ■ Often responds well to the blend method or short-wave diathermy method using an insulated or gold needle. ■ Special care is required with spacing between needle insertions and the level of current used. ■ Responds well to phoresis (see page 345) if applied before or after treatment.
Moist skin	■ High levels of moisture in the epidermis and dermis. ■ Conducts electrical current easily. ■ The current levels and intensity need to be monitored and adapted because of the ease with which it conducts electrical current. ■ The blend method is most effective because this skin type causes a faster chemical reaction to take place. ■ If short-wave diathermy is used, take care to prevent the current from backing up the follicle to the skin's surface as this causes surface burns.

Moisture gradient

The moisture gradient is the amount of moisture present in the skin and the follicle. It varies:

- throughout the epidermis
- from one area of skin to another
- from person to person.

The thicker the epidermis the more moisture there is present. In skin with a thick epidermis it is the lowest part of the follicles which tend to be the most moist. When the hair is in the anagen stage of growth, it is at its most moist as it is attached to the blood supply. The level of moisture within skin tissues will affect the methods, techniques and needles chosen.

Treatment considerations	How the moisture balance affects treatment
Treatment time	- Skin containing more moisture is more elastic and pliable resulting in a faster treatment. - Needle penetration is easier which is beneficial to both the client and therapist. - Moist skin may not be as reactive during and following treatment as other skin types so individual treatment sessions are longer which gives end results with fewer treatments.
Treatment reactions	- If there is more moisture, the skin produces more **frothing** during treatment which can appear on the surface of the skin.
Technique used	- You might use a 'blend, treat and leave' technique on skin with more moisture (see page 361). - You could use the blend method (see page 361) with the fastest and lowest levels of current.
Needles	- You would use an insulating needle with the short-wave diathermy method to prevent heat rising and causing blisters if there is too much sebum on the skin. - The diameter of the needle can be easily and accurately matched to the diameter of the hair with moist hair so insertion is easier than with dry skin. - Choose a gold needle for sensitive or dehydrated skin where insertion is more difficult due to the lack of moisture in the skin. - Gold needles reduce erythema. - Insulated needles reduce erythema and oedema by preventing the heat rising. They are suitable for use with short-wave diathermy.

Ethnic groups

Different ethnic groups possess different skin tones, skin types and hair growth (eg type, shape, depth and amount of hair growth). This will impact directly on electrical epilation treatments. Each skin type (Caucasian (white), Afro-Caribbean, Asian oriental and Mediterranean (olive)) skins should be treated individually on their own merits.

Afro-Caribbean skin

Whenever possible use the blend or galvanic methods so that the heat produced is kept to a minimum and doesn't cause any pigmentation issues.

- Hair growth is usually curly or distorted so short-wave diathermy would not be suitable.
- Use a two-piece gold needle for accuracy and sensitivity.
- If short-wave diathermy is the only method available for use, use an insulated needle so that the current is concentrated at the tip of the needle. This reduces the chance of a surface reaction.
- Afro-Caribbean skin is extremely sensitive to heat but it is very difficult to detect erythema. Therefore, you should perform short treatments and needle insertions should be spread out to prevent over-heating the skin tissue.

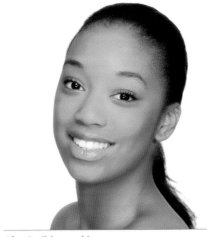

Afro-Caribbean skin

Asian and Mediterranean skin

- Use the blend method in combination with a gold needle to avoid sensitivity and adverse reactions.
- If short-wave diathermy is used, use the minimum levels of intensity possible and an insulated needle to reduce surface reaction.
- Asian/olive skin can be sensitive to heat and may have pigmentation variations.
- It can be difficult to detect erythema so short and well-spaced insertions are recommended.
- Avoid over-treatment of the area and allow sufficient time in between appointments for healing.

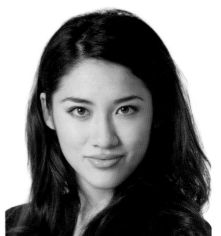

Asian skin

Oriental skin

- Oriental skin is prone to pigmentation marks and can become **pitted** if over-exposed to heat.
- It is sensitive so a gold needle should be used if possible.
- It can be difficult to detect erythema so short and well-spaced insertions are recommended.
- Leave sufficient time in between appointments.
- The pores are often small and tight so a small-sized short needle (size 2 or 3) is usually required (see page 357).

Oriental skin

Pitted
Having hollow indentations

Types of hair and hair growth rate

The type of hair and hair growth rate will affect the method of electrical epilation you use and the intensity and timing of the treatment. There are three types of hair:

- lanugo
- vellus
- terminal.

Within each of these types, the hair can be curly, straight or have compound hairs (see page 343).

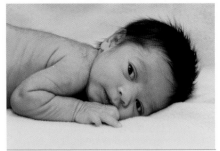

Lanugo hair on the back of a newborn baby

Vellus hair

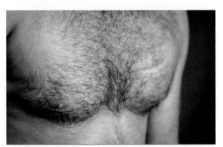

Terminal hair on a man's chest

Medulla
The innermost layer of the hair. It is made up of loose connected **keratinised** cells. The medulla is not always present. It can be **intermittent** or continuous within the hair which creates air pockets that reflect light and give the hair its sheen

Keratinised
Describing cells that have become hard, flat and dead. This is caused by the production of a protein called keratin and the **degeneration** of the nucleus of each cell

Intermittent
Occurring irregularly

Degeneration
Deterioration

Anagen
The active growth stage in the hair growth cycle

308 PROVIDE ELECTRICAL EPILATION

Lanugo hair
This is soft fine hair that covers a baby in the womb. It disappears a few months after birth and is replaced by vellus hair. Lanugo hair does not have a **medulla**.

Vellus hair
This is the fine, soft downy hair that is found all over the body with the exception of the palm of the hands and soles of the feet. These hairs do not usually grow more than 2cm in length. Generally they do not contain a medulla or dermal papilla unless they develop into terminal hairs (eg as a result of a medical condition).

Terminal hair
At birth this type of hair is found on the scalp, eyelashes and eyebrows. During hormone changes (ie puberty) terminal hair can replace vellus hair in certain areas. This type of hair is coarse and long. It has a well-developed root and bulb with a strong blood supply. The hair follicle extends deep into the dermis during **anagen** growth. Terminal hair is visible:

- on the scalp
- under the arms
- on the legs
- in the bikini line area
- on the face.

Terminal hair has three layers:
- cuticle
- cortex
- medulla.

Terminal hair can be subdivided into three types:
1 asexual: terminal hair that is present at birth
2 ambisexual: terminal hair growth at puberty
3 sexual: eg hair growth due to the male hormone androgen.

Hair growth rates
The rate of hair growth/regrowth will have an effect on the frequency of treatments. The rate of hair growth/regrowth varies depending on the type of hair, area of growth and hormonal factors, for example. The table below gives some average rates of growth/regrowth – but note this can vary considerably from individual to individual.

> **HANDY HINT**
> You might want to recap on the hair growth cycle by referring to pages 50–51 of the Anatomy and Physiology chapter.

Type of hair	F = Female M = Male	Regrowth time
Upper lip (vellus)	F	8–9 weeks
Upper lip (terminal)	F/M	4–6 weeks
Chin (vellus)	F	6–7 weeks
Chin (terminal)	F/M	5–6 weeks
Bikini line (terminal)	F	5–6 weeks
Eyebrows	F/M	5–6 weeks
Underarms (terminal)	F/M	7–8 weeks
Neck/nape (terminal)	F/M	5–6 weeks
Breast (terminal)	F	7–8 weeks
Chest (terminal)	M	6–7 weeks
Abdomen (terminal)	F	8–9 weeks
Fingers, toes (terminal)	F/M	6–8 weeks

Types of hair growth

The type of hair growth will influence:

- the method of electrical epilation
- the intensity of treatment
- the timing of the treatment.

Compound hairs

A compound hair is where the hair follicle has two or more dermal papillae. As a result at least two hairs grow from the same follicle. When using a direct current (either galvanic or blend), treat the larger hair with the current as this may affect both hairs. If only the larger hair is removed, and you are using the blend method, after completion of the treatment try to remove the hair gently using tweezers. If you are unable to remove the hair using tweezers, assess the condition of the skin and treat it again if appropriate.

Tombstone hairs

A tombstone hair is one that has been epilated during the early anagen stage before it has reached the skin's surface and therefore remains trapped in the skin. When a telogen hair is removed, the follicle can therefore sometimes contain a trapped anagen or tombstone hair. Tombstone hairs are dark and thick in appearance and don't have a root bulb. Tombstone hairs may just lift from the follicle with no traction and often don't require electrical epilation.

Embedded hairs

The hair doesn't come through the skin and remains embedded in the skin. These can be seen as small bumps on the skin. Embedded hairs are caused by friction on dry skin (eg tight-fitting clothes rubbing an area). If the hair is not infected, ease the hair out so that it is showing on the skin's surface. Epilate if appropriate. Allow the natural hair growth and healing processes to take place.

INDUSTRY TIP

It is important to choose the correct electrical epilation method for each type of hair (vellus and terminal) and each type of hair growth (ie fine, curly, straight, single or compound) as it will affect the success of the treatment.

HANDY HINT

Compound hair growth is also known as pili multigemini.

Ingrowing hairs

Ingrowing hairs grow under the surface of the skin. They can be caused by hair breakage, friction or dead skin cells blocking the pore. If the hair is not infected treat it in the same way as an embedded hair.

Curly hairs

The hair follicle has been distorted by waxing or plucking or is naturally curly or curved. The only electrical epilation methods that will offer successful results are the galvanic or blend methods. Lye (or sodium hydroxide), which is a liquid formed by the chemical process that takes place during epilation, can flow around the curves of the follicle.

Hypertrichosis

Hypertrichosis causes **superfluous** hair growth. It is the excessive growth of coarse, terminal hair for a particular age, gender and race. It can affect both men and women and describes a general overgrowth of terminal hair affecting the entire body surface. Not considered hormone dependent it results primarily from ethnic or genetic predisposition to hair growth.

Causes of hypertrichosis are:

- genetics/hereditary factors – hereditary tendency for heavy hair growth
- not hormone dependent.

Hirsutism

Hirsutism is excessive hair growth on the face and body, usually in females. It may also be accompanied by other male characteristics. It is caused by an excess of the male sex hormone, androgen, in the blood. This causes **dormant** hair follicles to grow hair and existing vellus and terminal hairs to grow larger. It often occurs where there is a hormonal imbalance (eg tumour of the adrenal or pituitary glands), ovarian problems or the menopause.

Causes of hirsutism include:

- stress, anxiety and worry
- hormonal imbalance
- natural hormonal changes (eg puberty, pregnancy and the menopause)
- disease or disorders of the endocrine system:
  - conditions affecting endocrine glands (eg pituitary, thyroid or adrenal) or tumours or cysts on certain endocrine glands
  - removal or partial removal of certain glands, eg hysterectomy or the removal of one ovary
- drugs – reaction to certain drugs (eg cortisone or testosterone)
- problems with the ovaries (eg polycystic ovary syndrome)
- systemic illness.

Changes in hair growth

Hair growth and changes in hair growth can be caused by a number of different factors such as:

- **congenital** factors
- topical stimulation
- systemic changes.

Superfluous

Unwanted hair growth. It doesn't necessarily mean excessive hair growth

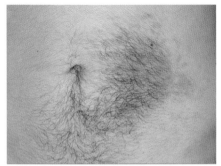

Hypertrichosis on the abdomen of a young man

Dormant

Inactive

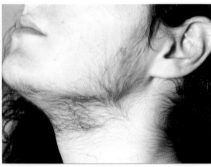

Hirsutism

HANDY HINT

Unwanted hair growth can be divided into two categories:

- hypertrichosis – due to genetic or racial factors which make an individual more likely to have heavy growth
- hirsutism – due to factors affecting the endocrine system which alter the hormone balance in the body.

  Note: hirsutism can be broken down into two further types:

  1 normal systemic
  2 abnormal systemic (see page 345).

Congenital

Present from birth

Congenital factors

Genetics will determine hair growth, hair colour and the type and the amount of hair we have.

Topical stimulation

Topical stimulation (eg plucking, threading and waxing of hormonally influenced areas) can cause excess hair growth over time, as can friction, eg from plaster casts.

Systemic changes

Normal systemic hair growth can be stimulated by hormonal changes. Abnormal systemic hair growth are primarily endocrine disorders: see the table below.

Normal hair growth	Abnormal hair growth
Puberty	Cushing's syndrome
Pregnancy	Achard-Thiers syndrome
Menopause	Adrenogenital syndrome
Medication (eg contraceptive pill, antidepressants)	Acromegaly
Stress	Polycystic ovary syndrome
	Anorexia nervosa

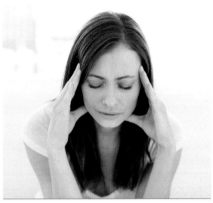

Stress can cause hormonal changes leading to hair growth

ANAPHORESIS AND CATAPHORESIS

Anaphoresis can be used as a preparatory treatment and cataphoresis can be used as an aftercare procedure.

Procedure	Description	Effect
Anaphoresis	■ A roller or electrode acts as a negative electrode on skin. This causes production of sodium hydroxide (or lye) which is alkaline. ■ Lye causes vasodilation of the blood vessels – brings blood, fluid and nutrients to the upper layers of the skin.	■ Opens pores. ■ Relaxes the tissues. ■ Increases erythema. ■ Makes insertions easier.
Cataphoresis	■ A positive electrode is used on the skin. ■ Creates a mild acidic reaction. ■ Neutralises the lye created during anaphoresis. ■ Causes vasoconstriction.	■ Closes pores. ■ Calms inflammation. ■ Soothes nerve endings. ■ Restores natural pH. ■ Has a **germicidal** effect on the skin.

Germicidal

Destroys germs

CONTRA-INDICATIONS TO ELECTRICAL EPILATION TREATMENTS

In addition to general contra-indications given on page 215 in Chapter 303, the following conditions will prevent an electrical epilation treatment taking place unless medical approval has been given.

Contra-indication	Restricts/prevents	Reason
Cardiovascular conditions	Prevents unless GP referral given	■ Conditions and medications are complex and varied. ■ GP referral needs to be obtained prior to treatment.
Pacemakers	Prevents	■ High frequency currents may affect the rhythm of a pacemaker. ■ In the worst case scenario this might result in a cardiac arrest. ■ Some models are insulated and may allow treatment but written approval from the GP and manufacturer is required.
Haemophilia	Prevents treatment of male clients	■ Male haemophiliacs' blood does not clot so if the skin is pierced it will not stop bleeding. ■ The blood of female carriers of haemophilia clots normally so they are not contra-indicated.
HIV or AIDS (human immunodeficiency virus or acquired immunodeficiency syndrome)	Prevents	■ Carries a high risk of cross-infection. ■ The body's ability to heal is restricted. ■ No insurance cover available.
Hepatitis A and B	Prevents	■ Chances of cross-contamination are high.
Roaccutane (acne medication)	Prevents	■ The medication has a thinning and peeling effect on the skin. ■ Electrical epilation should not be given for six months after the client has finished taking it due to skin sensitivity. ■ Even after six months, the skin could still be sensitive so take more care with current levels.
Keloid scars	Prevents	■ Electrical epilation could make the problem worse.
Bacterial, viral and fungal infections (eg bacterial (impetigo), viral (herpes simplex) and fungal (ringworm))	Restricts – prevents if in area to be treated.	■ Risk of cross-infection. ■ Skin is not healthy.
Other skin conditions (eg acne, psoriasis, eczema, cuts, abrasions)	Prevents/restricts	■ Risk of cross-infection from open wounds. ■ Skin is not healthy.
Bruising, swelling, oedema, sunburn	Prevents/restricts	■ Risk of further skin damage.

Contra-indication	Restricts/prevents	Reason
Diabetes	Prevents unless controlled by diet. If client is taking any medication for diabetes this will prevent treatment.	• Diabetic's skin heals at a slower rate. • The client is more prone to infection. • GP permission may be required.
Epilepsy	Prevents/restricts	• Electrical current could trigger an epileptic fit. • If controlled by medication and GP approval has been given, treatment may proceed with care.
Loss of sensation (eg from Bell's palsy, stroke, desensitised nerves)	Restricts	• Lack of feeling means the client is unable to give feedback regarding sensation. • Skin could potentially be over-treated or damaged.
Anticoagulant drugs (eg warfarin, heparin or asthma)	Prevents	• Might slow the healing process. • Risk of blood spotting as blood thinners prevent treatment.
Steroid medication (applied to skin or taken by mouth eg asthma inhalers)	Restricts	• Steroid medication might thin the skin. • Skin might be very sensitive. • Take care when selecting the amount of current and method to use.
Cancer	Prevents	• Radiotherapy and chemotherapy affect the immune system. • The rate of healing is affected. • More vulnerable to infection. • Most state that cancer remains a contra-indication for three to five years following the 'all-clear'.
Metal plates/pins	Prevents/restricts	• If present near the treatment area they could cause a galvanic burn due to a build-up of heat in the metal plate or pin.
Minor/young person	Prevents/restricts	• Currently, parental consent and GP approval are required if under 16 years of age (in the UK) and 18 years of age (in Scotland). • Hormonal imbalances can correct themselves during adolescence and hair growth will be affected.
Pregnancy	Restricts	• Hair growth can change during pregnancy due to the hormonal imbalances. • Excessive growth may disappear naturally as the hormones stabilise. • Do not treat abdominal areas or breast areas because of increased tenderness and swelling. • Do not use the blend method below the décolletage due to the direct current movement pattern through the body. • Do not treat during the first trimester (the first three months) because the foetus is still in the very early stages of development.

Contra-indication	Restricts/prevents	Reason
Moles	Prevents unless qualified in advanced electrolysis at Level 4	▪ Due to potentially increased melanoma risks electrical epilation is not recommended.
Hearing aid implants	Prevents/restricts – implants prevent treatment, detachable hearing aids restrict treatment	▪ Electrical currents may disable and damage hearing devices implanted deep within the ear.
Phlebitis/thrombosis/ varicose veins	Restricts	▪ Treatment can be adapted to avoid the affected area. ▪ If treatment is required on the affected area the condition should be treated by a medical practitioner prior to treatment.
Dermographia (sensitivity to skin friction)	Prevents/restricts	▪ Could cause severe swelling of the tissues during and after treatment. ▪ Treatment would depend on the severity of the condition and the area to be treated.
Lupus	Prevents	▪ Skin healing will be compromised.

Anti-coagulant

Drugs that prevent the blood from thickening

Dermographia

A sensitivity to any form of skin friction. Sufferers are usually born with the condition

Lupus

An incurable illness where the immune system produces far too many antibodies which circulate through the bloodstream. The antibodies cause reactions that result in inflammation. It is mainly suffered by females. Two major symptoms are joint and muscle pain and a constant feeling of extreme tiredness

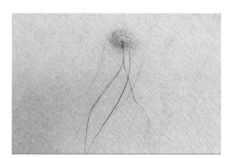

Hairs on moles can only be treated by therapists qualified at Level 4

INDUSTRY TIP

The advanced electrolysis qualification covers treatment of hairs in moles.

INDUSTRY TIP

If you notice any changes to a mole, advise the client to seek medical advice.

HANDY HINT

If a client is wearing a hearing aid, they should remove it prior to treatment otherwise it will give off a high-pitched noise. Remember that the client will be temporarily deaf.

INDUSTRY TIP

As an extra precaution it is recommended that therapists working in an at-risk environment have a hepatitis vaccination from their doctor.

ADAPTING THE TREATMENT

There are many conditions (eg non-medicated diabetes and skin that is hypersensitive or dehydrated skin weakened by chemical peels or medication) that are not necessarily contra-indications.

You need to make a judgement call and a professional decision based on the facts of each individual client. It may be that a GP referral is all that is needed to meet the requirements of the insurance company. You could also consider different ways of modifying the treatment, eg:

▪ carrying out treatments over a longer time scale

▪ a shorter treatment time

▪ greater spacing between individually treated hairs

▪ different methods and techniques.

For example, a cold sore is infectious and therefore a contra-indication. However, if a client requires electrical epilation in the bikini line area or under the arm, this would not be a contra-indication. Even the neck area could be treated although great care should be taken if working on the chin as contamination and cross-contamination is a real possibility. You should also consider healing after the treatment. If the client has a cold sore then they may be generally unwell which might affect their recovery from the treatment.

PRODUCTS FOR ELECTRICAL EPILATION TREATMENTS

PRE-CARE PRODUCTS

Pre-care products are used to clean and sanitise the area prior to treatment.

Pre-care product	Use
Skin sanitiser	▪ Ensures that the treatment area is clean and free of germs prior to treatment.
Antiseptic wipes	▪ Individually wrapped antiseptic wipes for cleaning the treatment area.
Hand sanitiser	▪ Water- and soap-free antibacterial handwash. ▪ Can be used to 'wash' gloved hands to ensure high standards of cleanliness.

AFTERCARE PRODUCTS

Aftercare products soothe the treatment area after treatment. They are designed to prevent infection and assist with the healing process.

Aftercare product	Use
Gels/lotions/creams	▪ Some prevent infection (eg witch hazel and creams containing triclosan). ▪ Others aid healing (eg aloe vera). ▪ Gels are most popular and are easy to apply. ▪ Creams are easily absorbed into the skin. ▪ Cooling on the skin. ▪ Can and should be purchased by client for continued use at home.
Tinted creams	▪ Reduce the appearance of erythema which may result following treatment.

EQUIPMENT AND TOOLS

Equipment/tools	Description/use
Couch 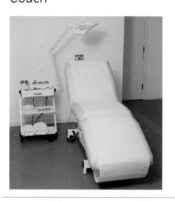	▪ Adjustable therapy couch. ▪ Protected with couch roll. ▪ Make sure your posture is correct and comfortable. ▪ Make sure the client is positioned correctly and comfortably.
Trolley 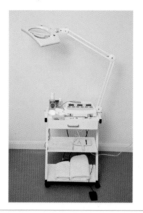	▪ Clean trolley. ▪ Set up in an organised way for treatment. ▪ Trolley should have sufficient space for all your tools and equipment.
Autoclave 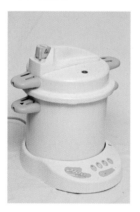	▪ For sterilising metal tools/equipment. ▪ Uses steam to sterilise equipment. ▪ After a treatment, wash equipment (eg tweezers and chuck caps) with hot soapy water (a soft toothbrush is ideal) to remove any microscopic particles of tissue fluids, inner root sheaths or skin cells that may have become attached to the instruments. ▪ Then rinse and place into the autoclave for sterilising.
Magnifying lamp 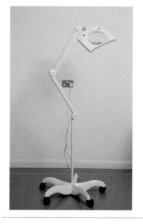	▪ Essential for clear vision. ▪ Magnifies and illuminates the treatment area. ▪ Enlarges the appearance of the hair and pores which helps with getting the correct insertion angle. ▪ Acts as a barrier between the client and therapist protecting the therapist from any splatters of blood or body fluids when working in intimate areas.

INDUSTRY TIP

A good-quality magnifying lamp is worth its weight in gold. The eye muscles are the only muscles that do not improve and tone with exercise. They can become strained resulting in dry eyes, headaches and deterioration of the eyesight.

Equipment/tools	Description/use
Epilation unit 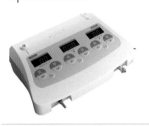	■ Produces an electrical current, either short-wave diathermy, galvanic or a blend of both.
Electrode 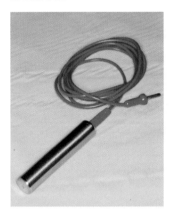	■ A metal bar (a positive/indifferent electrode) attached to the epilation unit. ■ Needed to complete an electrical circuit if using the galvanic or blend method.
Needle holder (switched and unswitched) 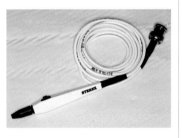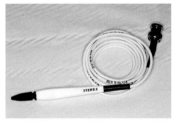	■ The needle holder is the means by which the current travels down the needle. ■ There are two types: switched or unswitched. ■ Switched needle holders are controlled by a button that is operated by the index finger. ■ Unswitched needle holders are controlled by use of a foot pedal.
Chuck caps 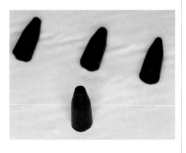	■ Used with some needle holder designs. ■ They fit on the top of the needle holder and holds the shaft of the needle in place. ■ Made from a mixture of ground glass and plastic (so can be put into an autoclave).

HANDY HINT

Refer back to Chapter 306/307 for information on electrical currents and electrodes.

HANDY HINT

Occasionally the chuck cap opening can shrink when it is put in an autoclave. This makes it difficult to load two-piece needles. Using pointed tweezers, gently place the closed tweezer tips into the chuck cap opening and make small circular movements to gently enlarge the opening. Chuck cap openings stretch fairly easily with a little pressure.

308 PROVIDE ELECTRICAL EPILATION

Equipment/tools	Description/use
Needles A two-piece needle	- Minute, highly polished medical grade stainless steel probes. - Inserted into the hair follicle. - Electrical current passes down the needle when the current is released once it meets the dermal papilla. - Vary in length, type, material and sizes. - You need to select the most suitable needle for the area being worked on.
Sharps box 	- A yellow-coloured secure container for disposal of used needles and contaminated waste. - Needles and contaminated waste are collected by a special company that is licensed to dispose of and incinerate the waste.
Epilation tweezers 	- Have a fine point allowing them to target specific hairs (eg to pick up an individual dark hair which has been epilated from a dense batch of lighter hair). - Have a few pairs of high-quality tweezers available to allow you to continue treatments whilst those you have already used are sterilised.
Gloves 	- Non-latex and powder-free gloves. - Protects the therapist and client from any contamination which may occur due to blood-spot/needle-stick injuries.
Consumables (eg cotton wool, tissues, face masks) 	- Needed throughout the treatment.

Equipment/tools	Description/use
Sanitiser 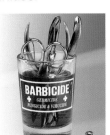	■ Fluid used for keeping instruments (eg tweezers) sterile.
Towels 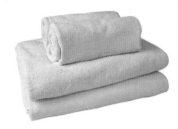	■ To cover the client to keep them warm. ■ To protect the client's modesty.
Mirror 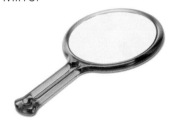	■ For use in consultation before treatment and to show client results after the treatment. ■ Ideally should have magnification function.

HANDY HINT

Refer back to the consultation section on pages 337–338 to remind yourself about the importance of using a mirror for electrical epilation treatments.

NEEDLE HOLDERS

The needle holder is the means by which the current travels down the needle.

There are two main types of needle holder:

■ switched
■ unswitched.

Switched needle holder

Switched needle holders are controlled by a button that is operated with the index finger. When the button is pressed, the current is able to flow.

The benefit is that the current remains in the needle holder and is quick to flow when the button is pressed.

Unswitched needle holders

Unswitched needle holders are controlled by use of a foot pedal. When the foot pedal is pressed, the current is able to flow. The needle holder is a smooth pen (with no button).

The benefits of this type of holder are:

■ the hand remains totally steady as no movement is required (ie the index finger is not required to press the button)

INDUSTRY TIP

Hair retardant products are also available. These are designed to slow down hair growth and regrowth. Some clients find these helpful but if they stop using them regularly the hair will grow back.

INDUSTRY TIP

Some needle holders have detachable cables. Needle holders and cables should be treated with care. Always have spare ones to hand as their lifespan is limited when in constant use.

HANDY HINT

Cables are manufactured with BNC (Bayonet Neill Concelman) connectors to fit specific brands of machines or with banana-style connectors to fit older-style machines or different brands.

- less risk of repetitive strain injury, carpal tunnel syndrome or other similar hand and arm conditions as there is no hand movement
- the needle holder can be held in a more flexible way for use in areas that are hard to reach.

Most modern epilators have the option of using both.

CHUCK CAPS

Chuck caps are caps which are screwed gently onto the tip of the needle holder. They protect the shank of the needle and hold the needle in place during treatment. They are usually made from ground glass and plastic which means they can be placed in an autoclave as they are able to withstand its heat.

The following steps show how to load a needle into the needle holder.

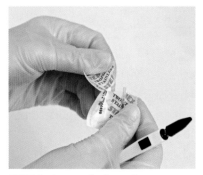

STEP 1 – Loosen chuck cap. Tear open needle packet and withdraw, holding the plastic protective sleeve.

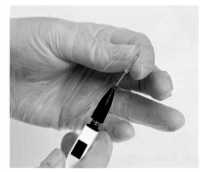

STEP 2 – The needle, together with its protective sleeve, is inserted fully into the chuck and needle holder.

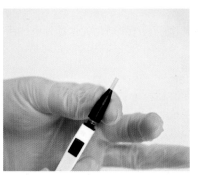

STEP 3 – Tighten the chuck cap, observing the depth of the loaded needle and reposition it as required.

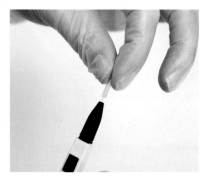

STEP 4 – Once the chuck cap is fully tightened, recover the plastic sleeve with a twist and a pull.

NEEDLES

Needles are available in different sizes, lengths and types. They are made from stainless steel and can then be coated with either 24-carat gold or a medical-grade insulation material.

All epilation needles come pre-sterilised and are disposable. They are packaged in individual wrappers which show the:

- batch number
- size of the needle
- use-by date.

Some needles are sterilised by gamma radiation while others are sterilised with ethylene oxide gas. Most have a five-year shelf life.

All needles have a:

- shank
- shaft
- tip.

Shank

This is the large metal section that is inserted into the needle holder. It conducts the current.

Shaft

This is the wire needle that is inserted into the hair follicle. It is smooth and highly polished to allow easy insertion.

Tip

This is the smooth rounded part of the needle. This is the first part of the needle to enter the hair follicle.

TYPES OF NEEDLE

The majority of needles are manufactured from medical-grade stainless steel which is strong, smooth, rust free and can be easily polished.

One-piece needles

These are manufactured from one piece of metal and are more rigid than two-piece needles. They are ideal for **advanced electrolysis** and for use by experienced electrolysists. They are not usually recommended for hair removal. However they can be useful when treating fine vellus hairs with short insertions or for use on very straight hair follicles. The needle narrows towards the end which allows a higher concentration of current at the tip.

Two-piece needles

Two-piece needles are made from two pieces of metal. The needle wire is pulled through the length of the shank and the two pieces are crimped together. This type of needle is strong and flexible. Two-piece needles flex when they meet resistance which allows the therapist to judge the accuracy of their insertion.

Two-piece needles are available in different shaft lengths – short is 0.48cm and regular is 0.63cm. The length is shown on the packaging with an S for short or R for regular.

They are also available in different shank sizes – F and K. F is the standard size in the UK and has a larger diameter than K.

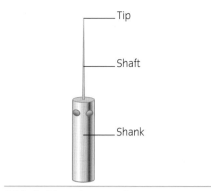

A labelled two-piece needle

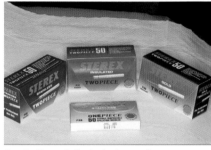

A selection of electrolysis needles

Advanced electrolysis
The treatment of skin blemishes such as facial thread veins, skin tags and spider naevi

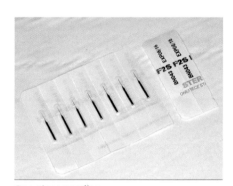

One-piece needles

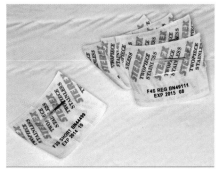

Two-piece needles

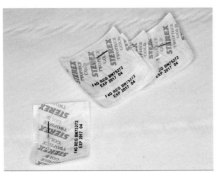
Gold needles

Hypoallergenic

Unlikely to cause allergic reaction

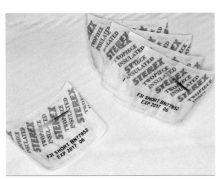
Insulated needles

Gold needles

A gold needle is a stainless steel needle that is coated with 24-carat gold. The benefits of gold needles are:

- Smoother insertion – gold is a very smooth metal which allows the needle to glide into the follicle. This results in less erythema and more comfort for the client.
- A more comfortable treatment – gold is a good conductor of electricity which sometimes allows the current to be reduced, resulting in less erythema and a more comfortable treatment for the client.
- Gold is **hypoallergenic** and therefore suitable for those with allergies to other metals and those with sensitive skins.
- Reduced trauma to the skin so healing is quicker.
- Results can be achieved more quickly – as the treatment is more comfortable for the client, each treatment session can last for a longer amount of time. As a result, fewer sessions are required and results are achieved in a shorter amount of time.
- Flexibility for the client – as there is less erythema, the client can book a treatment at a time that suits them without fear of obvious erythema afterwards.

> **HANDY HINT**
> As there is less erythema with a gold needle, a client will be more likely to follow the correct aftercare advice and less likely to use inappropriate products to cover up the erythema after their treatment.

> **HANDY HINT**
> Offering gold needles will contribute to profitability. Gold is slightly more expensive than stainless steel so a small additional charge will help with making a healthy profit.

Insulated needles

Insulated needles are stainless steel needles that are coated with a medical-grade insulation material. Only the tip of the needle is left exposed. They are recommended for use on sensitive skin. They are only suitable for use with short-wave diathermy as the insulation material deteriorates if it comes in contact with the lye (sodium hydroxide) produced in the galvanic and blend methods. The benefits of using insulated needles include the following:

- They prevent the heat generated in short-wave diathermy from rising up the needle to the surface of the skin. Instead the heat stays at the base of the hair follicle where it is required.
- A more comfortable treatment – the treatment is more comfortable because the heat does not rise to the surface of the skin.
- Less erythema on the surface of the skin as the heat is kept at the base of the hair follicle.
- Faster healing time – skin trauma is limited to the area of treatment and minimal.

NEEDLE DIAMETERS

It is important to ensure that you use the correct diameter of needle to make sure that the treatment is effective. The diameter of the needle must be equal to the diameter of the hair that is being treated. The diameter of the needle affects the heating pattern produced at the tip. Therefore it is very important to select the correct needle size.

Through experience you will learn which needle to use on each type of hair. To begin with it is easy to just look at the hair and place the needle next to it. If you select a needle that is too large it will not fit comfortably into a smaller hair follicle.

Needles are available in six different sizes (diameters):

Needle size	Use
2	Used on fine, vellus, facial hair.
3	Used for fine, shallow, terminal facial hair.
4	Used for average terminal hairs on the face and body.
5	Suitable for use on coarse terminal hair. Most commonly used on the body.
6	Used on thick, coarse hair (eg pubic hair).
10	Not used for hair removal. Used for advanced electrolysis techniques.

WHY DON'T YOU ...

treat one side of an upper lip with a stainless steel needle and the other side of the upper lip with a gold needle. Compare:

- the skin reaction
- how easy each insertion was.

Make a note of the client's comments about sensitivity and feel.

HANDY HINT

The smaller the size of needle, the thinner it is.

HANDY HINT

Size information is clearly stated on needle packaging.

HANDY HINT

The size is the diameter of the needle in thousandths of an inch, eg size 3 is three thousandths of an inch in diameter.

INDUSTRY TIP

Needle stick injuries

In the event of a needle stick injury you should:

- remove gloves and apply pressure at the point of the injury to encourage bleeding
- immerse the area in warm running water as soon as possible and wash it thoroughly with antibacterial soap
- dress the area to cover and protect the wound
- apply a fresh pair of disposable gloves before continuing with further treatment
- load a new needle and chuck cap
- dispose of any blood waste in the yellow clinical waste bin
- record the injury in the salon's accident book
- visit your doctor for further advice if required.

INDUSTRY TIP

For safe effective treatment the diameter of the needle needs to match the diameter of the hair. It might therefore be necessary during the course of the treatment to change the needle for a larger or smaller size.

In this part of the chapter you will learn about:

- methods of electrical epilation
- probing techniques
- how to carry out an electrical epilation treatment
- contra-actions to electrical epilation treatments
- home-care and aftercare advice for electrical epilation treatments.

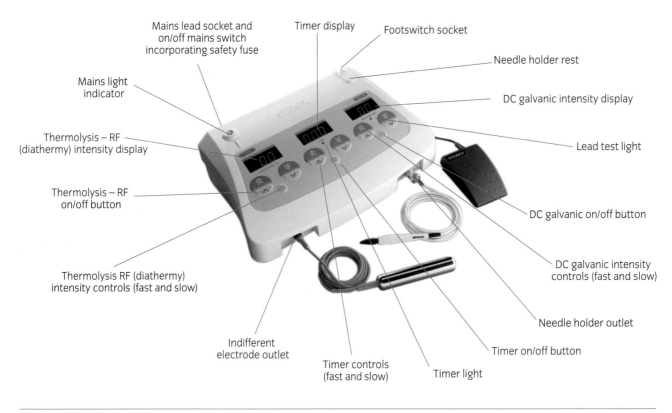

Mains lead socket and on/off mains switch incorporating safety fuse

Timer display

Footswitch socket

Needle holder rest

Mains light indicator

DC galvanic intensity display

Thermolysis – RF (diathermy) intensity display

Lead test light

Thermolysis – RF on/off button

DC galvanic on/off button

Thermolysis RF (diathermy) intensity controls (fast and slow)

DC galvanic intensity controls (fast and slow)

Needle holder outlet

Indifferent electrode outlet

Timer on/off button

Timer controls (fast and slow)

Timer light

An epilator

METHODS OF ELECTRICAL EPILATION

There are three methods of electrical epilation:

- galvanic (uses direct current)
- short-wave diathermy or thermolysis (uses an alternating current)
- blend (uses a mixture of direct current and alternating current).

The method chosen will depend on the client's hair and skin type. Electrical epilation is only effective when the hair is in the anagen stage of hair growth (ie the active growth stage where the dermal papilla is still attached to the blood supply).

The initial method may change over a course of treatments. During a course a variety of methods can be used for their different benefits – either at the same time on the same area or on different areas of the face or body.

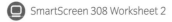 SmartScreen 308 Worksheet 2

GALVANIC METHOD

Galvanic epilation uses a direct current (see page 293 in Chapter 306/307) that flows from a positive electrode to a negative electrode. During galvanic epilation the client needs to hold an **indifferent electrode** to complete the electrical circuit. The needle holder is the negative electrode (cathode) and the indifferent electrode is the positive electrode (anode).

When a direct current is passed through the saline solution (water (H_2O) and salt ($NaCl$)) found in the hair follicle, the salt and water break down into their chemical elements and form different substances. These substances are:

- sodium hydroxide ($NaOH$)
- chlorine gas (Cl_2)
- hydrogen gas (H_2).

Sodium hydroxide (also known as lye) is a caustic agent that causes tissue destruction. It is the lye that destroys the hair bulb and cuts off the blood supply to the hair. The amount of lye needed varies according to the hair type. Fine hairs are likely to require about 15 units of lye and very coarse hairs may require 80 units of lye.

This method of electrical epilation was the first method used and is very effective but slow. Each hair takes a minimum of ten seconds to treat.

Indifferent electrode

The electrode held by the client that completes the circuit

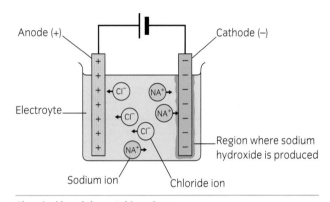

Chemical breakdown taking place

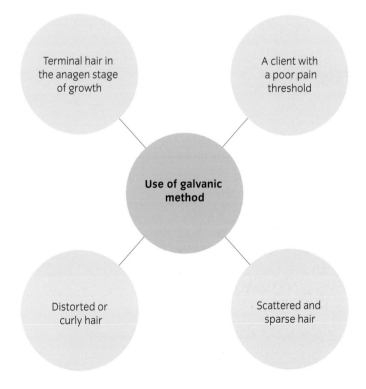

HANDY HINT

If a client has a poor pain threshold, the galvanic method can be used at a low level of current over a longer time (eg 30–60 seconds per hair) for a more comfortable treatment.

Alternating current

Current that changes direction – it flows one way and then in the opposite direction

Coagulation

Turning a liquid into a solid

SHORT-WAVE DIATHERMY METHOD

Short-wave diathermy uses an **alternating current** with very high frequency (2–30MHz or 2–30 million cycles per second) and low voltage (see page 292 in Chapter 306/307). The high-frequency current creates vibrations which agitate (or disturb) the tissues. This agitation within the tissues causes friction which produces heat. It is the build-up of heat at the base of the hair follicle that causes the destruction (**coagulation**) of the tissue.

Short-wave diathermy is the fastest method of electrical epilation but said to be the least effective. It is precise and is focused on the dermal papilla so it doesn't damage any surrounding tissue.

INDUSTRY TIP

Short-wave diathermy is a good method to use on a new client before the regrowth pattern is established and because the hairs being treated are unlikely to be in the anagen growth stage.

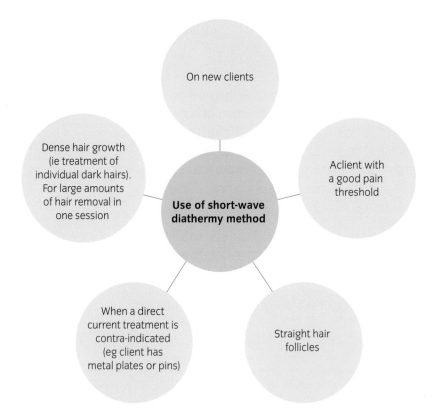

The reaction of an alternating current on the skin (as used in the short-wave diathermy or thermolysis method of electrolysis) follows a pattern starting with the current and ending with either coagulation or cauterisation of the tissues as the flow chart below illustrates. To achieve a safe treatment, with no detrimental effect on the skin, the desired result in hair removal is coagulation of the dermal papilla, which when repeatedly treated in this way results in the eventual destruction of the hair. Cauterisation is used in advanced electrolysis techniques to achieve highly specific and desired results.

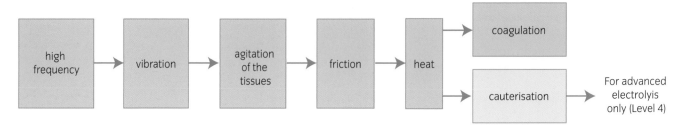

BLEND METHOD

This is a mixture of both short-wave diathermy (alternating current) and galvanic (direct current). Lye is produced as a result of the direct current used in galvanic and the alternating current used in short-wave diathermy produces heat. The heat speeds up the reaction of the lye. As lye is heated it becomes more effective and is capable of reaching every part of the lower hair follicle.

There are three different treatment techniques that can be used with the blend method:

- a higher level of current for a shorter period of time (ie relatively high levels of current for five seconds)
- a lower level of current for a longer period of time (ie slightly lower levels of current for six seconds or more)
- 'treat and leave'.

HANDY HINT

'Treat and leave' technique

A group of hairs is treated and then left for a while before removal. Using a low level of current, treat the hairs in one area. Leave them in the follicle to allow the lye to take effect and repeat this part of the procedure in another area. Return to the original area and remove the hairs with tweezers. As the lye has taken effect, the hairs should lift out easily. This procedure can be carried out on different areas.

Clients who are well into a treatment plan (ie with plenty of anagen hair)

Dark terminal hair

A client with a low pain threshold

Use of blend method

Clients with a good level of moisture in the skin and hair follicle

Where the hair is not too dense

HANDY HINT

Good levels of moisture in the skin and hair follicle encourage the production of lye resulting in a more effective treatment.

HANDY HINT

This method is slower than short-wave diathermy. However it offers less regrowth and is therefore actually quicker in the long term.

PROBING

STRETCHING THE SKIN

It is important to make sure that you insert the needle correctly to ensure an effective treatment. Before inserting the needle, you need to make sure that you have stretched the skin to allow for easy insertion:

- The two-finger stretch – during insertion, stretch the skin using the index (1) and middle finger (2) of the hand not holding the needle holder.

- The three-finger stretch – similar to the two-finger stretch but with the addition of the ring or fourth finger (3) of the hand holding the needle holder to assist with stretching the skin. This technique opens up the follicle to allow easy entry.

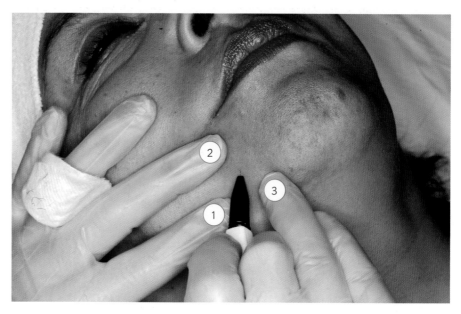

Whenever possible, aim for a steady supportive, three-way stretch position to make sure that your probing is accurate and that the treatment is as comfortable for the client as possible.

HANDY HINT

For comfort, avoid downward pressure. Instead, try to use a gentle pulling pressure.

INDUSTRY TIP

Do not remove the hand creating the two-finger stretch. It should stay on the client at all times.

INDUSTRY TIP

Tweezers – best practice

- Avoid moving on and off the client.
- Place epilated hairs onto a collection point.
- Keep the fingers close together and the hand as relaxed as possible to avoid tension in the arm and shoulders.

INSERTING THE NEEDLE (OR PROBING)

- Insert the needle parallel to the hair growth. As a guide, look at a small group of hairs in the area to see the direction of growth for that area. However take care to observe closely as each hair is individual.

- Study carefully the angle of the hair at pore level as it leaves the follicle. This is the angle of insertion. Once you have established the direction of hair growth and the angle of the hair, you can insert the needle.

- Position the needle parallel to the hair and slide it into the follicle. Using either the two- or three-finger stretching technique, depending on the area, insert the needle gently being sure not to apply any force. Make sure that you don't cause any depression or puckering of the skin. When you feel a slight resistance to the needle, you have reached the correct depth and the current can be applied. Remember to keep observing the skin for any reaction or loss of colour in the area – these are signs of incorrect probing.

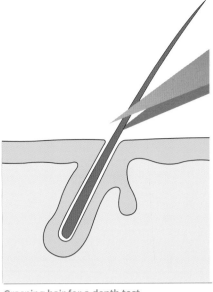
Grasping hair for a depth test

ACTIVITY

Carry out a depth test on yourself. Using tweezers, carefully grasp a hair at the very base and pluck it out. Using a magnification lamp, observe how much of the hair was below the surface of the skin and the stage of growth the hair is at. Place the hair on a tissue. Try to find a hair in each of the stages of growth and note the depth of the hairs.

INCORRECT PROBING

Inaccurate probing could result in:

- an ineffective treatment
- damage to the surrounding tissues
- over-stretching the follicle
- blood spotting
- damage to the sebaceous glands
- permanent scarring
- discomfort for the client
- a loss of confidence in the therapist
- legal action.

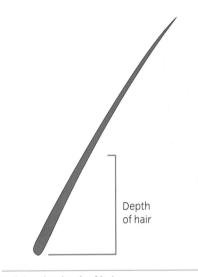
Judging the depth of hair

It is therefore very important to make sure your probing is accurate. If any skin damage is caused adequate healing time must be allowed before any further treatment is given.

Incorrect probing	Effect of incorrect probing
1 Probing is too deep 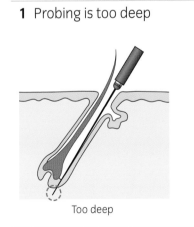 Too deep	- Will hurt the client and may rupture a capillary, resulting in a blood spot. - Destruction of the follicle will not take place and skin damage may occur. - Bruising can occur and if eyebrow hair is probed deeply could result in a black eye. - Scabs can also be caused by probing too deeply.

Incorrect probing	Effect of incorrect probing
2 Probing is too shallow 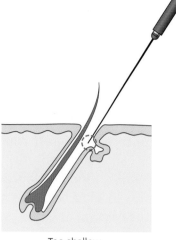 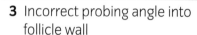 Too shallow	■ Could cause skin damage (eg surface burns). ■ **Blanching** which may cause permanent hypo- or hyper-pigmentation. ■ Client will experience pain and discomfort both at time of treatment and following treatment. ■ The treatment will be ineffective.
3 Incorrect probing angle into follicle wall 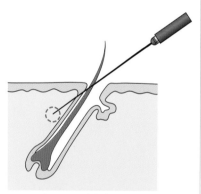 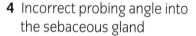 Probing into folicle wall	■ Will cause surface burns and capillary damage. ■ The treatment will be ineffective. ■ Discomfort to the client. ■ Blanching and bruising could occur. ■ Could result in the formation of scabs. ■ Blood spotting.
4 Incorrect probing angle into the sebaceous gland 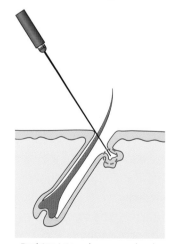 Probing into sebaceous gland	■ An uncomfortable, ineffective treatment. ■ Could result in tissue damage and potential infection of the sebaceous gland. ■ Sebum can seep onto the skin's surface leading to dehydration and surface burns.

Incorrect probing	Effect of incorrect probing
5 Applying the current whilst inserting or removing the probe – current released into the incorrect area 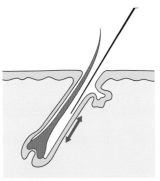 Needle movement	■ Blanching (which may result in temporary or permanent hyper- or hypo-pigmentation). ■ Increased discomfort for the client both during and after treatment. ■ Healing time extended. ■ An ineffective treatment with only partial destruction of the follicle (as the current has been released into the surrounding tissue).
6 Needle is too small for hair follicle and doesn't match diameter of the hair – probe moves from side to side and current spreads into surrounding tissue 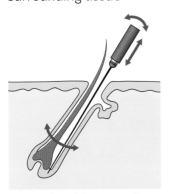 Needle point movement	■ An uncomfortable, ineffective treatment. ■ Will result in skin damage as the dermal papilla has not been targeted and electrical current has spread into the surrounding skin. ■ If using short-wave diathermy the heat can escape to the surface of the skin causing blanching (and therefore the risk of permanent hypo- or hyper-pigmentation). ■ Causes discomfort to the client. ■ Risk of using a higher intensity to try to find working point.

CARRYING OUT AN ELECTRICAL EPILATION TREATMENT

Before you begin the treatment:

■ Fully prepare the room and work area. Make sure that all tools and equipment are sanitised and sterilised and that the work area is clean and tidy.

■ Carry out a thorough consultation, explaining the treatment and allowing the client the opportunity to ask questions. Prepare the client and ask them to remove jewellery from both the area to be treated and their hand if they are going to be holding an indifferent electrode.

■ Wash and dry your hands thoroughly and apply a pair of gloves. Sanitise the gloves using antibacterial hand sanitiser.

■ Position the magnifying lamp over the treatment area. Sanitise the treatment area using an antiseptic wipe.

■ Assess the hair growth pattern and direction.

- Load the needle holder in front of the client so the client can see that you are using a fresh sterile needle.
- Place the tweezers in one hand and the needle holder in the other and switch on the magnifying lamp.

Remember to position yourself so that you are comfortable and so that you can reach the equipment easily, without having to over-stretch. If you are right-handed, sit on the right-hand side of the client. If you are left-handed, sit on the left-hand side of client. You can move around to access difficult treatment areas. The pictures below show the correct stance for the main treatment areas with a right-handed practitioner.

The following images show epilation being carried out on different parts of the body.

Lip

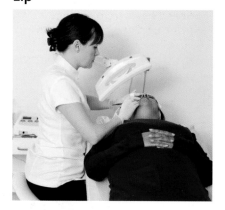

Chin

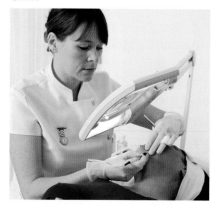

Face

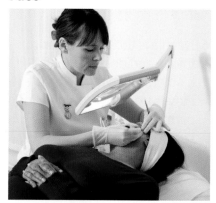

Eyebrow

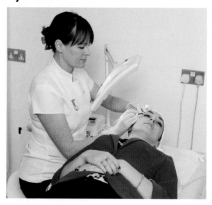

Underarm

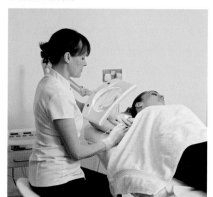

Breast

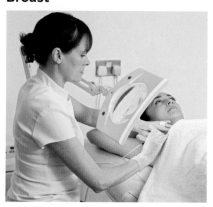

Bikini line

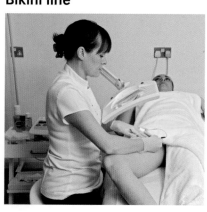

Abdomen

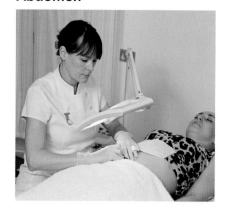

Leg

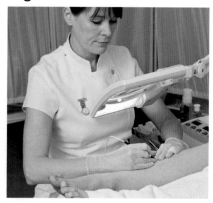

The step by steps below show the techiniques required to perform electrical epilation.

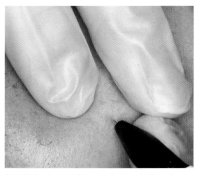

STEP 1 – Insert the needle (probe) and allow the current to flow for the required number of seconds. Remove your finger from the button or foot from the foot pedal and remove the needle.

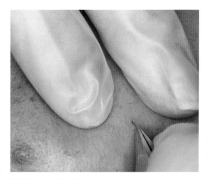

STEP 2 – Gently slide the hair out using a pair of tweezers.

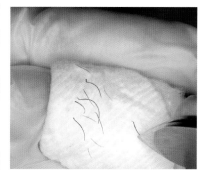

STEP 3 – Place the epilated hair on a cotton pad. If the hair does not slide out easily, check the accuracy of your probing and the depth of insertion. If the probing is accurate there are a number of options depending on the current being used (see industry tip box).

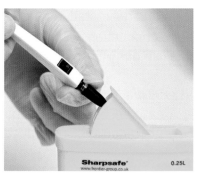

STEP 4 – At the end of treatment, dispose of the needle by loosening the chuck cap on the needle holder and tapping the used needle into the sharps box.

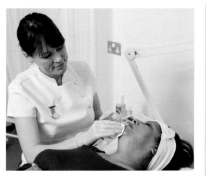

STEP 5 – Wipe the treatment area over with sanitiser and apply aftercare lotion/gel/cream to a piece of cotton wool and then gently wipe over the treatment area.

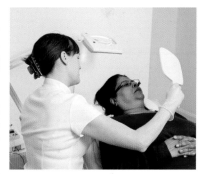

STEP 6 – Show the client the results in a mirror and show them the removed hairs on the cotton pad.

INDUSTRY TIP

Short-wave diathermy

- Increase the intensity of the current in line with the manufacturer's instructions and try another hair. If there is no adverse skin reaction, repeat this procedure until the hair can be removed from the follicle without traction. Remember to keep observing for any skin reaction.
- Increase the time of current release (but not the intensity) from one second to one and a half seconds up to a maximum of two seconds.

Blend

- Increase the time or the current intensity as appropriate.
- Try using the 'treat and leave' method (see page 361).

Galvanic

- Increase the time or the current intensity as appropriate.
- Alternatively, try using the 'treat and leave' method (see page 361).

HANDY HINT

Always remember to switch off the epilation unit and take the indifferent electrode from the client if using blend or galvanic.

HANDY HINT

Industry-standard sharps boxes have openings that are designed to prevent the chuck cap falling in.

Once you have finished the treatment:

- Provide aftercare advice (both verbal and written) and take the client back to reception so they can rebook if they wish to.
- Dispose of waste in the correct manner – contaminated waste in the sharps box and general waste in a lined bin with a lid.
- Sanitise and sterilise the work area and equipment in preparation for the next client.

CONTRA-ACTIONS

A contra-action is an adverse reaction that can happen during or after treatments. The table below lists the contra-actions that might occur during or after an electrical epilation treatment and the action that should be taken if they do.

Contra-action	Cause	Action required
Blanching of the skin (see industry tip box)	<ul><li>Insertion is too shallow so the electrical current is released too close to the skin surface and burns the skin.</li><li>The intensity of the current is too high.</li><li>The length of time that the current is applied for is too great.</li><li>The needle used is too small in diameter allowing heat to rise to the surface of the skin.</li></ul>	<ul><li>Keep the area dry and use an antiseptic lotion. Recommend continued use of a product containing aloe vera to aid cellular renewal and regeneration.</li><li>If hypo-/hyper-pigmentation results it may fade over time (although it can be permanent).</li><li>Once healed exfoliate the area regularly, massage the area to encourage the blood supply and use good-quality skin products to promote healing.</li></ul>
Excessive oedema	<ul><li>An allergic reaction to the nickel content of the epilation needle or products used.</li><li>Insertion too deep – particularly on the eyebrows.</li><li>Insertions too close in an area of dense hair growth.</li><li>Intensity too high.</li><li>Length of treatment too great.</li></ul>	<ul><li>Apply a cool compress.</li><li>Use a soothing aftercare product.</li><li>Increase space of insertions on areas of dense hair or sensitive skin.</li><li>Keep within the time limits for the treatment and treat sensitive areas for less time.</li><li>Use gold needles as they are hypoallergenic.</li></ul>
Excessive erythema	<ul><li>Intensity of the current is too high.</li><li>Current applied for too long.</li><li>Over-working an area (ie spacing is too dense).</li><li>Insertions are too deep or too short.</li></ul>	<ul><li>Apply a cool compress.</li><li>Use a soothing aftercare product.</li><li>The use of gold needles or insulated needles is recommended.</li></ul>

Contra-action	Cause	Action required
Blood spotting or bleeding	<ul><li>Incorrect insertions. Insertions too deep.</li><li>Forcing the needle through the skin and not following the line of the follicle into the skin.</li><li>The needle used is too large which can damage the sides of the follicle and create bleeding.</li></ul>	<ul><li>Stem any flow by applying slight pressure using a fresh cotton bud.</li><li>Ensure accurate insertions using the correct diameter of needle.</li><li>Perform a depth test to judge the depth of the hair if in doubt.</li></ul>
Pitting	<ul><li>Over-treatment over a period of time.</li><li>Repeatedly inaccurate insertions.</li><li>Insertions too deep.</li><li>Current applied when inserting or removing the needle.</li><li>Needle used is too large a needle.</li><li>Level of current used is too high. Current applied for too long. Continued use of short-wave diathermy on unsuitable hairs (eg curly or distorted follicles).</li></ul>	<ul><li>Therapist needs to change their technique and ensure they do regular CPD.</li><li>Keep the area dry and use an antiseptic product.</li><li>Once healed exfoliate the area regularly, massage the area to encourage the blood supply and use good-quality skin products to promote healing.</li></ul>
Bruising	<ul><li>The needle has penetrated through the base or side of the follicle resulting in damage to a superficial capillary.</li></ul>	<ul><li>Apply pressure immediately to prevent blood spreading under the skin.</li><li>Carry out a depth test if in doubt (eg eyebrows require very superficial insertions).</li><li>Ensure the correct diameter needle is being used.</li><li>Check accuracy of insertions.</li><li>Be gentle with an elderly client or client with sensitive skin.</li></ul>
Weeping follicles	<ul><li>Too much galvanic current has been used causing excessive chemical decomposition of the skin tissues.</li></ul>	<ul><li>Apply a cold compress and a good antibacterial aftercare product.</li><li>If a blister forms ensure it stays dry and clean. Do not irritate, pop or pick a blister.</li><li>Use a lower intensity current or use for a shorter length of time.</li></ul>
Bending or damaging the needle	<ul><li>Incorrect angle of insertion of the needle.</li><li>Damage to needle as a result of knocking it against equipment (eg magnifying lamp).</li></ul>	<ul><li>Replace the needle immediately.</li><li>Never try to straighten.</li><li>Find out the cause and put it right (eg if the needle was damaged on the magnification lamp, move the lamp).</li></ul>

Pitting

Severe skin damage caused by the collapse of the skin surrounding a follicle. Over-treatment, over a period of time, may have caused the collagen to collapse and the elastin framework in the dermis to be permanently weakened. It appears as an indentation or 'hole' in the skin

Contra-action	Cause	Action required
Hyperhidrosis (excessive sweating)	■ Clients may be nervous. ■ Illness. ■ Recent exercise. ■ Hot weather conditions. Hot flushes (menopause).	■ Allow clients time to compose themselves and offer them a glass of cold water. ■ Reduce the temperature of the treatment room but making sure it is still comfortable. ■ Gently wipe the skin (if appropriate). ■ Ensure current levels are as low as possible. ■ If using short-wave diathermy, use an insulated needle to help prevent the heat rising.
Palpitations	■ Can be caused by a variety of medical conditions. ■ Can be triggered by stress or panic.	■ Stop treatment and try to calm the client. ■ Loosen clothing with client's permission and offer gentle reassurance. Provide the client with a cold glass of water. ■ Raise the couch into a more upright position and adjust your working angle.

Palpitations

Rapid heartbeats experienced when an individual is stressed or panicked

 SmartScreen 308 Handout 8

> **HANDY HINT**
>
> With the blend or galvanic methods mild oedema around the hair follicle that has been treated can occur due to the chemical reaction. This usually disappears very quickly.

> **HANDY HINT**
>
> Hyperhidrosis can affect the accuracy, speed and ease of insertion and excess moisture may reduce the effectiveness of the current.

HOME-CARE AND AFTERCARE ADVICE

Following an electrical epilation treatment, you should give your client suitable aftercare advice. This will help the client maximise the benefits of the treatment and help to prevent any adverse reactions. Recommend that the client:

■ avoids touching the treatment area for 12–24 hours to avoid contamination – the area will be sensitive and susceptible to infection

■ avoids wearing make-up on the treated area for 24–48 hours

■ cleanses the skin gently using non-perfumed cleansers or soap-free products and uses the recommended aftercare product a minimum of twice a day to promote healing

■ avoids using tweezers, wax or electrical tweezers as this will stimulate the hair growth encouraging it to become thicker and coarser

■ avoids using bleach or any depilatory creams on the treatment area as this could infect and sensitise the area

■ trims hairs with scissors in between treatments as this does not affect hair growth or if absolutely necessary shave between services

- avoids heat treatments (eg saunas) for 24–48 hours after treatment as they might result in irritation, oedema, erythema, soreness or even infection
- avoids excessively hot baths or showers for 24–48 hours after treatment
- avoids exposing the treated area to UV light
- avoids swimming for 24–48 hours because the pores are open
- avoids products containing **AHAs** or chemical peels for two weeks before any treatment
- avoids perfumed products in the treated area for 24–48 hours
- avoids wearing restrictive clothing in the treated area for 24–48 hours
- reports any scabs or pustular infection to the salon and to not pick or rub the skin as this may lead to scarring
- applies aftercare products using a fresh cotton wool pad following the manufacturer's instructions.

HANDY HINT

Recommending aftercare products provides you with a good retail opportunity.

AHAs

Alpha hydroxy acids that exfoliate the skin

WHY DON'T YOU...
try the various aftercare products for yourself and see how they make your skin feel.

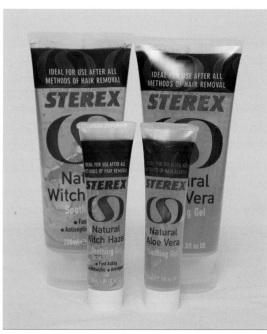

Electrolysis aftercare products

My client is transgender (male to female). She has male pattern facial hair growth (a beard) which is strong, coarse, dense terminal hair. Initially, she was having a two-hour treatment once a week. She began taking prescribed female hormones which helped a little in weakening the hair on the body but made only an insignificant improvement to the coarse, dense facial hair.

To start with I used short-wave diathermy because it produced quick results within the time allowed and enabled me to treat a large amount of hair. This was the method the client requested. I find most transgender people are very knowledgeable about hair removal and electrolysis. The currents were initially about a quarter of the output of the machine and I used a size 5 needle.

I concentrated on removing the dark hairs only and I left the white hairs because they were less noticeable. The client decided that this was the best course of treatment. This had the benefit of naturally spacing out treatment within an area of dense hair growth and prevented over-treatment. The client's upper lip was her main concern so I concentrated on this area and spent any additional time removing areas at the side of the face.

My client shaved in between treatments. Although I advised her against this, it was necessary for her emotional well-being.

The client has now been having treatment for a year and the hair growth has been visibly reduced. She now comes for one hour every other week. Over time I have noticed that the hair growth has not only decreased but also the regrowth has become finer and lighter. I have been able to go down 2 needle sizes. Eventually I should be able to see her for short 'tidying-up' appointments using a size 2 or 3 needle every month.

My client's confidence has grown considerably as a result of having electrical epilation. The female hormones have also continued to make a huge difference to her appearance and she has become more confident and comfortable in her own skin. She has decided to proceed to the next stage in her journey and explore the option of sexual reassignment surgery. I have been privileged to help her on her journey to becoming a happier person who can hold her head up high and rejoice in her new-found confidence.

Use the questions below to test your knowledge of Chapter 308 to see how much information you have retained. These questions will help you revise what you have learnt in this chapter.

Turn to page 499 for the answers.

1 The three layers of the hair are:
  a Cuticle, dermis, epidermis
  b Cortex, cuticle, dermis
  c Medulla, cuticle, epidermis
  d Cuticle, cortex, medulla

2 Vellus hair is usually:
  a Fine and long
  b Dark and thick
  c Dark and long
  d Fine and downy

3 A prohibition notice can be issued if:
  a The salon presents a danger
  b The salon follows health and safety
  c The salon follows some health and safety
  d The salon does not offer epilation

4 Which **one** of the following would **not** prevent an epilation treatment?
  a A broken bone
  b Hepatitis A and B
  c Haemophilia
  d Severe diabetes

5 What is the chemical breakdown of saline?
  a $NaCl + CO_2$
  b $Na + Cl$
  c $H_2O + NaCl$
  d $CO_2 + H_2O$

6 When carrying out an epilation treatment on an area of very dense hair growth, which **one** of the following is it most important to treat?
  a All the hair
  b The dark hair
  c The finer hairs for comfort
  d The white hair

7 A photograph is taken before a course of treatments to:
  a Show the client the results
  b Show the other therapists
  c Help the therapist to remember who the client is
  d Show to other clients

8 The most suitable needle to use on a client with a nickel allergy is:
  a An insulated needle
  b A stainless steel two-piece needle
  c A stainless steel one-piece needle
  d A 24-carat gold plated needle

9 Hirsutism is:
  a Male pattern hair growth
  b Female pattern hair growth
  c Distorted hair growth
  d A lack of hair growth

10 Which **one** of the following is a technique used when utilising blend?
  a Higher for longer
  b Shorter for lower
  c Lower for longer
  d Higher for wider

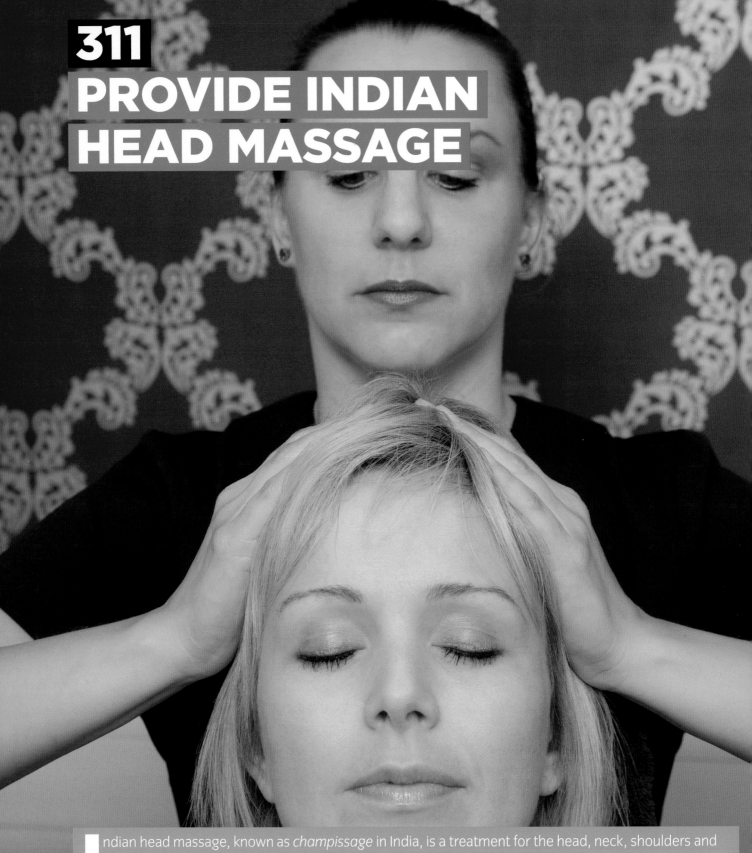

311
PROVIDE INDIAN HEAD MASSAGE

Indian head massage, known as *champissage* in India, is a treatment for the head, neck, shoulders and upper arms. It has been practised in India for centuries, and it is traditional in Indian families for massage to be given daily – especially to babies – to help them bond with their mothers. The Indian head massage techniques used in the West have been adapted from the traditional eastern version, which is based on Ayurvedic principles. Ayurveda (meaning 'science of life') is an ancient system of medicine, which focuses on keeping the whole body healthy and keeping the mind, body and spirit in balance. There are three vital energies called *doshas* (*vata*, *pitta* and *kapha*), which can be affected by diet, lifestyle, seasons, the time of day and stress levels. This in turn causes an imbalance in the energy flow or life force of the body (*qi* or *chi*).

In this chapter you will learn to:

- prepare for Indian head massage
- provide Indian head massage.

You should make sure you are familiar with the:

- structure, function, position and action of the muscles of the body
- location, function and structure of the bones of the body
- location, function and structure of the circulatory and lymphatic systems of the body.

PREPARE FOR INDIAN HEAD MASSAGE

PREPARATION OF THE THERAPIST

As a therapist you will be working in close proximity to the client throughout this treatment. It is very important that you are dressed and presented in a professional manner. See Chapter 301 for more information.

Before you start any treatment you should make sure you are fully prepared physically by doing the hand exercises in Chapter 305/309, and that you are mentally focused. The client is paying for your time and attention and you should avoid any distractions.

PREPARATION OF THE TREATMENT AREA

The treatment area should be fully prepared before the client arrives. You should make sure that all work surfaces have been cleaned and are tidy and organised. Make sure that any equipment or products that you need are ready and easily accessible before you start, so that you do not have to interrupt the flow of your treatment to go and get anything. Check that any equipment you require is plugged in and is in working order.

THE TREATMENT ENVIRONMENT

The client needs to be comfortable during their treatment. Additional information on preparing the treatment environment can be found in Chapter 305/309.

PREPARATION OF THE CLIENT

- The client should remove all jewellery, including earrings, necklaces and facial jewellery. Ask them to place these in their bag. If the client is removing glasses, ask them to place them in their bag or on the trolley in a safe place if they prefer. If the client is wearing a hairpiece, it will need to be removed before the treatment.
- Indian head massage is usually applied over light clothing. The ideal item of clothing for the client to wear is a T-shirt (advise the client about this when they book). Bulky clothing and collars are best avoided as they will get in the way.
- If the client is removing their outer clothing, make sure they understand what needs to be removed. Female clients can leave their bra on but just hook their arms out of the straps. They can then be given a towel or wrap to protect their modesty.

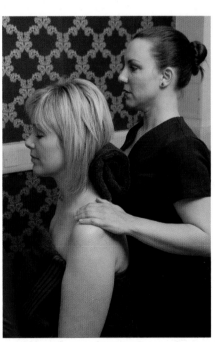

Make sure you are positioned correctly before starting the treatment

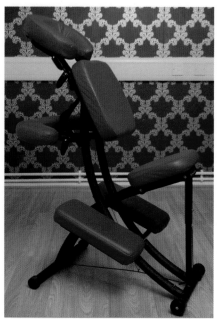
INDUSTRY TIP

Clean oil off work surfaces and containers quickly, as oil residue is sticky and is a great breeding ground for bacteria.

- Provide the client with a sterile comb so that they can comb through their hair – or you may prefer to do this as part of the treatment ritual. It is important to do this before you start to remove any loose hair and to make sure the hair is tangle free.

- Position the client on a chair or stool. If they are going to rest on a couch, this should be positioned in front of them. You should encourage the client to sit up for the first part of the treatment until you need to work on the face and scalp – if they lean forward this will make it difficult for you to access them without overreaching and straining your back.

- It is important that both the client's feet remain in contact with the ground during the treatment. You need to consider both the height of the client and your ease of access so that you are both comfortable before you start.

- The client should rest their hands unfolded in their lap.

EQUIPMENT AND PRODUCTS

Couch

A treatment couch may be useful for the client to rest up against during treatment. Pillows can be placed at the end of the couch for the client to lean forward on to.

Treatment chair

A height-adjustable chair will be required. This should have a low back so that the client's upper back is accessible and no arms to allow the therapist full access to the client during treatment. The chair should also have no wheels so that the client remains in a fixed, secure position throughout the treatment.

An Indian head massage treatment chair

INDUSTRY TIP

If you have a large bust, you may find using a pillow rolled over at the end more comfortable than having the client rest their head back into your chest during the treatment of the face and scalp.

INDUSTRY TIP

Try to avoid using make-up remover wipes, as these often contain mineral oils that can cause skin congestion. Many clients and therapists use them because they are quick and easy and seem more economical, but in the long term they are not always cost-effective or beneficial to the skin.

Trolley

The trolley should have at least two shelves and be positioned within easy reach. Position all the products you know you will need on the top shelf so you can access them easily. The trolley should be cleaned with a suitable cleaning product. Protect the surface with a piece of couch roll to mop up any oily residue.

Lined bin

This should preferably be a pedal bin, so you do not have to touch it with your hands. Use it to dispose of waste as soon as possible and prevent any cross-infection.

Towels

A freshly laundered towel will be required for the client to rest on. A rolled towel or prop is also needed to place behind the client's neck for support while you are treating the head and face. The client will also need a large towel to wrap around themselves.

Skincare products

As the client will be having their face treated as part of the Indian head massage, you will need cleansing products to remove their make-up before you start the treatment. Different companies offer training to support their own product ranges.

Massage oils and creams

A selection of massage mediums is available, including various carrier oils and creams. See Chapter 305/309 for more about the different massage mediums.

Consumables

You will also require some consumables:

- cotton wool to remove cleanser
- tissues
- couch roll to protect towels and maintain hygiene
- spatulas, to decant products hygienically.

Accessories

The following accessories will be useful:

- Comb or brush – to comb or brush through the client's hair at the start and finish of the treatment. This will help to make sure you can get your hands through the hair during the treatment and will also remove any loose hair before you start. These items should be sterilised before and after use to avoid cross-infection.
- Hair clips – if the client has long hair, it is a good idea to clip it out of the way while you work on the back, neck, shoulders and arms.

Treatment oils

There are a variety of oils that may be used during Indian head massage treatment – these are not only used to help with contact during treatment but also for their particular properties. Make your choice according to the client's treatment objectives, hair and skin type, allergies and preferences. It is important to carry out a patch test (see Chapter 303) if you have any concerns about product allergies. For skin types and conditions and how to recognise them, see the Anatomy and Physiology chapter.

Treatment product	Uses	Hair/skin type
Sesame oil	<ul><li>Traditional oil widely used in India, due to its anti-inflammatory and nourishing properties.</li><li>May help reduce swelling and muscular aches and pains.</li></ul>	<ul><li>Dry hair and skin</li><li>It is thought that sesame oil can help to delay the onset of grey hair</li></ul>
Olive oil	<ul><li>A rich, nourishing oil.</li><li>Anti-inflammatory.</li></ul>	<ul><li>Dry or dehydrated skin</li></ul>
Mustard oil	<ul><li>Traditional Indian head massage oil which is strong-smelling.</li><li>Has a warming effect on tissues; good for use in winter.</li><li>May cause sensitisation in some clients due to the heat produced.</li></ul>	<ul><li>Good for muscular aches and pains, joint stiffness and sporty clients</li><li>More suitable for male clients</li></ul>
Coconut oil	<ul><li>Semi-solid at room temperature, this oil needs warming before use – this can be done by working into the hands.</li><li>Has a pleasant aroma.</li></ul>	<ul><li>Dry, brittle, over-processed or coarse hair</li><li>Skin/hair in need of moisturising and softening</li></ul>

Treatment product	Uses	Hair/skin type
Grapeseed oil	■ A light-textured oil with very little aroma. ■ Mixes well with thicker oils to give a better working consistency.	■ Suitable for all skin types, but particularly sensitive or oily skins
Almond oil	■ A light, nourishing oil. ■ Reduces pain and stiffness. ■ Has a high vitamin E content.	■ Suitable for all skin types, but particularly dry and mature skins
Cream	■ Can be used on clients who do not like the feel of oil on their skin. ■ Can be used on the face and chosen according to skin type.	■ Different types according to product
Powder	■ Ideal if a client does not want oil in their hair. ■ Apply to the hands only, to help them slide easily through the client's hair.	■ Oily hair

THE CONSULTATION

A detailed consultation to establish the client's priorities and needs must take place before every treatment. For more information on the consultation process, see Chapter 303.

Contra-indications to Indian head massage

A description of each of the following conditions can be found within the relevant system in the Anatomy and Physiology chapter. You should be familiar with all of the contra-indications to this treatment.

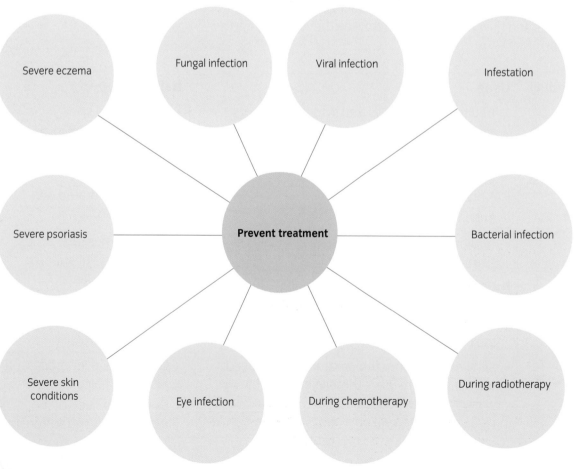

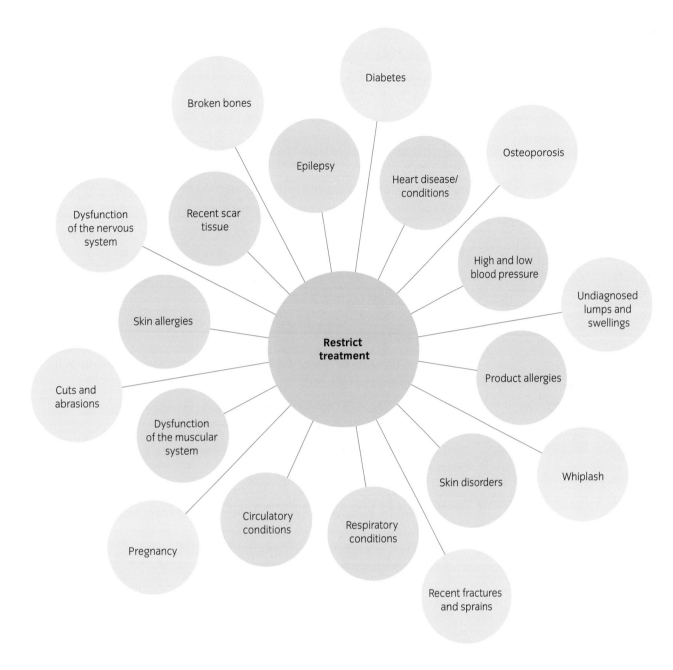

PROVIDE INDIAN HEAD MASSAGE

SmartScreen 311 Handout 1

Indian head massage can be performed with the client fully clothed, so it is considered a non-invasive treatment. It is a great introductory treatment for clients who have never had a massage and may feel embarrassed about undressing. It is also a very portable treatment – all you need is a chair or stool, so it can be performed in virtually any environment, for example at a desk in an office.

THE PHYSICAL, PHYSIOLOGICAL AND PSYCHOLOGICAL EFFECTS OF TREATMENT
A detailed list of physical, physiological and psychological effects can be found in Chapter 305/309. However, there are some specific benefits related to Indian head massage, shown in the following table.

Benefit	Explanation
Improved skin and hair texture	■ Techniques used will desquamate the skin. ■ Oils and creams will nourish and condition the skin and hair, especially if left on for some time after the treatment. ■ Improved circulation will improve the skin and hair growth.
Improved scalp condition	■ An increase in circulation will help bring nutrients to the cells. ■ Techniques used will desquamate the scalp.
Improved muscle tone	■ Stimulating techniques will cause the muscle fibres to contract, causing a very temporary change in muscle tone.
Improved memory	■ Stimulating techniques will help improve circulation and stimulate the scalp.
Improved concentration	■ Stimulating techniques will help improve circulation and stimulate the scalp.
Reduced tension headaches	■ Techniques used will help to aid relaxation, which will in turn reduce tension headaches.
Reduced tinnitus	■ Tinnitus is a ringing or 'shushing' sound in the ear – it is believed that relaxation helps to reduce it.
Improved sleep patterns	■ General relaxation of the body and mind will help sleep patterns.
Reduced sinus problems	■ Congested sinuses will benefit from the increased circulation over the face and scalp and pressure point massage will stimulate the flow of energy in the area.

INDIAN HEAD MASSAGE TECHNIQUES

The massage movements used during an Indian head massage treatment are effleurage, petrissage, tapotement, frictions and vibrations (see Chapter 305/309 for more detailed information on these). There are also some techniques that are used specifically in Indian head massage, shown in the following table.

Technique	Application	Effects
Champissage – tapotement	This is a traditional movement. Hold the hands together as if praying, with the thumbs overlapped for support. Strike the skin with the fingertips in a tapping action.	This is a stimulating movement; the effects are similar to hacking
Petrissage – chopping	Hold the hands flat to the skin side by side. Slide the hands together, chopping and pushing the skin tissue up in between them.	Similar to tapotement
Pressure points	This is usually applied to the scalp and face. Apply pressure using either the thumbs or fingertips (one or more) systematically over the skin's surface. Apply pressure and hold it in time with the breath. Breathe in, apply pressure, hold, breathe out and then release the pressure.	Stimulating to both the circulatory and the lymphatic systems

MARMA POINTS

Marma points are specific points located throughout the head and body where energy flows. Pressure is applied to these during treatment to help balance the flow of energy.

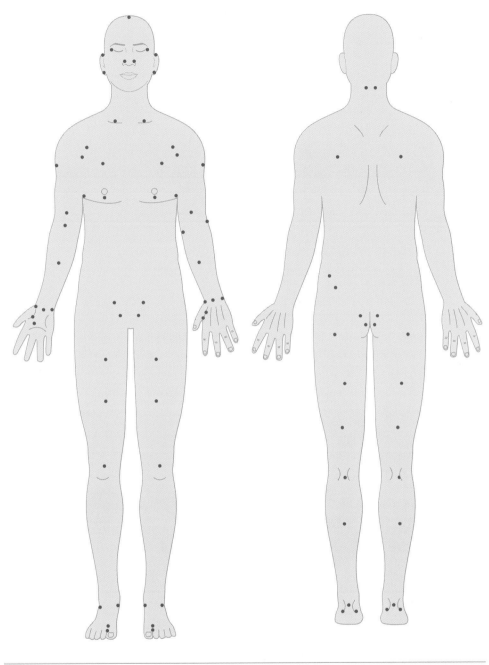

Marma points of the body

TREATMENT TIMING

A commercial Indian head massage treatment is usually between 30 and 45 minutes long, depending on the routine. On-site massage, for example in an office, may be shorter.

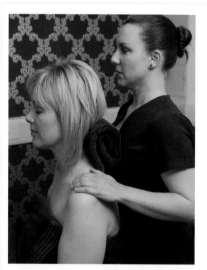

MEETING TREATMENT OBJECTIVES

The techniques that you use will need to be altered and applied according to the objectives of the treatment. Details of the treatment objectives for all massage treatments can be found in Chapter 305/309. Below are some that relate specifically to Indian head massage.

- Relaxation – increase effleurage and keep techniques slow and flowing, in particular any petrissage techniques. Reduce tapotement and frictions, keeping them near the start of the treatment.
- Sedation – movements should be slow and rhythmical. Repetitive stroking and effleurage will also help to sedate both physically and mentally. Avoid tapotement techniques unless carried out very early in the treatment.
- Stimulation – increase the use of tapotement and frictions to stimulate the client both physically and mentally. Keep movements brisk and firm.
- Invigoration – make techniques firm, brisk and bracing to enliven and revitalise the client both physically and mentally.

INDIAN HEAD MASSAGE

GROUNDING SEQUENCE

The following is a suggested treatment routine. Once you are ready to start, excuse yourself to wash your hands. Return and proceed to cleanse the client's face. Leave a few minutes before you start to balance and ground both yourself and the client. This is shown in the following four steps.

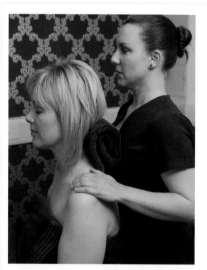

STEP 1 – Stand behind the client. Place both hands on the client's shoulders, then ask the client to take a deep breath and exhale slowly. Do this three times.

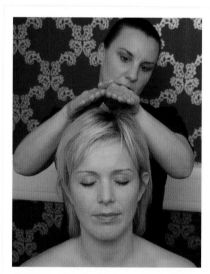

STEP 2 – Place both hands over the top of the head, with a gap between them. This will be over the crown chakra. Take deep breaths for one minute.

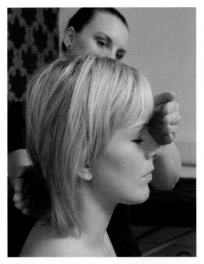

STEP 3 – Stand to the side of the client and place one hand on the occipital bone and one hand over the third eye chakra (centre of the forehead). Hold for one minute.

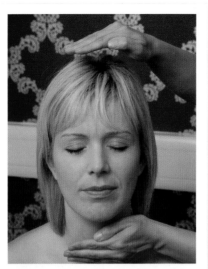

STEP 4 – Stand behind the client and place both hands in front of the throat and over the throat chakra. Hold for one minute.

HANDY HINTS

Make sure you tell the client the benefits that the oil will have on their hair. It is a really excellent conditioner and will help strengthen the hair shaft. Make sure you give the client clear instructions on how to remove the oil from their hair following treatment.

Application of oil

Gently rake your fingers or a comb through the client's hair. Place the fingers together with the thumb to form a circle and place on the crown of the head. Pour warm oil into the finger circle using a container with a funnel, or a squeezy applicator. This will enable you to control the application and will prevent the oil running down the face. Work the oil through the hair and over the treatment area.

If the hair is long, clip it up on the top of the head out of the way.

INDIAN HEAD MASSAGE ROUTINE

The following 30 steps show an example of an Indian head massage routine.

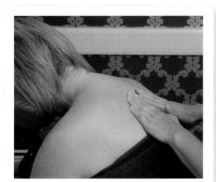

STEP 1 – Start with sweeping effleurage to the client's upper back, including the neck and shoulders. Repeat this six times.

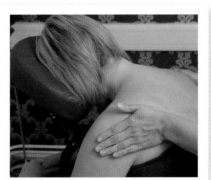

STEP 2 – Apply hand kneading to the upper back, including the shoulders.

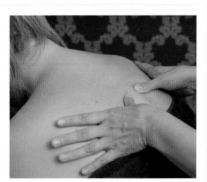

STEP 3 – Apply thumb kneading to the erector spinal muscles on the upper back.

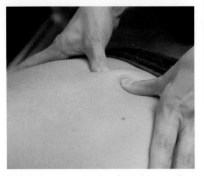

STEP 4 – Next, use thumb circles on either side of the client's spine.

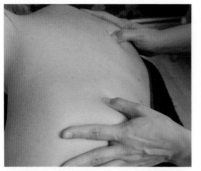

STEP 5 – Then apply thumb kneading to the shoulder area.

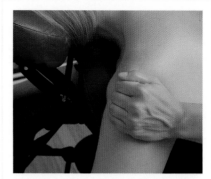

STEP 6 – Follow with palm effleurage to the shoulder area.

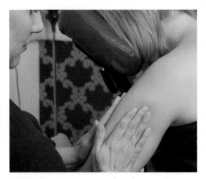

STEP 7 – Moving onto the client's arms, perform effleurage on the upper arm area.

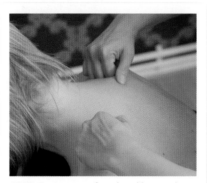

STEP 8 – Next, perform knuckling on the trapezius.

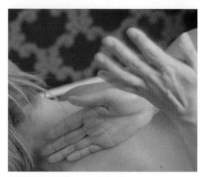

STEP 9 – Follow with hacking movements to the upper trapezius.

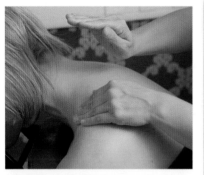

STEP 10 – Moving to the upper shoulders, apply cupping.

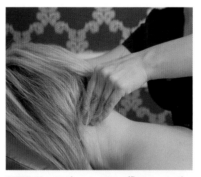

STEP 11 – Apply sweeping effleurage to the neck.

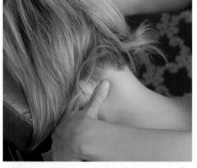

STEP 12 – Move on to thumb kneading of the neck.

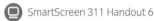 SmartScreen 311 Handout 6

HANDY HINTS

Do not overload the hair with oil; it only needs a superficial coating, saturating the hair will be a waste. Do however make sure that the ends of the air are covered well as this is often the area that suffers the most from dryness.

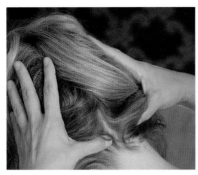

STEP 13 – Next, apply thumb pressure on the pressure points at the base of the skull.

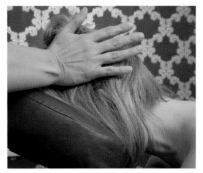

STEP 14 – Follow with flat hand effleurage to the scalp.

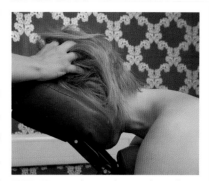

STEP 15 – Use finger raking on the scalp.

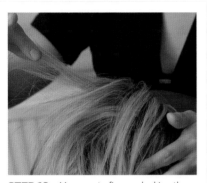

STEP 16 – Move on to finger plucking the hair.

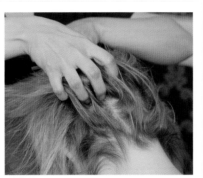

STEP 17 – And then hair raking.

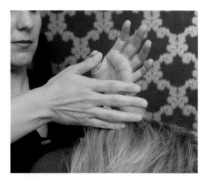

STEP 18 – Next, apply hacking to the scalp, but make sure you apply only light pressure!

HANDY HINTS

It is really important that you do not have rings on your hand as you will find that the client's hair will get caught and this will pull the hair making it an uncomfortable experience for the client.

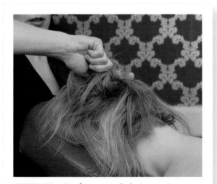

STEP 19 – Perform gentle hair tugging.

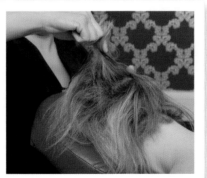

STEP 20 – Follow with gentle hair twists.

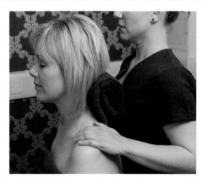

STEP 21 – Place your hands on the client's shoulders and ask them to take two to three deep breaths.

HANDY HINTS

Some clients find it hard to relax. Encourage the client to keep their eyes closed by instructing them to do so. This will help to encourage the client to relax and avoid distractions that might be in the treatment room.

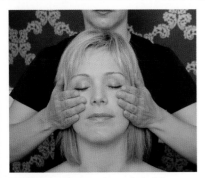

STEP 22 – Next, apply gentle facial pressure, with your fingers and palms flattened.

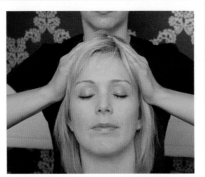

STEP 23 – Apply the same gentle pressure to the scalp.

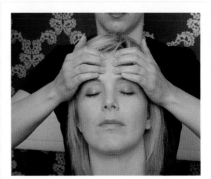

STEP 24 – And the forehead.

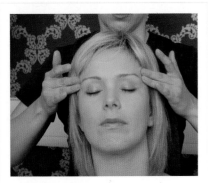

STEP 25 – Using two fingers, gently press the pressure points on the temples.

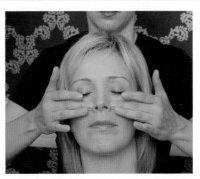

STEP 26 – And then to the pressure points on the sinus area using one finger on each side this time.

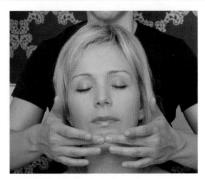

STEP 27 – Apply the same movement to the jaw.

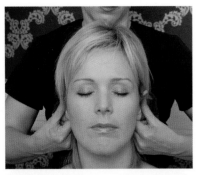

STEP 28 – Then use your thumbs to gently press the pressure points on the ears.

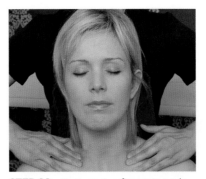

STEP 29 – Next, use two fingers to apply pressure to the pressure points on the clavicle.

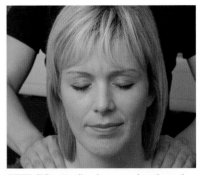

STEP 30 – Finally, place your hands on the client's shoulders to finish.

 SmartScreen 311 Handout 9

When you have finished, step back from the client so that you move out of their personal space. Check they are feeling alright and offer them a drink of water. Allow the client to relax for a few minutes and gather their thoughts.

CONTRA-ACTIONS

A contra-action is an adverse, usually unwanted, reaction that happens either during or as a result of a treatment. Therefore you need to be aware of what to look out for and how to deal with a reaction if one occurs. In Chapter 305/309 you will find a list of contra-actions and actions to take, which will also be applicable to Indian head massage. The contra-actions for pre-blended oils also apply to those used in Indian head massage.

HOME-CARE AND AFTERCARE ADVICE

There is a comprehensive list of aftercare and home-care advice in Chapter 305/309. In addition to this, some advice is specific to an Indian head massage treatment.

SPECIFIC HOME CARE FOR INDIAN HEAD MASSAGE

Advise the client to leave the oil in the hair for as long as possible to condition and nourish it. They should sleep with a towel over their pillow to prevent staining.

To remove the oil from the hair, advise the client to wet their hair and then place some shampoo in the palm of their hand, add water and mix it with the fingers. They should then apply the diluted shampoo to the hair and scalp.

For information on client feedback and evaluation, see Chapter 305/309.

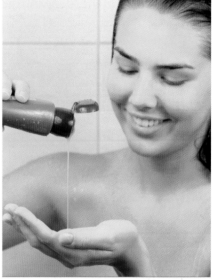

Informing the client how to wash the oil out of their hair is an important part of Indian head massage aftercare

TEST YOUR KNOWLEDGE

Use the questions below to test your knowledge of Chapter 311 to see how much information you have retained. These questions will help you revise what you have learnt in this chapter.

Turn to page 499 for the answers.

1 Which **one** of the following describes a marma point?
   a Nerve ending
   b Energy wheel
   c Chakra site
   d Pressure point

2 Mustard oil is used to do which **one** of the following?
   a Calm and soothe the skin
   b Decongest the skin
   c Warm the tissues
   d Reduce sensitivity

3 Which **one** of the following is a contra-indication to Indian head massage treatment?
   a Scar tissue
   b Baldness
   c Impetigo
   d Alopecia

4 Which **one** of the following is a traditional Indian head massage medium?
   a Grapeseed oil
   b Almond oil
   c Olive oil
   d Sesame oil

5 Following an Indian head massage treatment, how long should a client be advised to leave the oil on their hair?
   a 2 hours
   b 8 hours
   c Overnight
   d A month

6 What is the colour of the root chakra?
   a Red
   b Orange
   c Yellow
   d Green

7 Indian head massage is part of which tradition?
   a Native American
   b Chinese
   c Ayurvedic
   d Western

8 Which three chakras are balanced at the beginning of an Indian head massage?
   a Crown, third eye and throat
   b Third eye, heart and solar plexus
   c Solar plexus, crown and third eye
   d Heart, throat and crown

9 Which one of the following describes coconut oil in its natural form when cooled?
   a Gel
   b Wax
   c Semi-solid
   d Solid

10 Which **one** of the following is a traditional Indian head massage technique?
   a Pressure point
   b Hacking
   c Frictions
   d Champissage

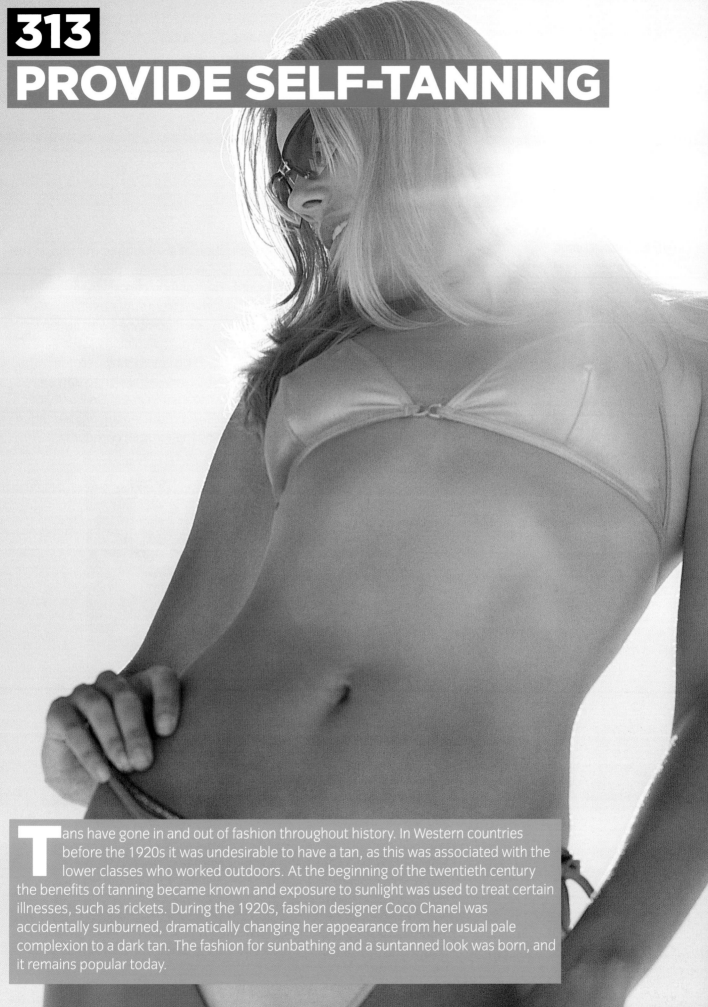

313
PROVIDE SELF-TANNING

Tans have gone in and out of fashion throughout history. In Western countries before the 1920s it was undesirable to have a tan, as this was associated with the lower classes who worked outdoors. At the beginning of the twentieth century the benefits of tanning became known and exposure to sunlight was used to treat certain illnesses, such as rickets. During the 1920s, fashion designer Coco Chanel was accidentally sunburned, dramatically changing her appearance from her usual pale complexion to a dark tan. The fashion for sunbathing and a suntanned look was born, and it remains popular today.

In this chapter you will:

- be able to prepare for self-tanning treatments
- be able to provide self-tanning treatments.

You should make sure you are familiar with the:

- structure and functions of the skin.

WHAT IS SELF-TAN?

Dihydroxyacetone (DHA)
The main ingredient in self-tanning solutions, made from sugar beets and sugar cane

Self-tanning is achieved by the application of a solution to the skin, in the form of a liquid, cream, gel or spray lotion – by hand, with a spray gun and compressor or in a spray booth. The solution contains **dihydroxyacetone (DHA)**, which is derived from sugar beets, sugar cane and glycerol. When applied to the skin it combines with amino acids to form chemical compounds known as melaninoids, which are brown in colour. This property of DHA was discovered by German scientists in the 1920s when they found it caused the skin to darken. Further research in the 1950s by Eva Wittgenstein at the University of Cincinnati confirmed that by consistently reproducing the pigmentation effect, the DHA did not penetrate beyond the stratum corneum.

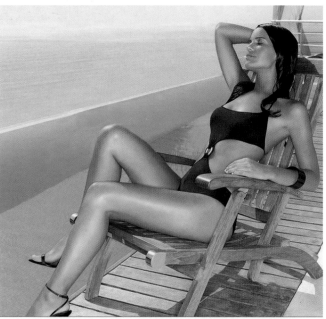

The suntanned look continues to be popular today

PREPARE FOR SELF-TANNING TREATMENTS

PREPARATION OF THE THERAPIST

You should present yourself in a professional manner and in line with salon policy. For more about this, see Chapter 301.

You will also be working in close proximity to the client throughout this treatment, and personal protective equipment (PPE) appropriate to the treatment must be worn.

A tanning solution is a chemical which can stain the skin and clothing, as well as irritating the **respiratory tract**. This is because it can be inhaled (breathed in), and this can be a particular problem if a therapist is carrying out lots of treatments. Make sure you have the PPE listed below, whether you are performing a manual or a spray tan application – your employer should supply it.

Respiratory tract

The mouth, nose, trachea (windpipe) and lungs – together they form the body's breathing mechanism

PPE	Description
Gloves 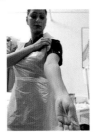	Disposable gloves that are talc and latex free, to protect the hands from discolouration.
Apron 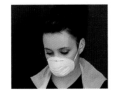	Plastic apron – wear this to prevent the tanning solution from staining your uniform.
Mask	Disposable face mask – this is optional. However, if you are using a lot of spray tan it will help prevent inhalation and protect the respiratory system.

INDUSTRY TIP

Alert your employer if stocks of PPE are getting low, so that nothing runs out.

INDUSTRY TIP

Some tanning products contain nut derivatives, which if used on a client with a nut allergy could prove fatal.

PREPARATION OF THE CLIENT

Carry out a thorough consultation before the treatment, making sure that the result of the patch test has been recorded (see Chapter 303). The patch test needs to be carried out at least 24 hours prior to the treatment, to make sure the client has no allergy to the product. You'll need to check the manufacturer's instructions for the correct timing.

During the consultation you should discuss the client's requirements, including the final colour choice. The higher the percentage of DHA in the product, the darker the tan result will be. If there is no percentage shown on a product, it will usually be labelled as light, medium or dark. Some suppliers will provide a printed colour guide to help the client choose.

Explain to the client fully what the treatment includes, and give them the opportunity to ask questions. Client care and communication are particularly important when discussing a tanning treatment – remember that this may be their first treatment, and they may feel a little self-conscious or nervous about it. Allow the client plenty of time to ask questions and reassure them at every stage of the treatment. Remain professional and mature at all times, as the client will be in a state of undress and may feel vulnerable.

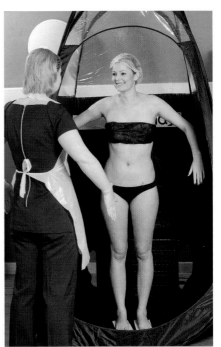

A therapist showing a client how to stand in order to get an even tan from the treatment

313 PROVIDE SELF-TANNING

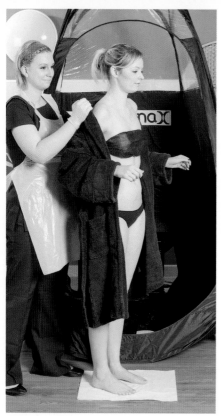

Therapist assisting client prior to spray-tanning treatment

INDUSTRY TIP

Ask the client to apply a base coat of nail polish to fingernails and toenails prior to the treatment, as this will prevent staining of the nails.

When they book the treatment, you should advise the client to do the following:

- Remove all make-up prior to the treatment.
- Remove all perfumed products, including body lotions and anti-perspirant/deodorant.
- Exfoliate the skin 24 hours prior to tanning – using an oil-free exfoliator.
- Apply moisturiser to dry areas such as knees, elbows and heels 24 hours before treatment.
- Carry out any hair removal such as waxing or shaving 24 hours before spray tanning.
- Wear loose black clothing (no silk).
- Bring flip-flops with them to wear after the treatment.

Once the treatment requirements have been established, the following steps should be taken:

- Ask the client to take out their contact lenses or remove their glasses, if wearing them.
- Ask the client to remove all jewellery and other accessories.
- Cleanse the face of any make-up.
- Provide protection for hair, hands and feet.
- Provide the client with disposable briefs or ask them to put on their own clothing, eg a bikini.
- Provide the client with a mask – this is optional, but it is advisable if the client has a respiratory condition such as asthma. The client should place the mask in front of their nose and mouth during the tanning treatment.

Check that the client has their hair protector on properly – it should be behind the ears so that the tan will reach them, and should not be too low down on the forehead or the back of the neck as this will cause a demarcation line.

ACTIVITY

It is necessary to have had a patch test to ensure you are not allergic to the tanning solution before carrying out the following activity. Prepare your skin, then, using the three different shades of tan, take a cotton bud and apply a small amount of each to an area on your body such as the arm. Let it fully develop and then record the results by taking a photograph. This will give you a full understanding of how the different tan strengths look when fully developed.

PREPARATION OF THE TREATMENT AREA

All tools and equipment need to be disinfected before and after treatment to reduce the risk of cross-infection.

- The treatment area needs to be wiped down using a disinfectant, and trolleys and therapy couches will need protecting with disposable couch roll.
- Flooring needs to be of a type that can be wiped clean using hot water and disinfectant; carpet is not suitable in the treatment area, as it

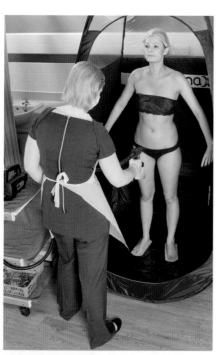

A well-prepared treatment area during a spray-tan treatment

cannot be cleaned properly. It is also advisable to have a dark-coloured floor rather than cream or white, due to the staining which will occur from prolonged use of tanning ingredients in the area.

- Where possible, use disposable foot mats for the client to stand on – these are slightly weighted so they will not blow around like tissue paper would. Adhesive foot-shaped disposable cardboard cut-outs, available in left and right shapes, stick to the client's feet throughout treatment and are ideal. These prevent discoloration of the soles of the feet, which can often happen during tanning treatments, as well as providing hygienic foot protection to reduce the risk of cross-infection.

- There needs to be adequate ventilation to allow for exchange of oxygen and to prevent a build-up of tanning solution in the air. This will also prevent the odour of the tanning solution from lingering.

- Lighting should be bright and even so that it does not cast any shadows – this will help you achieve an even application of the tanning products. Some tanning tents now have plastic windows in them to allow more light in.

- The room needs to be warm enough for the client to feel comfortable throughout their treatment. If it is too hot, this may cause the client to perspire and could affect the consistency of the end result.

- The room in which the treatment is taking place needs to be private, as the client will be in a state of undress.

- If music is playing it needs to be at a noise level acceptable to all, and appropriate for all clients from young to mature.

- A lidded, lined waste bin should be in the room for disposal of any waste products, eg tissue or cotton wool. This waste bin should be emptied between clients into a bin liner, which will be sealed and placed in the outside bin every evening.

- Have cleaning products available to wipe over the treatment area between clients.

- The spray-tan unit needs to be dismantled and cleaned in accordance with the manufacturer's instructions between clients. This prevents different coloured tanning solutions mixing together to produce an undesirable result. As the tanning solution contains DHA, which is a sugar, if the spray-tan unit is not cleaned thoroughly the mechanism will become blocked, which will prevent it working correctly and may lead to a spotting effect during application. The spray-tan compressor also needs to be portable appliance tested (PAT) annually, and have a label displaying this.

- Test that the spray gun is working before the treatment begins; this can be done by placing water in the spray gun and switching the compressor on. This will also clear the gun of any tanning solution.

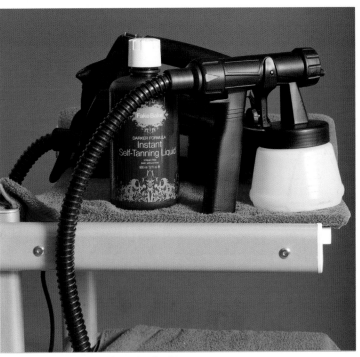

A spray-tan unit with self-tanning liquid

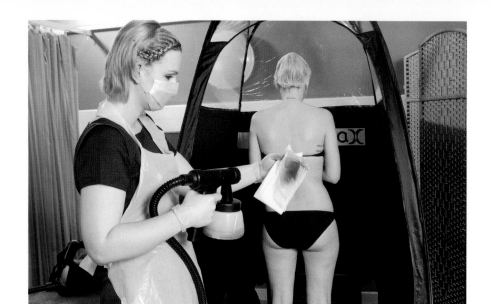

Always test the spray gun before starting the treatment

THE CONSULTATION

Complete a client consultation card, as this will help protect you in case of legal action, by showing what procedures you followed. Filling it in also provides you with an opportunity to inform your client of what a tanning treatment involves but, most importantly, it ensures that all contra-indications have been discussed and eliminated.

- Always greet the client by name, introduce yourself, smile and be sincere. Show the client to a private area, which should be quiet and relaxing.
- Make clear to the client that you need to do a consultation, which will involve you asking some questions that will help you to decide on the best treatment plan for them.
- Using open questions during the consultation will help you to gather as much detail as possible. Also include personal details such as name, address and contact number and record these clearly on the client consultation card.
- Allow the client to ask any questions they like at any time so that they feel confident in the treatment process.
- Explain what the treatment involves, how long it will take and, if relevant, what home care and aftercare are required.
- During the consultation a brief skin analysis should be conducted to determine whether the skin is sensitive, mature or dehydrated, as these conditions may affect the choice of tan (see the Anatomy and Physiology chapter for more about skin types and conditions).
- Keep a record of the treatment for future reference.

ACTIVITY

Some clients may be interested in other tanning methods. Make a list of the advantages and disadvantages of self-tanning compared with UV tanning.

CONTRA-INDICATIONS

It is important to check for any contra-indications that may prevent or restrict treatment. These are described in the following tables.

Prevent	Reason
Skin diseases such as impetigo (bacterial), ringworm (fungal), shingles (viral), scabies (infestation)	Risk of cross-infection.
Severe skin disorders, eg severe eczema or psoriasis	The condition could be worsened.
Eye infections, eg conjunctivitis	Risk of cross-infection, and the condition could be worsened.
During chemotherapy or radiotherapy	Medication will alter the effects of the treatment, and these clients should also avoid unnecessary exposure to chemicals.

Restrict	Reason
Skin disorders, eg rash	May irritate.
Undiagnosed lumps and swellings	May aggravate the condition, and the underlying issue is unknown.
Recent fractures and sprains	Work around any dressing/bandages.
Product/skin allergies	Allergic reaction may occur.
Respiratory disorders	The condition may be aggravated; ensure the client has any necessary medication with them.
Broken bones	Will stain the cast.
Recent scar tissue	May irritate.
Cuts and abrasions	May irritate.
Contact lenses	During a spray tan the mist may settle on the lenses.
Pregnancy (especially during the first three months)	Hormonal changes may affect the colour of the tanning treatment.

 SmartScreen 313 Worksheet 1

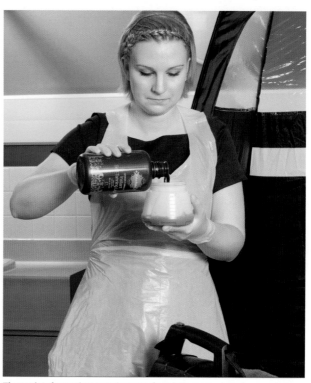

Therapist decanting tanning product into spray-tanning container

Compressor

A machine used to supply air or other gas at increased pressure

Turbine

Something that pushes air forward

There are a large number of products and equipment designed for tanning treatments. New products and machinery are being constantly developed to help improve the process and achieve the ultimate streak-free natural-looking tan. Spray-tan machinery is becoming smaller, lighter and less noisy as **compressor** units have been exchanged for **turbine** units.

Along with the equipment, products and tools on pages 397–400 you will also need:

- a record card
- cotton wool
- tissue/couch roll
- a lined bin
- sanitising/sterilising fluid.

Certain essential products, tools and equipment are used in all treatments.

Product, tools and equipment	Description	Use
Therapy couch	Cushioned treatment couch	May be used for the client to lie on during hand application of tan or during exfoliation treatment.
Cleanser	Oil-free solution	Used to remove any barriers from the skin prior to treatment.
Exfoliator	Mitt form or cream/liquid	Removes dead skin cells, especially around drier areas such as knees and elbows, and helps to achieve a more even colour.
Pre-tan moisturiser	Oil-free solution	Applied to areas where the tan may 'grab' such as knees, elbows and heels; helps give a more even coverage.

Product, tools and equipment	Description	Use
Barrier cream	Thick protective cream	Applied to the palms of the hands and soles of the feet to prevent staining.
Tanning solution	Solution which contains DHA in varying percentages to achieve differing depth of colour	Liquid for spray tan and cream for hand application; applied all over the treatment area to achieve a healthy tan.
Spray-tan tent and spray-tan booth	Two types: ■ pop-up tent which can be folded away after use ■ mechanical booth in which the client stands	The client stands in the tent while the therapist spray tans them. The client stands in the booth and a pre-measured dose of tanning solution is automatically sprayed on to them.
Spray-tan compressor	A pump which produces a stream of compressed air; sometimes called a pig due to its shape	Releases the spray tan, which is being pushed along a hose by the compressor.

Product, tools and equipment	Description	Use
Spray-tan gun	Gun-shaped, with a trigger	Forces the tanning solution out of the gun to give a fine mist application to the face/body.
Air hose Air hose	Plastic tubing	Attaches the spray-tan gun to the compressor.
Protective hair covering	Disposable fabric cap	Protects the client's hair from the tanning solution.
Disposable underwear	Disposable fabric briefs which are available as a brief, g-string or boxer short; also available as a backless bra	Prevents the client's own clothing from being damaged by the tanning solution/products.
Sole protectors	Woven fabric or card foot shapes which stick to the client's feet	Reduce the risk of staining to the feet during spray-tan application.

Product, tools and equipment	Description	Use
Consumables 	Cotton wool, cotton buds and tissues	Used to remove cleansers and excess tan from areas such as eyebrows and the palms of the hands.
Disposable gloves 	Latex- and talc-free gloves	Prevent staining of the therapist's hands.
Sanitising products 	Solutions such as witch hazel, pre-tan wipes	These are used to clean the area prior to treatment, if there is no shower available; usually in a wipe form.

It is essential to make sure that all tanning equipment is working before you carry out the procedure. You need to keep it well maintained and cleaned in order to prevent the spray gun getting clogged. Always clean your equipment according to the manufacturer's instructions and report any broken equipment to a manager.

MACHINE APPLICATION OF SELF-TAN

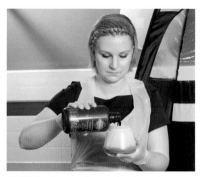

STEP 1 – Decant the product into the spray container.

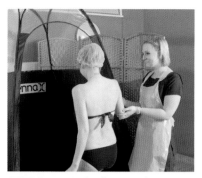

STEP 2 – Assist the client into the tanning tent.

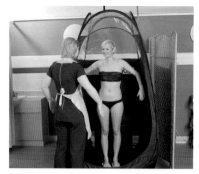

STEP 3 – Explain the tanning procedure to the client and advise them on how to stand during the treatment.

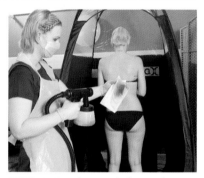

STEP 4 – Test the spray before application (using a tissue to see the density of the colour).

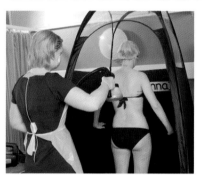

STEP 5 – Following training or manufacturer's instructions, apply the tan in a logical sequence on different areas of the body.

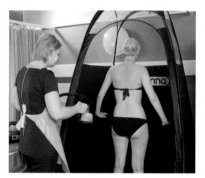

STEP 6 – Spray evenly across the treatment area, remembering not to go too close, to avoid dripping and a build-up of tanning product.

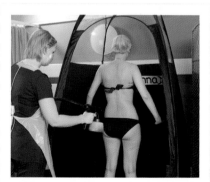

STEP 7 – Keen the gun at the correct angle during treatment to avoid uneven coverage.

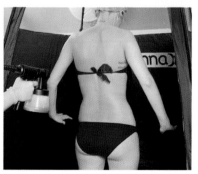

STEP 8 – Building the tan application slowly will be visible by the change in colour.

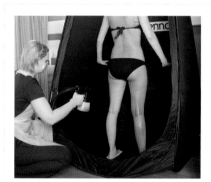

STEP 9 – Moving over body parts, always keep consistent depth of colour on each area.

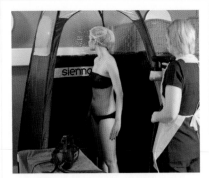

STEP 10 – Make sure the client is facing away, to avoid inhalation of the product.

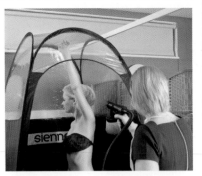

STEP 11 – Cover all areas of the body. Remember to adapt the depth of colour to show natural tan areas.

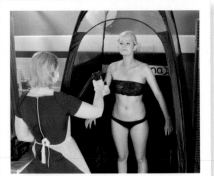

STEP 12 – Moving in a sequence will make sure that you do not miss an area, keeping an eye on the overall effect.

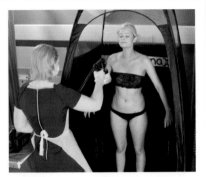

STEP 13 – Ask the client to close their eyes when working over the face area, to avoid stinging and watery eyes.

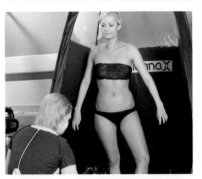

STEP 14 – Double check for even coverage to make sure no area has been left out.

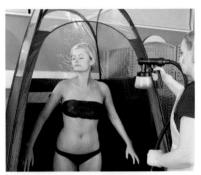

STEP 15 – Make sure you include the client's ears and protect their hair throughout the treatment. Ask the client to breathe our rather than in at this point.

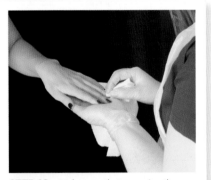

STEP 16 – Make sure that you wipe the client's finger nails at the end of the treatment, to avoid build-up of colour or staining.

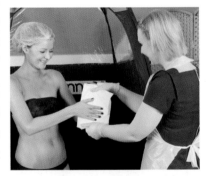

STEP 17 – Rub tissues between the client's palms to avoid yellow staining once the tan has developed.

INDUSTRY TIP

Keep diagrams to hand that show the positions the client will need to be in during treatment. Show the client these during the consultation so that they understand what is required of them.

To ensure an even application, make sure that you:

- always hold the spray gun straight and at right angles to the body
- always follow the same routine
- always spray lightly on hands, elbows, knees and feet
- never spray too close to the body – the manufacturer's instructions should suggest the best distance to spray from.

HAND APPLICATION OF SELF-TAN

Always follow the manufacturer's instructions to ensure that you achieve the optimum effect – these will vary between products. Wear gloves to prevent your skin getting stained where there is contact with the product.

The product may be applied with the client lying down or standing, depending on the available facilities and their preference. The procedure for manual treatment application should be carried out as follows:

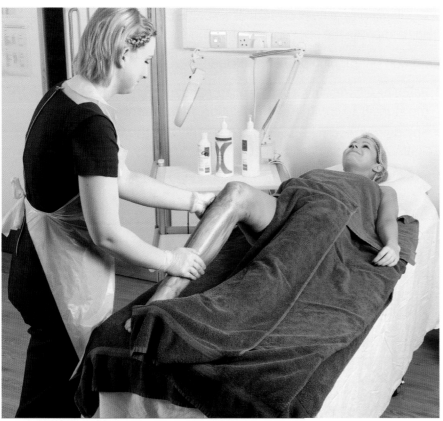

A therapist applying the tanning product by hand

1 Exfoliate the skin thoroughly.
2 Remove the exfoliator by either cleansing with sponges or asking the client to take a shower (the skin should then be dried).
3 Apply moisturiser to the feet, ankles, knees, elbows and wrists (moisturiser lightens the results, and should only be applied if recommended by the manufacturer), and barrier cream to the palms of the hands and the soles of the feet.
4 The application of the tan should be methodical. Ensure that all body parts are covered and that you have achieved an even application.
5 Any tanning product must be removed from the client's eyebrows and nails, the palms of their hands and the soles of their feet.
6 Use buffing mitts if recommended by the manufacturer to gently rub away any streaky patches.
7 Allow time for the product to dry thoroughly.
8 Ensure that the client is happy with the result and understands the aftercare advice.

Look in beauty magazines or on the Internet, and see how many brands of self-tanning products you can find. Check which ones have associated retail products to go with the self-tan.

TROUBLESHOOTING

If the client is not prepared properly, or too much tanning product is applied, the tan application may become streaky or patchy. There are tanning remover wipes that you can use to remove excess, and these should be used as soon as you notice any problem areas. However, if your client complains of streakiness, suggest to them that exfoliation will help to improve the appearance of the finished tan.

Common self-tanning problems include:

- Patchiness/streaking – use exfoliator and blend tanning solution with moisturiser to create a 50/50 solution, then reapply.
- Splodging/splatting – if you do over-spray and the tan forms 'splats', lightly dab with a tanning mitt.
- Green patches where deodorant has not been removed – these should wash off with a shower.
- Any uncovered cuts and abrasions will absorb the tanning solution and become darker and more noticeable.
- Discoloration of bleached/highlighted hair – the client will need to consult a hairdresser to rectify the hair colour.

HOME-CARE AND AFTERCARE ADVICE

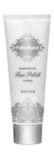 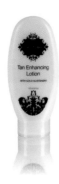 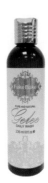

It is important to advise the client what to do after their treatment, as the development time of a spray tan can be up to 24 hours. If they do not follow the aftercare advice, the treatment result may be affected.

Advise the client to:

- avoid contact with water for at least six hours, or overnight if possible
- pat the skin dry after bathing rather than rubbing it
- avoid touching the skin
- wear loose dark clothing
- avoid any activity which may cause perspiration for 12 hours
- avoid swimming for 12 hours – chlorine and sea water will fade the tan prematurely

- moisturise daily using the recommended products
- exfoliate the skin as the tan fades to keep it even; if this is not done a build-up of dead skin cells will cause patchiness
- be aware that the tan may stain delicate fabrics
- re-book for the next tanning appointment in approximately seven to ten days.

CONTRA-ACTIONS

Contra-actions are rare, but they do happen. It is the therapist's job to ensure that the client is aware of contra-actions and how to deal with them.

Contra-action	Comments
Irritation/allergic reaction	An allergic reaction may occur if the client has an allergy to a product used during the treatment. Remove the product straight away and apply a cool compress. If the problem persists for longer than 24 hours, ask your client to seek medical advice.
Skin allergy	If a skin allergy occurs, advise your client to remove the product straight away and consult their GP, and to let the salon know the outcome.
Skin/hair discoloration	Hair discoloration is most common on bleached or very blonde hair. If this happens, advise the client to shampoo their hair straight away to prevent staining. If the skin discolours and the tan becomes patchy, advise your client to exfoliate to remove the patchiness.

CLIENT FEEDBACK

It is important to gain feedback from the client. If you have prepared the skin and applied the product correctly, this feedback should be positive. Some manufacturers recommend that their cream tan is applied quite thickly, which will not reflect the end result once the guide colour is washed off. Make sure the client is aware if this is the case, as part of their consultation, so it does not come as a shock. Show the client an area where the tan has not been applied, such as the demarcation line of their underwear, so they can compare the depth of colour. Ask open questions to ensure that you get a clear idea of the client's opinions about the result. You want their feedback to be constructive to help you improve. If the client is happy with their tan, hopefully they will come back to the salon and ask for you. Always thank the client for their feedback, whether negative or positive.

METHODS OF GAINING FEEDBACK

Feedback can be gained by:

- asking questions verbally
- observation – is the end result as smooth and even as can be expected (depending on the products being used), with no streaks or patches?
- handing out written questionnaires.

An excellent and very simple method of reviewing client satisfaction is to see how many of your clients re-book.

COMPLETING RECORDS

You must keep records of the treatments you carry out. The make, type and percentage of tan used should be noted, along with any adaptations and anything that the client specifically requested. Contra-actions should also be noted if they occur. These client records must be stored safely and confidentially in line with the Data Protection Act (see the Legislation chapter), and will useful for reference on future visits.

TEST YOUR KNOWLEDGE

Use the questions below to test your knowledge of Chapter 313 to see how much information you have retained. These questions will help you revise what you have learnt in this chapter.

Turn to page 499 for the answers.

1 What is the sugar that makes the tanning solution work?
   a AHD
   b ADH
   c DHA
   d HAD

2 What are the three parts of a spray-tanning unit?
   a Hose, solution, booth
   b Compressor, booth, gun
   c Solution, hose, compressor
   d Gun, hose, compressor

3 Which of the following cells create pigment in the skin?
   a Erythrocytes
   b Melanocytes
   c Leucocytes
   d Phagocytes

4 What is tanning solution absorbed into?
   a Sebaceous glands
   b The epidermis
   c Sweat glands
   d The dermis

5 How long does the application of a spray tan, including drying time, usually take?
   a 10 minutes
   b 15 minutes
   c 20 minutes
   d 60 minutes

6 Which of the following would restrict a spray-tan treatment?
   a Impetigo
   b Ringworm of the body
   c Shingles
   d Cuts and abrasions

7 What is the layer of the epidermis that is shed during exfoliation called?
   a Stratum lucidum/clear layer
   b Stratum germinativum/basal layer
   c Stratum corneum/horny layer
   d Stratum spinosum/prickle cell layer

8 Which of the following is **not** a method of tanning?
   a Using a sunbed
   b Applying exfoliator
   c Using a self-tanning lotion
   d Sunbathing in the sun

9 A professional spray tan usually fades within how many days?
   a 1–2
   b 3–5
   c 7–10
   d 12–13

10 Which **one** of the following is a contra-action to a spray tan?
   a Streaking
   b Itching
   c Uneven patches
   d Stained soles

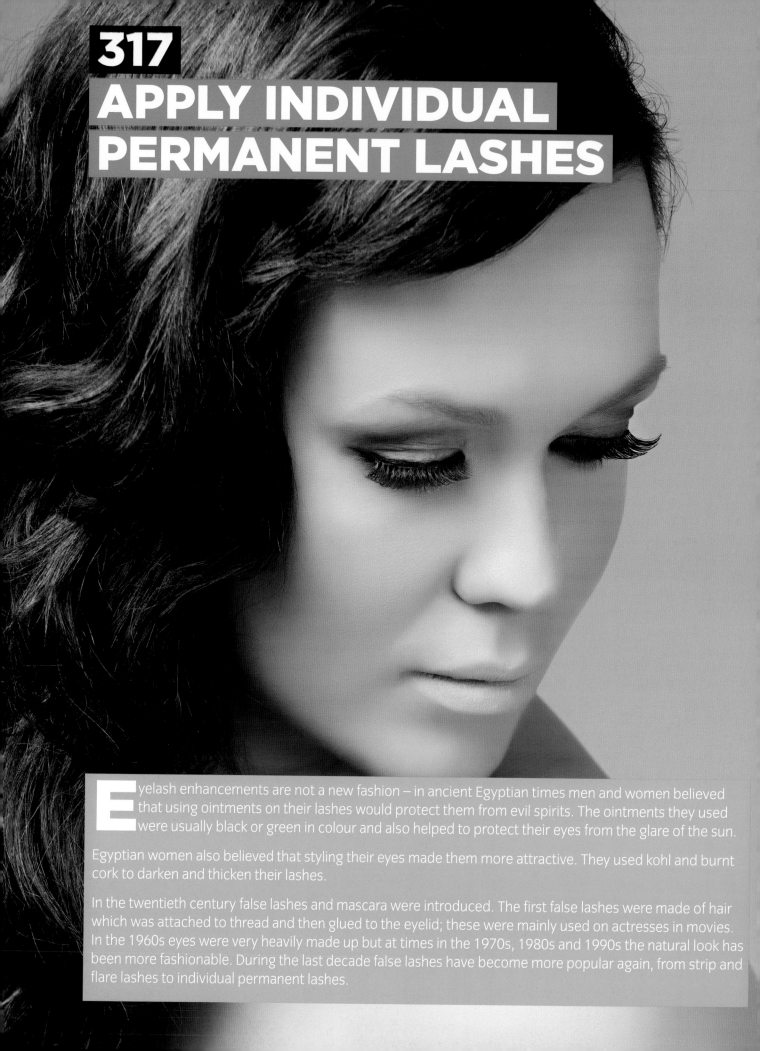

317
APPLY INDIVIDUAL PERMANENT LASHES

Eyelash enhancements are not a new fashion – in ancient Egyptian times men and women believed that using ointments on their lashes would protect them from evil spirits. The ointments they used were usually black or green in colour and also helped to protect their eyes from the glare of the sun.

Egyptian women also believed that styling their eyes made them more attractive. They used kohl and burnt cork to darken and thicken their lashes.

In the twentieth century false lashes and mascara were introduced. The first false lashes were made of hair which was attached to thread and then glued to the eyelid; these were mainly used on actresses in movies. In the 1960s eyes were very heavily made up but at times in the 1970s, 1980s and 1990s the natural look has been more fashionable. During the last decade false lashes have become more popular again, from strip and flare lashes to individual permanent lashes.

In this chapter you will:

- be able to prepare for individual permanent lash treatments
- be able to provide individual permanent lash treatments.

You should make sure you are familiar with the:

- structure of the hair and hair growth cycle
- main diseases and disorders of the hair.

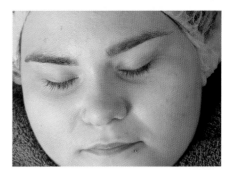

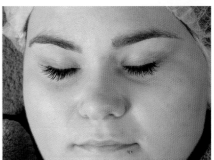

A client before and after an individual permanent lash treatment

PREPARE FOR INDIVIDUAL PERMANENT LASH TREATMENT

PREPARATION OF THE THERAPIST

For this treatment you will be working in close proximity to the client, so personal hygiene is very important. You must make sure that your uniform is clean, your breath is fresh, any long hair is secured away from the face and your nails and hands are clean. For more about your own presentation, see Chapter 301.

PREPARATION OF THE CLIENT

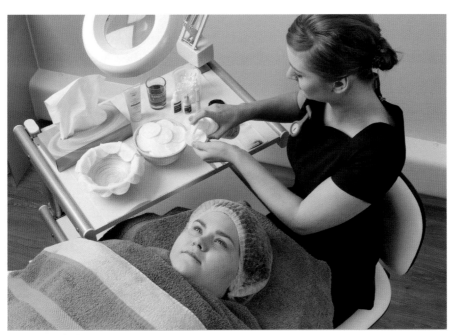

A client ready for treatment

The application of permanent lashes can take up to two hours and the client will be in a semi-reclined position during the treatment. It is very important to make sure the client is comfortable at all times and that they are positioned at the correct height for you to work on them without straining your back. Once the consultation has taken place and the style of lash has been established, the lash area needs to be prepared according to the manufacturer's instructions. However, as a guide, the eye make-up remover you use should be non-oily, as an oil-based one will create a barrier which will stop the lash enhancements sticking to the natural lash. Once the eye area is cleansed, wipe over with damp cotton wool and let it dry. If necessary, blot dry with a tissue. Some manufacturers will also recommend the use of a degreasing product as a final step.

PREPARATION OF THE TREATMENT AREA

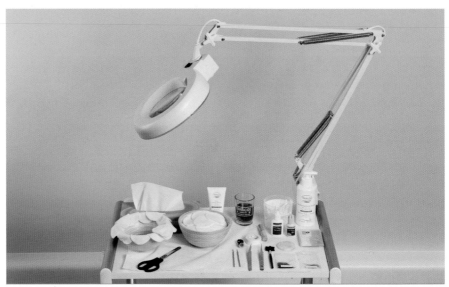

Trolley layout for a permanent lash treatment

- Suitable lighting is very important while performing lash treatments. A clear view is required throughout to ensure that the chosen product is applied in a correct, safe and effective manner. The treatment room needs to be at an appropriate temperature, so that both you and the client are comfortable.
- Good ventilation is required so that the room smells fresh, and to allow for exchange of oxygen. You may become sleepy if the room is stuffy.
- The room needs to be warm enough for the client to feel comfortable throughout their treatment, but if it is too hot this may cause them to perspire and could affect the consistency of the products.
- If music is playing it should be at a noise level acceptable to all and appropriate for both young and mature clients.
- Privacy is a very important aspect of the client feeling comfortable throughout their treatment. Make sure that the treatment room door is closed and remember never to leave your client on their own in the treatment room.
- All tools should be sterilised using the most suitable means. Use an autoclave for small metal tools such as tweezers.
- The therapy couch or chair must be disinfected before and after use, and can be protected for the duration of the treatment by placing disposable couch roll on it.
- Use a tiered trolley to place products and tools on. It needs to have wheels so that you can move it around and position it next to you to allow for easy access to the products/tools you will need during the treatment. It should be made of a material which is easily cleaned.
- You will need a supply of sterilised tweezers for this treatment.

THE CONSULTATION

The consultation is very important, as it is necessary to find out what type of look the client wishes to have before application – whether they want to appear natural or somewhat enhanced or achieve a dramatic effect. A portfolio of before and after pictures is an ideal way to show the client the effects it is possible to achieve. Allow the client plenty of opportunity to ask questions, and if possible have a list of frequently asked questions and answers to show the client – there may be something on the list that they would not have thought about. The desired length of the lashes should be discussed, but do explain that it is not possible to select the exact length of lashes to be used until the treatment starts and they can be measured against the client's natural lashes.

During the consultation you should also check that the client has had a patch test to ensure that they are not allergic to any of the products used during eye treatments. The patch test should include testing for adhesive, micropore tape, eye patches and solvent. Each test must be carried out in accordance with the manufacturer's instructions for the product, including the procedure and timings, eg 24 hours prior to the treatment. Record the results of the patch test on the client record card. Interpreting the results is important; they will be either a positive or a negative reaction to the products.

- Positive – the skin will appear irritated and inflamed, and swelling may occur. Ask your client to seek medical advice and do not continue with the treatment.
- Negative – the skin will appear normal with no reaction. If this is the case you can continue with the treatment.

ACTIVITY

Create a list of frequently asked questions and answers. Ask friends, family and colleagues what they would like to know before and after having the treatment to get ideas.

Information to record before, during and after the treatment:

- the client's name, contact details and date of birth
- the date of the treatment
- the occasion, eg wedding
- type of lashes required, eg natural, enhanced or dramatic
- type of adhesive used
- lash length and thickness used
- lash colour used
- approximate quantity used
- any reactions – eg nervous client, client kept opening their eyes
- contra-indications or contra-actions
- the cost of the treatment
- aftercare advice, detailing when the client needs to return for maintenance/infills
- the client's signature and yours – BEFORE the lash application commences.

INDUSTRY TIP

Ask the client's permission to take before and after photos of the treatment, and use them to build a portfolio. This will be helpful when you want to get a job in the industry, as you can show it to potential employers as well as clients. You could even design a permission slip that the client can sign to say that you can use their image in your portfolio.

INDUSTRY TIP

Very fair-haired clients will benefit from a lash tint in advance of the individual lash application.

If during the consultation you find that the client cannot wear permanent lashes, you can offer an alternative treatment. Below are other possible treatments for the lashes.

- Perming – this treatment takes about an hour to carry out and gives a curl to the natural lash. Unlike when using lash curlers, the curl is permanent until the lashes finish the growth cycle and are lost.
- Eyelash and eyebrow tinting – this is the application of a dye to the natural lashes and eyebrows in order to add definition. Changing their colour gives the illusion of thicker, fuller lashes.
- False flare lash extensions – these are a small cluster of around five synthetic lashes, which can be applied to the client's natural lash. They are heavier and less natural-looking than permanent lashes, and do not require a medical-grade glue, resulting in a much shorter duration of wear.
- Strip lashes – these come in pairs and are applied to the edge of the eyelid. They are available in a variety of lengths, styles and thicknesses, and give a dramatic effect. They should be removed each night with care, and can be reused.

ACTIVITY

Research the different styling of lashes throughout the years, and use the Internet to help you find images. Make a chart to record your findings.

ACTIVITY

Compare flared and individual lashes – price, application time, how long they last, what is available, skill level needed to apply them and so on. Record your findings.

CONTRA-INDICATIONS

During the consultation, you need to establish whether there are any contra-indications which will prevent or restrict treatment. It is important to remember that only a medical professional can give a diagnosis. You should advise the client to get anything which appears to be a contra-indication checked by their GP.

As this treatment concerns the eye area, most contra-indications will relate to the eyes.

Contra-indication – preventing treatment	Description
Conjunctivitis 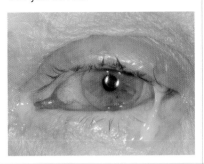	An inflammation of the membrane covering the eye. The eyes may be itchy and red, and pus may be present.
Dry-eye syndrome 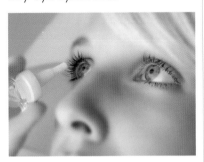	The eyes feel dry and the client will need to apply eye drops every hour or so. Lashes may irritate and the eye drops may dissolve the adhesive bond on the artificial lashes.
Eye infections 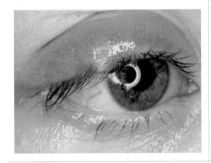	Varies depending on the infection. There is a risk of cross-infection.
Alopecia 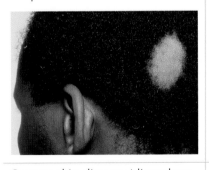	This is hair loss which can be triggered at any time, so each permanent application must be assessed separately. It may be that there are no hairs present to attach lashes to, or the application may trigger alopecia, resulting in the lashes (natural and artificial) falling out.
Severe skin disease/disorders 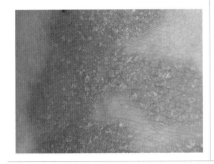	These include psoriasis, eczema and dermatitis. Depending on their severity, the treatment may cause further irritation to occur.

Contra-indication – preventing treatment	Description
Trichotillomania 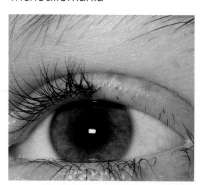	This is a condition where the client pulls their own hair out, from the head, eyebrows and lashes. The client may cause further damage by pulling the lash extensions out.
Skin/product allergies 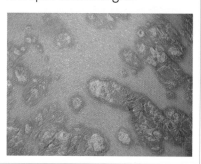	The client should not react to the adhesive, as it does not come into contact with their skin; however the gel pads, micropore tape or the gloves the therapist is wearing may cause an allergic reaction. Check for allergies during the consultation.
During chemotherapy 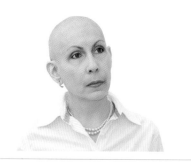	This may result in hair loss including the lashes. Even when lashes remain application should be avoided as the extensions will further damage the already weakened lashes.

The following contra-indications should also be taken into consideration, with the treatment either not being carried out, or restricted and modified as necessary:

- fungal, bacterial and viral infections
- during radiotherapy
- cuts and abrasions in the area
- infestations
- epilepsy
- diabetes
- high/low blood pressure
- undiagnosed lumps and swellings.

PRODUCTS AND EQUIPMENT

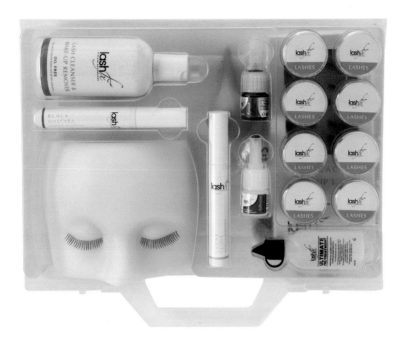

A professional permanent lash kit

A selection of products is required to carry out this treatment to a professional standard.

Product	Use
Non-oily eye make-up remover	To cleanse the eye area without leaving an oily barrier.
Adhesive	A professional adhesive which is suitable for use around the eyes. It is incredibly strong, so care must be taken during application. Do not apply too much, otherwise the client's eyes may stick together.

Product	Use
Anti-wrinkle gel patches	Placed over the lower lashes during treatment, to protect the under-eye area and also to prevent the upper and lower lashes sticking together during the treatment.
Adhesive remover	Used for the removal of excess adhesive or for lashes which have been positioned incorrectly and need to be removed and reapplied.
Sterile eye wash	To flush out the eye if anything enters it.
Professional sealer	Helps to seal the lashes and prolong their life.

Lashes	Effects
J curl	Natural lash curl
C curl	Enhanced curve
D curl	Dramatic curl
Rainbow lashes Designed lashes	Lashes come in a variety of colours and effects to create a fun look, give instant glamour or add impact for a special occasion. Gem lashes and feather lashes are other varieties that can be used.
Y-type lashes	These offer a speedier application time and fewer are needed – however, they do not always look quite as natural, and are really only suitable for naturally thick lashes due their weight.
Different diameters This is a W-lash which comes in sizes of 10, 11 and 12mm	Most lash companies will supply lashes of all lengths in different diameters. The diameter will affect the end result – the thickest lashes should be reserved for the most dramatic effect on naturally strong lashes.

ACTIVITY

Practise separating lashes on a strip lash using tweezers and magnifiers. This is quite tricky and needs lots of practice.

EQUIPMENT

You will need the following general equipment for this treatment:

- cotton wool
- pillow
- magnifying lamp
- mirror
- head band
- scissors.

The specialist equipment needed to perform the treatment is detailed in the following table.

Equipment	Use
Adhesive cup 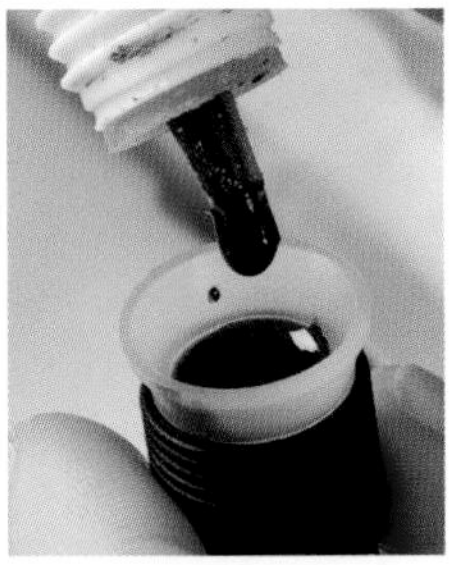	A small cup that holds a small amount of adhesive to prevent it drying out before it can be used.
Cup ring 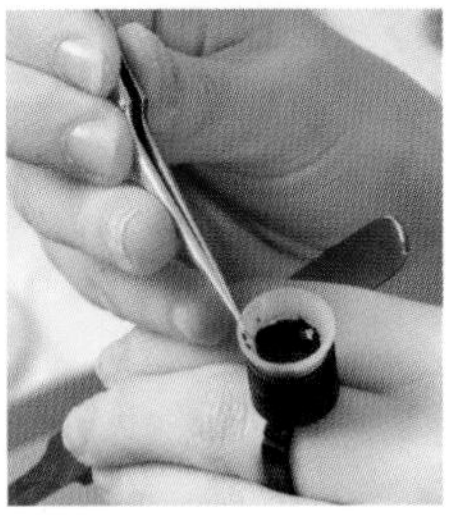	A small ring which is placed on the fingers or thumb – the adhesive cup sits in it.
Adhesive stone	A flat, smooth stone which the adhesive can be placed on as an alternative to an adhesive cup and ring. Usually made of jade, it helps to keep the adhesive cool, therefore stopping it from setting too quickly, before it can be used.
Disposable eyelash combs 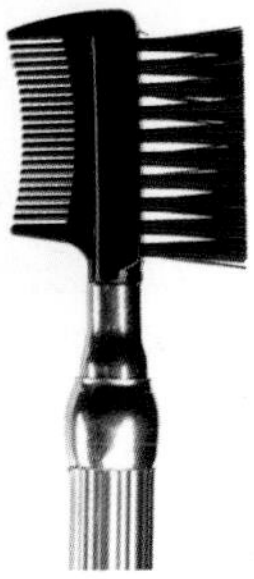	Used to comb through the lashes before, during and after the treatment.

Equipment	Use
Micropore tape	If the lashes are not already on pre-taped strips, they will need to be taken out of their container and placed on the micropore tape to enable the correct lash to be chosen for quick application. Micropore tape can also be used to hold back the upper layers of lashes to enable a layering effect.
Eyelash blower	A small rubber blower which is squeezed over the eyelashes to help the adhesive dry.
Tweezers	Needlepoint tweezers are required to separate the lashes, and for the application of the lash.

PROVIDE INDIVIDUAL PERMANENT LASH TREATMENTS

APPLYING LASHES

Once the consultation has taken place and you, the treatment area and the client are prepared, lash application can begin. Each brand of lashes will have its own routine for you to follow, which will help you to apply the lashes safely and achieve a great look for your client. However, here is a general description of the techniques required for applying lashes.

Position the client comfortably with support cushions where necessary (bear in mind the two-hour treatment time) and sanitise your hands.

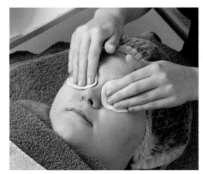

STEP 1 – Cleanse the eye area with a recommended eye make-up remover.

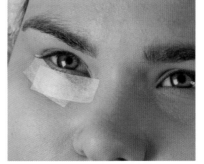

STEP 2 – Comb through and separate the lashes, then allow them to dry. Apply adhesive eye shield.

INDUSTRY TIP

Comb through the lashes again, straightening any tangles and loosening and removing any lashes that are ready to be shed.

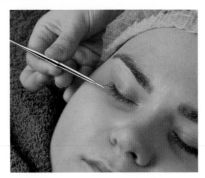

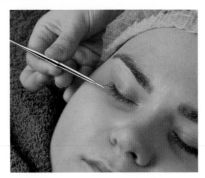

STEP 3 – Size up the permanent lashes next to the natural lash to assess the length, width/thickness and curve required.

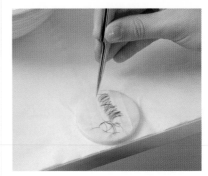

STEP 4 – Prepare a selection of the chosen lashes according to the manufacturer's instructions.

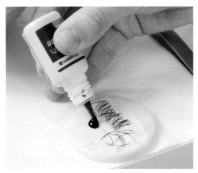

STEP 5 – Dispense the required adhesive.

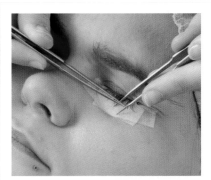

STEP 6 – Commence application by isolating a natural lash, holding the tweezers at a 45° angle in your non-working hand.

HANDY HINT

Cover the surface of the isolated hair with adhesive by stroking the glue from the single lash extension along it (avoid contact with the skin of the eyelid).

HANDY HINT

Work from eye to eye to allow the adhesive to dry; this also allows you to position the lashes in the same places on both eyes.

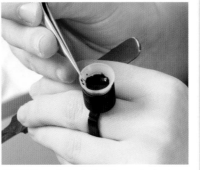

STEP 7 – Select a lash to be applied using the 'working' tweezers, and dip it into the adhesive.

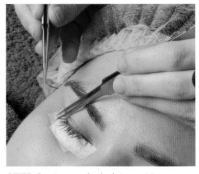

STEP 8 – Secure the lash in position, leaving a 0.5–1mm gap from lash line to lid.

INDUSTRY TIP

Once you've applied a lash, and before the adhesive is fully set, check the positioning to make sure the lash is pointing in the same direction as the natural lash. If there is any excess adhesive it can be removed at this stage using a disposable micro-brush. Do not brush along the lash, as this may remove it if the adhesive is not dry.

INDUSTRY TIP

If you are right-handed, apply the lashes to the back of your left hand, position the adhesive pot on your left thumb and also use this hand with the tweezers to isolate the natural lash. Use your right hand to dip the lash into the adhesive and then apply it. If you are left-handed, reverse the method.

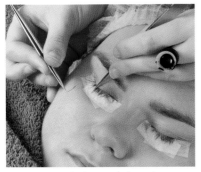

STEP 9 – Apply the next lash. Lashes should be positioned at spaced intervals along the lash line in order to achieve a balanced look and avoid adjacent lashes sticking together during application.

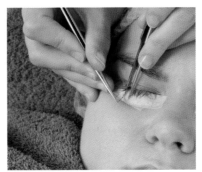

STEP 10 – On completion, comb the lashes through gently, avoiding the root area.

INDUSTRY TIP

Lashes can be layered to create a fuller effect. This can be done in two ways – the first is to use micropore tape to hold back the uppermost lashes. This is then repeated with the next layer of lashes. The individual lashes are then applied to those natural lashes closest to the inner upper lid. The layers of micropore tape are removed in reverse order, and extensions applied to the released lashes. The second method is to ensure that, when isolating lashes, they are selected from the different natural layers.

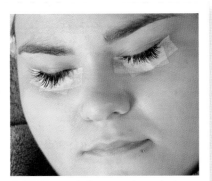

STEP 11 – Apply the protective sealer to coat the adhesive and lash, to improve longevity. Remove the eye shield.

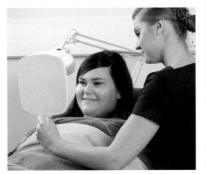

STEP 12 – Provide the client with a mirror to see the finished result.

HANDY HINT

Discuss aftercare advice and book the client in for a maintenance appointment.

ADAPTING THE LASHES TO SUIT THE CLIENT'S FACIAL CHARACTERISTICS

Naturally curly lashes

These will require a shorter lash extension, as a maximum bonding area is recommended. Use 'C' lashes.

Strong, healthy lashes

These can take extra-thick lash extensions if desired, which should only be applied to strong, healthy lashes that are naturally thick, so that they can carry the weight.

Deep-set eyes

Use slightly longer lashes so the extra length makes the eyes more noticeable. However, they should not be so long that they irritate the upper eye area if they eyes are very deep-set. Choosing the straightest lashes available will help you avoid this.

Round eyes

Lashes used on round eyes should be shorter at the inner corner and gradually extend in length toward the outer eye.

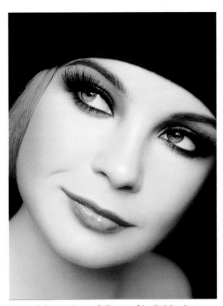

A model wearing a full set of individual permanent lashes

CLIENT FEEDBACK

When the treatment is finished it is important to gain feedback from the client to make sure they are happy with the treatment and the finished results. This can be achieved by asking the client to complete a written questionnaire, or verbally, by asking them open questions. Peer evaluation by a more senior member of staff will ensure that you gain useful feedback, including tips on what you did well and how you can improve in the future.

MAINTENANCE AND REMOVAL OF PERMANENT LASHES

To keep the lashes looking their best the client should return every two to three weeks to have loose lashes removed and new lashes applied. You should advise the client of this during the initial consultation.

In rare cases the client may not like the feel of permanent lashes, or they may simply decide they no longer wish to wear them; in this case you need to be able to remove them. It is extremely important that you tell the client not to try to remove the lashes themselves, as this may lead to the natural lashes being pulled out.

REMOVAL OF INDIVIDUAL LASHES

- Position the client comfortably with support cushions where necessary (bear in mind the two-hour treatment time) and sanitise your hands.
- Cleanse the eye area with a recommended eye make-up remover.
- Put a small amount of adhesive remover into an adhesive cup, then dip a micro-brush into the remover.

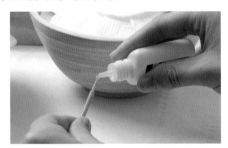

- Using two micro-brushes – a dry one underneath the lash and one dampened in adhesive remover on the top – stroke along the lash to be removed. This dissolves the adhesive and helps with the removal of the lash.
- When all the lashes have been removed, wipe the eye area with damp cotton wool to remove any remaining adhesive or adhesive remover. If the adhesive remover enters the eye it will become sore and the eye will need flushing out.

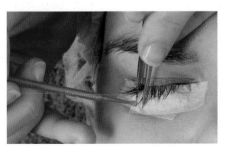

- Advise the client that the eye area may feel tender for a couple of hours. If any tenderness persists they should seek medical attention.

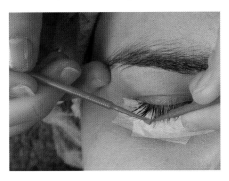

HOME-CARE AND AFTERCARE ADVICE

Once the lashes have been applied, the client needs to know how to look after them to prolong their life. The client should be advised to:

- avoid getting the lashes wet for at least two hours after application
- avoid heat treatments including hot water in the area for 48 hours
- avoid oil-based products, as these may break down the adhesive bond.
- avoid waterproof mascara, as it requires removal with an oil-based product
- avoid using an eyelash curler as it will loosen the lashes
- always pat the eye area dry; do not rub as this will loosen the adhesive bond
- return for maintenance appointments every two to three weeks
- not remove the lashes themselves – a special adhesive remover needs to be applied to avoid breakage of the natural lash
- seek medical attention in the event of an allergic reaction.

CONTRA-ACTIONS

A contra-action to this treatment will usually be a result of an allergic reaction. If this happens during the treatment, stop it immediately. The cause of the allergy needs to be found – you cannot assume that it is the lashes, as it may be the gel pads or the cleansing products used during the process. The reaction may be made worse if you try to remove the lashes. Advise the client to seek medical attention, and if possible give them a list of ingredients and some remover to supply to the medical practitioner.

Stinging or watery eyes

These may be just natural reactions, or they may be caused by sensitivity to the adhesive. Gently blot the eyes frequently, as the tears will affect how well the lashes adhere. Adhesive for sensitive eyes is available, but usually has a weaker set. If the watering is excessive, the treatment may have to be stopped, with a careful explanation to the client. Shorter sessions could be booked, or partial sets of lashes applied.

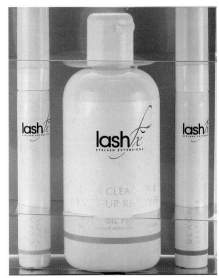

Professional lash care products

TEST YOUR KNOWLEDGE

Use the questions below to test your knowledge of Chapter 317 to see how much information you have retained. These questions will help you revise what you have learnt in this chapter.

Turn to page 499 for the answers.

1 What is the maximum length a permanent lash can be when applied to natural lashes?
   a ¼ longer
   b ⅔ longer
   c ½ longer
   d ¾ longer

2 Following a treatment, how often should a client return to the salon for maintenance to their individual permanent lashes?
   a Every two to three weeks
   b Weekly
   c Monthly
   d Never

3 Eyelash extensions are suitable for all clients. True or flase?
   a True
   b False

4 The J-curl permanent lash is described by which **one** of the following?
   a Dramatic
   b Natural-looking
   c Enhanced
   d Colour coded

5 What is the approximate number of permanent lashes that are applied per eye?
   a 30
   b 40
   c 50
   d 60

6 Which **one** of the following would prevent a permanent eyelash treatment?
   a The client wearing glasses
   b Contact lenses
   c Trichotillomania
   d Tinted eyelashes

7 Before application or removal of permanent lashes, which **one** of the following should the lower lashes be covered with?
   a Wet cotton wool
   b A gel pad
   c Micropore tape
   d Dry cotton wool

8 Which **one** of the following is the best method of sterilising tweezers?
   a An autoclave
   b A UV cabinet
   c Alcohol-based sanitiser
   d Soap and water

9 What type of tweezers are used for the application and removal of permanent lashes?
   a Automatic
   b Slant-edge
   c Needlepoint
   e Round-tip

10 Which glue should be used to apply semi-permanent lashes?
   a Flare lashes glue
   b Latex glue
   c Semi-permanent lash glue
   d Hair extension glue

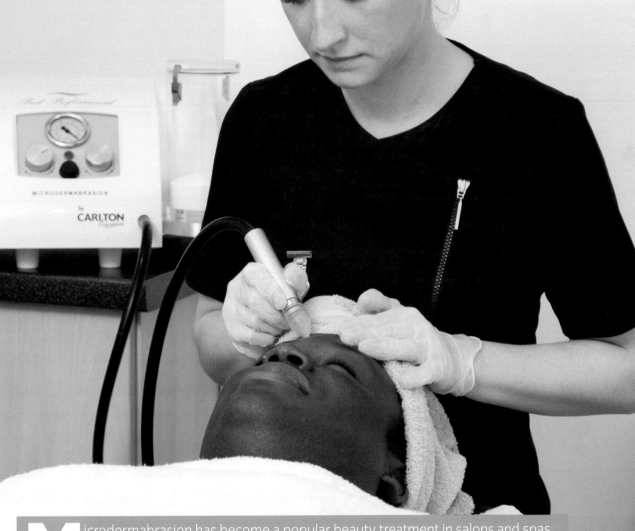

321
APPLY
MICRODERMABRASION

Microdermabrasion has become a popular beauty treatment in salons and spas. It is used to improve the condition of the skin on the face and body. It gently removes the surface layers of the skin to leave it feeling soft and smooth and looking brighter. Whilst it is quite an easy treatment to carry out, it is important to have proper training as if it is done incorrectly it can cause damage.

This chapter covers the skills and knowledge required to perform microdermabrasion treatments on different skin types and conditions and how to provide clients with advice to maintain the benefits of the treatment.

In this chapter you will learn how to:

- prepare for skin treatment using microdermabrasion
- provide skin treatment using microdermabrasion.

WHAT IS MICRODERMABRASION?

Micro
Very small

Dermabrasion
(Derm-ah-bra-zhun) Removal of layers of the skin by mechanical means

Abrade
To scrape

> **HANDY HINT**
>
> Brush up on your knowledge of the skin for this unit – see pages 20–46 in the Anatomy and Physiology chapter.

Microdermabrasion exfoliates the skin. It is used for improving the appearance of the skin and treating various skin conditions. It is a very popular treatment because it has an immediate effect but it also has long-term effects due to the stimulation of the skin's repair functions.

Currently, there are two popular methods of microdermabrasion:

- Crystal microdermabrasion – very small crystals are sprayed onto the skin, at a variable pressure, to exfoliate the skin. The crystals and exfoliated skin cells are removed by a vacuum.
- Diamond microdermabrasion – an abrasive substance is used to smooth out the top layers of the skin. Instead of using crystals to exfoliate the skin, a hand piece containing diamonds or other particles is passed over the skin. The diamond tip abrades the skin and, in a similar way to crystal microdermabrasion, the exfoliated particles are then removed by vacuum through the same hand piece. This is a newer procedure which is gaining popularity.

Most microdermabrasion machines will come with the option of using either crystals or diamond tips.

PREPARATION OF THE WORK AREA

There should be a high standard of cleanliness in the work area. Prior to a treatment being carried out:

- Disinfect all equipment within the work areas, such as the trolley, lamps, couch and electrical equipment.
- Check the temperature of the treatment area – it should be warm enough that the client feels comfortable but not too hot to cause flushing of the skin.
- Carry out all necessary electrical safety precautions and tests.

> **HANDY HINT**
>
> Your work area should be well ventilated. The lighting should be bright enough to see the skin clearly but not too bright. Ensure the music isn't too loud and that the aromas are pleasant. You want to create a relaxing environment.

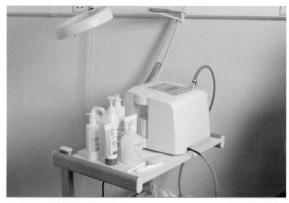

A clean and tidy work area

> **HANDY HINT**
>
> Make sure that electrical equipment has been PAT tested and that it is still valid.
> - Ensure that wires are not causing a trip hazard.
> - Keep water away from the machine in case of accidental spillage.

PREPARE THE CLIENT FOR MICRODERMABRASION

Prepare the client by:

- asking them to remove their jewellery (eg earrings, necklace or any facial piercings) from the treatment area
- positioning them on the treatment couch – making sure they are comfortable and that you can easily access the area to be treated
- checking that their expectations are realistic and that they are fully aware of the microdermabrasion process.

EQUIPMENT AND TOOLS

CRYSTALS

The most successful and most commonly used crystals for crystal microdermabrasion are **aluminium oxide** (corundum crystals). This is because in terms of hardness they are second only to diamonds which makes them excellent for abrading the skin.

Other types of crystals that are used include:

- magnesium oxide crystals
- sodium bicarbonate (baking soda) crystals
- sodium chloride (salt) crystals
- occasionally nut shells or fruit stones (generally labelled as organic grains).

Aluminium oxide crystals are the most commonly used in microdermabrasion because they are hard enough to provide the level of exfoliation needed and because they are the best crystals for use with the equipment. The other crystals listed above provide less effective exfoliation and may clog up the machine.

DIAMONDS/SILICON CARBIDE

Silicon carbide is often used in place of diamonds for diamond microdermabrasion.

Silicon carbide is a very hard manufactured **crystalline** material made from silicon and carbon. It comes as a powder.

Although silicon carbide is more commonly used than diamonds, the name diamond microdermabrasion is used because it sounds more attractive. Silicon carbide heads are less expensive than diamond heads so they can be disposed of and replaced more frequently.

Aluminium oxide

A natural metal compound found in the earth

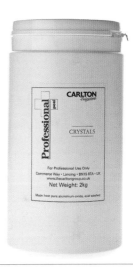

Microdermabrasion crystals

Crystalline

Having the structure of crystals

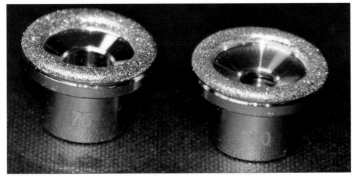

Silicon carbide heads

COMPONENTS OF THE DIFFERENT TYPES OF MICRODERMABRASION MACHINES

A microdermabrasion machine is made up of:

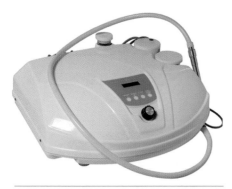

Crystal machine

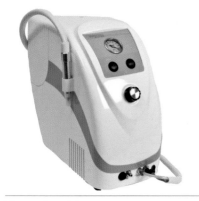

Diamond machine

Crystal machine	Diamond machine
Two tubes: ■ one for clean crystal spray ■ one for used crystal removal.	Single tube connected to machine and hand piece.
Operating buttons, eg: ■ on/off button ■ crystal settings ■ vacuum settings ■ anti-clog button.	Operating buttons, eg: ■ on/off button ■ vacuum settings.
Hand piece: ■ made from metal or glass ■ attached is a nozzle that targets the crystals onto the skin.	Hand piece: ■ made from metal or plastic ■ attached is the diamond head that is used on the client's skin.
Pressure gauge: ■ shows how much pressure is being applied to the skin from vacuum suction.	Pressure gauge: ■ shows how much pressure is being applied to the skin from vacuum suction.
Vacuum/air pump: ■ pulls and raises a small section of skin whilst pumping the crystals through the tube onto the skin ■ vacuums away the used crystals, skin and debris into the used crystal container.	Vacuum/air pump: ■ pulls and raises a small section of skin whilst pumping the crystals through the tube onto the skin.
Clean crystal container.	
Used crystal container.	

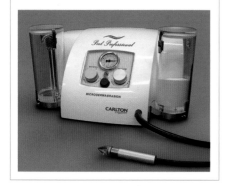

Vacuum

To collect particles (eg crystals) by suction

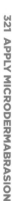

ADVANTAGES AND DISADVANTAGES OF THE DIFFERENT TYPES OF MICRODERMABRASION EQUIPMENT

The advantages and disadvantages of the different types of microdermabrasion equipment are shown in the table below.

Type of microdermabrasion machine	Advantages	Disadvantages
Crystal microdermabrasion	<ul><li>More hygienic as crystals are used once only and can be disposed of.</li><li>Crystals can penetrate into folds of the skin and wrinkles as they are fired under pressure.</li></ul>	<ul><li>Can be costly replacing crystals.</li><li>Concerns about risks from inhalation of crystals.</li></ul>
Diamond microdermabrasion	<ul><li>Less expensive as diamond head replacement (ie **consumables**) is required less frequently than crystal replacement.</li><li>No crystal residue to clear away after treatment.</li></ul>	<ul><li>Hygiene issues as diamond heads can be difficult to clean effectively.</li><li>Longer treatment or more repeat movements are necessary to penetrate into the folds of the skin and wrinkles as the diamonds are **static** on the hand piece.</li></ul>

PREPARATION OF PRODUCTS AND EQUIPMENT FOR MICRODERMABRASION

1 Make sure you have all the necessary tools and equipment in place:
   - microdermabrasion machine
   - crystals or a selection of diamond heads
   - disposable applicator heads (if using crystal microdermabrasion).

2 Prepare the machine according to the manufacturer's instructions, eg:
   - the new crystal container is three-quarters full
   - the container for the used crystals is empty
   - the disposable nozzle cap on the applicator is clean.

3 Test the machine to make sure it is in good working order.

4 Adjust the height of the couch to suit the client (eg to take into consideration the client's mobility and the areas of the body to be treated).

5 Cover the couch with a clean towel and/or disposable couch roll.

Consumables
Items that are used fairly quickly and that need to be constantly replaced

Static
Not moving; fixed

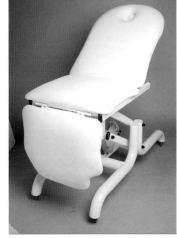
A treatment couch

INDUSTRY TIP
A fully adjustable couch is advisable to suit the needs of different clients. A fully adjustable couch also helps prevent postural problems for the therapist.

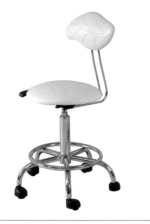

A therapist's stool

INDUSTRY TIP

A stool with castors allows you to move freely during the treatment.

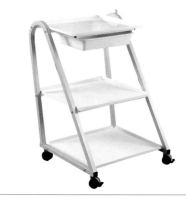

A stable trolley with enough shelves for storage

Vinyl

A type of plastic which provides a reasonable resistance to oil and grease. It is not as strong or as resistant to tearing as nitrile

Nitrile

A type of rubber with increased strength and resistance to oils and acids

HANDY HINT

One towel should be available for the therapist to make sure that their hands are dry when touching the microdermabrasion machine.

6   Adjust the height of the therapist's stool so that your posture is correct and your back is supported.

7   Ensure your trolley is stable and that it has enough shelves to put the equipment on the top and any products and water below to prevent any accidental spillage onto the machine.

8   Make sure you have clean towels or a gown to protect the client's modesty.

9   Ensure you have a waste bin for general waste and a yellow waste bag for disposing of the crystals.

10   Make sure you have the following personal protective equipment (PPE):

- **vinyl** or **nitrile** disposable gloves for therapist to prevent cross-infection (see industry tip below)
- a face mask for the therapist to avoid inhaling crystals (see industry tip on page 431)
- protective goggles for the client to prevent any loose crystals going into their eyes.

11   Prepare the trolley with the following equipment and products:

- tissues (for drying the client's skin)
- disposable sponges (for cleansing and mask removal)
- headband or bonnet (ideally disposable)
- cotton wool (used sparingly for eye make-up removal)
- selection of bowls (for water)
- spatulas
- mask brush
- skin cleanser
- serum
- ampoules
- mask (soothing and hydrating)
- moisturiser
- sun protection product.

INDUSTRY TIP

It is important to wear disposable protective gloves (vinyl or nitrile) when performing a microdermabrasion treatment. (Powder-free gloves are recommended to reduce the risk of potential allergies.) During the treatment, you are removing the skin's protection so the client's skin is more vulnerable to bacteria. Wearing gloves helps to reduce the risk of cross-infection. As there is a small risk of breaking the skin and causing blood spotting, gloves also protect the therapist from infection.

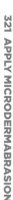

CONSULTATION

Consultation is a vital process during which you should assess the client's needs and objectives and their suitability for the treatment. More detailed information on the consultation process and communication techniques can be found in Chapter 303, Client care and communication in beauty-related industries (pages 212–215 and 206–211).

The consultation should be carried out in a comfortable and private area following industry codes of practice. The consultation techniques for assessing your client's skin should include:

- questioning: asking your client questions to establish the factors contributing to the skin's condition
- manual inspection: touching/feeling the skin to determine its condition
- visual inspection: looking at the skin closely to determine its type and condition.

SKIN ANALYSIS

It is important to carry out a skin analysis using visual and manual inspection techniques to assess the client's skin type, the pigmentation of the client's skin and any sun damage. This is because microdermabrasion can affect melanin. If the melanin in the skin is more active, there is a greater potential to cause unwanted pigmentation changes. Darker skins should be treated gently and gradually to avoid pigmentation problems.

A thorough skin analysis is important prior to any treatment. As microdermabrasion is an exfoliating treatment, when you are carrying out your skin analysis you need to assess whether the skin can withstand exfoliation and what adaptations should be made. You need to:

- assess the client's general skin type (ie dry, oily or combination)
- consider the client's skin's characteristics (ie dehydrated, mature skin, young skin, lacking in tone, wrinkles, blemishes (eg milia, pustules, comedones) and pigmentation variations)
- look at the client's skin tone (ie fair, medium or dark).

MANAGING CLIENTS' EXPECTATIONS

Microdermabrasion is a high-profile treatment, often used by and endorsed by celebrities. As a result, clients' expectations of the treatment might be unrealistic. It is therefore important to manage your clients' expectations. Microdermabrasion offers many benefits to many skin conditions but it can't miraculously turn back the clock.

THE CLIENT TREATMENT PLAN

During the consultation process, discuss and agree the treatment plan with the client in line with their needs and desired outcomes. Make recommendations to the client to get the best possible results from the treatment. Once you have discussed and agreed the treatment plan, summarise and confirm the client's objectives and the treatment process.

The thickness of the stratum corneum (outer layer of skin) will affect the level of exfoliation. Finer skins can't **tolerate** as much exfoliation.

INDUSTRY TIP

Most modern crystal microdermabrasion machines do not spray crystals into the air. However, there is a small risk of inhaling stray crystals. It is therefore advisable to wear a face mask during treatment.

INDUSTRY TIP

It is important to establish whether the client has any allergies to the products and equipment used in the treatment. It is also as important to find out whether the client has had an allergic reaction in the last two to four weeks even if the reaction is unrelated to the treatment. This is because the treatment stimulates **histamine** production so any treatment may cause the skin to react.

Histamine

The chemical the body produces when having an allergic reaction. It causes blood vessels to dilate and an inflammatory response in the tissues

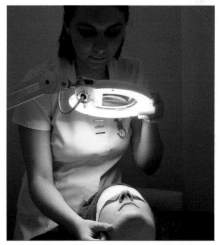

A therapist carrying out a skin analysis

INDUSTRY TIP

A mirror is a handy tool to use during a consultation. Allow the client to look in the mirror and point out to you exactly what they would like to improve.

Tolerate

Cope with

The following table gives information on the type of microdermabrasion treatment you should provide based on the client's skin type or condition.

Skin type or condition	Treatment using the crystal method	Treatment using the diamond method	Products
Dry skin	<ul><li>Light exfoliation only.</li><li>Low pressure and low crystal flow.</li><li>Use rapid movements with no repeat movements.</li></ul>	<ul><li>Use a low-grade abrasion head and low pressure.</li><li>Rapid movements with no repeat movements.</li></ul>	Nourishing and hydrating masks, serums and creams
Oily skin	<ul><li>Medium exfoliation.</li><li>Medium pressure and medium crystal flow.</li><li>Avoid any pustules.</li><li>Repeat movements if necessary.</li><li>Adapt speed of movement as required in each area.</li><li>Rapid movements in areas with finer skin.</li><li>Slower movements in areas of thickened skin.</li></ul>	<ul><li>Use a medium-grade abrasion head and medium pressure.</li><li>Avoid any pustules.</li><li>Adapt speed of movement as required in each area.</li><li>Rapid movements in areas with finer skin.</li><li>Slower movements in areas of thickened skin.</li></ul>	Hydrating, balancing, purifying and soothing masks, serums and creams
Combination skin	<ul><li>Light to medium exfoliation.</li><li>Low to medium pressure and low to medium crystal flow.</li><li>Adapt speed of movement as required in each area.</li><li>Rapid movements in areas with finer or drier skin.</li><li>Slower movements in areas of thickened skin.</li></ul>	<ul><li>Use a low- to medium-grade abrasion head and low to medium pressure.</li><li>Adapt speed of movement as required in each area.</li><li>Rapid movements in areas with finer or drier skin.</li><li>Slower movements in areas of thickened skin.</li></ul>	Hydrating, balancing and soothing masks, serums and creams
Mature skin	<ul><li>Light to medium exfoliation.</li><li>Low to medium pressure and low to medium crystal flow. Always support the skin during treatment to avoid dragging.</li><li>Adapt speed of movement as required in each area.</li><li>Rapid movements in areas with finer skin.</li><li>Slower movents in areas of thickened skin.</li></ul>	<ul><li>Use a low- to medium-grade abrasion head and low to medium pressure.</li><li>Always support the skin during treatment to avoid dragging.</li><li>Adapt speed of movement as required in each area.</li><li>Rapid movements in areas with finer skin, slower movements in areas of thickened skin.</li></ul>	Regenerating and hydrating masks, serums and creams

Skin type or condition	Treatment using the crystal method	Treatment using the diamond method	Products
Dehydrated	<ul><li>Medium to deep exfoliation.</li><li>Medium to high pressure and medium to high crystal flow.</li><li>Adapt speed of movement as required in each area.</li><li>Rapid movements in areas with finer skin.</li><li>Slower movements in areas of thickened skin.</li></ul>	<ul><li>Use a medium- to high-grade abrasion head and medium to high pressure.</li><li>Adapt speed of movement as required in each area.</li><li>Rapid movements in areas with finer skin.</li><li>Slower movements in areas of thickened skin.</li></ul>	Hydrating and soothing masks, serums and creams
Sensitive or fine skin	<ul><li>Not suitable for treatment.</li></ul>	<ul><li>Not suitable for treatment.</li></ul>	
Pigmented skin	Initial treatment:<ul><li>Light exfoliation only, low pressure, low crystal flow.</li><li>Use rapid movements with no repeat movements.</li></ul>Subsequent treatments:<ul><li>If no contra-actions occur: medium to deep exfoliation.</li><li>Medium to high pressure and medium to high crystal flow.</li><li>Adapt speed of movement as required in each area.</li><li>Rapid movements in areas with finer skin.</li><li>Slower movements in areas of thickened skin.</li></ul>	Initial treatment:<ul><li>Use a low-grade abrasion head and low pressure.</li><li>Rapid movements with no repeat movements.</li></ul>Subsequent treatments:<ul><li>If no contra-actions occur; medium- to high-grade abrasion head and medium to high pressure.</li><li>Adapt speed of movement as required in each area.</li><li>Rapid movements in areas with finer skin.</li><li>Slower movements in areas of thickened skin.</li></ul>	Hydrating, brightening and pigment treatment masks, serums and creams

CLIENT RECORD CARDS

It is important to complete a client record card with details of the treatment plan and note any modifications to the treatment. You may add to it during the treatment. You can also refer back to the information on the record card if the client has further treatments. If the client is having a course of treatments, you will be able to use the information to assess how successful the treatments have been and discuss the results with the client.

A client record card

SENSITIVITY TESTING

It is recommended that you carry out a sensitivity test 24 hours prior to the treatment:

- Cleanse the area to be tested.
- All the products that will be used during the treatment (eg cleanser, crystals and aftercare products (eg serum, mask and moisturiser)) should be applied to an area just behind the ear approximately 2cm x 2cm.
- Carry out a second sensitivity test using only the crystals (ie no products). This is because the products (eg cleanser etc) are the things most likely to cause a reaction.
- Ask the client to leave the area alone and return to the salon the next day for you to assess the reaction.
- Note any contra-actions that occur within 24 hours or any adverse reactions.

Contra-actions

- Mild erythema.
- Slight flaking of the skin.

Adverse reactions

- Severe or prolonged erythema.
- Swelling (oedema).
- Changes in pigmentation (**hyper-pigmentation** or **hypo-pigmentation**).

If no adverse reactions are seen after 24 hours, a full treatment may take place. If any adverse reactions are observed then the treatment should not go ahead. However, if adverse reactions are observed on the first test but not the second, treatment may go ahead using different products (after testing these).

Hyper-pigmentation
Increase in pigmentation in the skin

Hypo-pigmentation
Loss of pigmentation in the skin

CONTRA-INDICATIONS TO MICRODERMABRASION

In addition to the general contra-indications listed in Chapter 303 (page 215), there are a number of contra-indications that are specific to microdermabrasion:

Contra-indication	Restricts/prevents treatment	Reason
Vascular/fragile skin or acne rosacea	Prevent	<ul><li>The skin is very fragile and thin.</li><li>Cannot tolerate this type of exfoliation.</li></ul>
Cosmetic procedures (eg acid peels)	Prevent	<ul><li>The skin is already undergoing exfoliation.</li><li>It will be highly sensitised.</li><li>Cannot tolerate further exfoliation.</li></ul>
Roaccutane (medication for acne)	Prevent	<ul><li>Reduces sebum in the skin.</li><li>Skin is dry, thinned and highly sensitised skin during its use and for up to six months afterwards.</li><li>The skin cannot tolerate microdermabrasion.</li></ul>
Active viral lesions (eg herpes simplex or cold sores)	Prevent	<ul><li>High risk of cross-infection.</li></ul>
Cancer/chemotherapy and radiotherapy	Prevent	<ul><li>Microdermabrasion activates the circulation and lymphatic flow.</li><li>If cancerous cells are present there is a potential risk of mobilising them within the circulatory system.</li></ul>
Pregnant women	Prevents	<ul><li>Hormonal changes during pregnancy mean that the skin is more prone to hyper-/hypo-pigmentation.</li></ul>
Active acne lesions	Restricts treatment if only a few are present but would prevent treatment if they are more widespread.	<ul><li>Treatment would spread the bacteria and cause cross-infection.</li></ul>
Moles	Restricts treatment	<ul><li>If the nature of the mole is unknown, the client needs to seek medical advice prior to treatment.</li></ul>

Contra-indication	Restricts/prevents treatment	Reason
Fine or young skins	Prevent	■ Skin cannot withstand this kind of abrasion. ■ Skin doesn't need this kind of abrasion.
Haemophilia	Prevents	■ Blood clotting is reduced. ■ As there is a potential to cause bleeding you should not carry out microdermabrasion.
Tattoo	Restricts treatment – areas around the tattoo may be treated.	■ Deeper exfoliation over a tattoo may result in blurring and fading of the tattoo.

Haemophilia

A condition in which blood clotting is reduced

SKIN CANCER

Skin cancer is the most common type of cancer in the UK. A client may ask for a pigmentation mark to be removed. As a therapist, particularly one who provides microdermabrasion treatment, you are in a unique position to spot possible skin cancers. As a therapist you are not medically qualified to give a diagnosis of a skin condition. However, it is very important that you are aware of the key indicators of skin cancer and know how to direct the client to a medical expert without causing distress or alarm.

EFFECTS AND BENEFITS OF MICRODERMABRASION

The table below shows the effects and benefits of microdermabrasion treatments:

Effects	Benefits
■ Stimulates cellular renewal and circulation. ■ Removes dark, keratinised cells and debris.	■ Improves skin's health and appearance (ie brightens dull skin). ■ Restores and revives mature skin. ■ Reduces fine lines and wrinkles. ■ Refines and reduces scar tissue.
■ Smoothes out uneven texture.	■ Smoothes and restores the skin's texture.
■ Removes the surface layer of the epidermis so that pigmented areas will appear lighter.	■ Reduces hyper-pigmentation (eg age spots and sun damage).
■ Deep exfoliation: 　■ removes debris from the surface of the skin 　■ unblocks pores.	■ Deep facial cleansing.
■ Increases circulation and lymphatic flow, smoothing the skin.	■ Improves the appearance of cellulite.

ACTIVITY

Put together an information sheet or leaflet that could be used on a salon's website to promote microdermabrasion services.

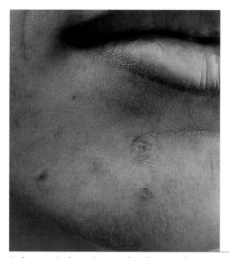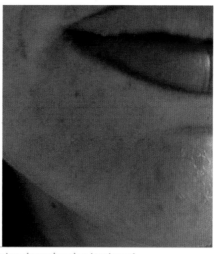

Before and after photos of a client undergoing a microdermabrasion treatment

WHY DON'T YOU...

look on the Internet or contact local salons offering microdermabrasion and find out how many use crystal microdermabrasion and how many use diamond microdermabrasion. Discuss the benefits of each method with your tutor.

INDUSTRY TIP

Microdermabrasion is an ideal treatment for male clients. Male skin tends to be naturally thicker than female skin and regular shaving can make the skin thicker and cause ingrown hairs. Microdermabrasion will remove keratinised cells and debris and stimulate cellular renewal making it an ideal treatment for men.

TREATMENT TIMES

The microdermabrasion process is relatively quick depending on the area to be treated. A session will usually last about 50–60 minutes; approximately 15–20 minutes of this time will be spent using the machine and the rest of the time will be for pre-cleansing and post-treatment care.

The number and interval of treatments will depend on:

- the required end result
- the skin's condition
- the skin's reaction to the treatment.

As a guide, clients are likely to have a course of between six and 12 treatments every seven to ten days in order to achieve the **optimum** results. Where deeper exfoliation has taken place, at least 10–14 days should be left between treatments to allow the skin time to heal and recover.

INDUSTRY TIP

Microdermabrasion offers a dramatic instant result and long-term effects. To meet the needs of different clients your treatment menu should include 'quick-fix' (a light instant 'polish') as well as a more intensive exfoliation option.

Optimum

The best possible; ideal

INDUSTRY TIP

It is quite common for salons to offer a faster 'quick polish' type microdermabrasion facial. This can be carried out in 30 minutes by excluding the **lymphatic drainage** prior to treatment and using cooling gel to finish the treatment rather than a treatment mask.

Lymphatic drainage

Specific movements that stimulate the circulation and lymphatic flow to help get rid of toxins and waste. This improves the skin condition and helps to regenerate the skin

CARRY OUT MICRODERMABRASION TREATMENTS USING THE CRYSTAL AND DIAMOND METHODS OF APPLICATION

Once you have completed the consultation and the client profile, you can start the treatment. You also need to make sure that the response to the sensitivity test doesn't prevent treatment. Before you start, ask the client to remove their clothes and jewellery and put them somewhere for safekeeping.

A client's first treatment should always be carried out lightly (ie on a low pressure setting with rapid movements) to assess the skin's reaction. The depth of treatment can be increased at future sessions as long as there are no contra-actions.

> **INDUSTRY TIP**
>
> Do not apply any products to the skin whilst you are using the microdermabrasion machine unless the manufacturer's instructions say you can do so. Any products used on the skin will be sucked up into the machine and might stop it from working.

> **INDUSTRY TIP**
>
> Keep water and moisture well away from the machine and the crystals. Imagine if you left a bowl of sugar or salt out in the open; any moisture in the air would cause the salt or sugar to clump together. This is exactly what will happen to the crystals if they are not kept in a sealed container away from moisture.
>
> The same applies to the crystals in the machine. If you work on wet skin or keep a steamer near the microdermabrasion unit, the moisture will get inside the machine and form clumps of crystals.

MICRODERMABRASION PROCEDURE

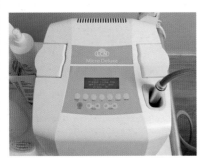

STEP 1 – Set up the machine (check that it is in working order prior to use).

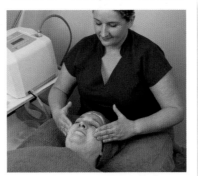

STEP 2 – Prepare the client's skin for the treatment procedure by cleansing with appropriate products for their skin type.

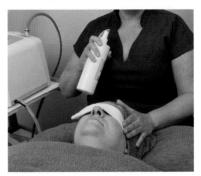

STEP 3 – Tone the skin using an appropriate product, ensuring that you protect the eyes of the client.

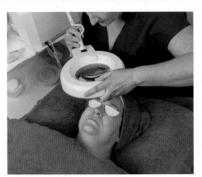

STEP 4 – Place eye pads onto the client's eyes. Check the client's skin for any identifying issues such as broken capillaries.

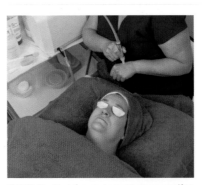

STEP 5 – Test the equipment on yourself to make sure that everything is working correctly and that it is at the correct level.

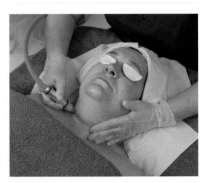

STEP 6 – Carry out the procedure following the manufacturer's instructions. Start with the client's neck. Use tissue to collect debris from the treatment.

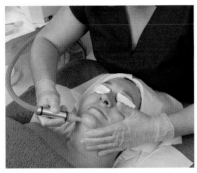

STEP 7 – Next work across the client's jaw line.

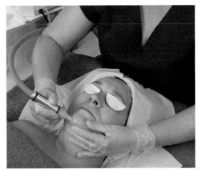

STEP 8 – Work across the chin area in small movements.

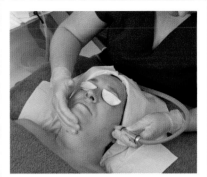

STEP 9 – Work across the cheek area in a continuous motion.

HANDY HINT

Diamond method

If you are using the diamond method, after step 4 put the appropriate diamond head in place on the hand piece. Select the appropriate head according to the client's needs, the desired outcome and the manufacturer's instructions. Diamond heads are available with varying sizes of particles; bigger particles for deeper exfoliation and smaller particles for more **superficial** exfoliation.

Superficial

Near the surface

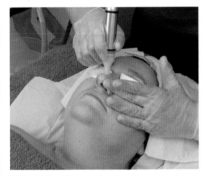

STEP 10 – Work across the nose area in smaller steps.

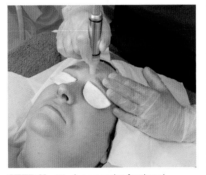

STEP 11 – Work across the forehead, looking at the skin reaction throughout.

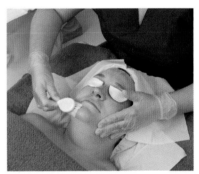

STEP 12 – Using a soft brush, remove dead skin cells/debris from the client's face.

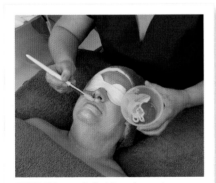

STEP 13 – Apply facial mask evenly over the entire neck and face area, placing eye pads over the client's eyes for comfort.

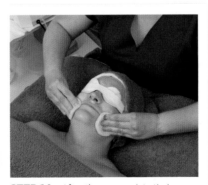

STEP 14 – After the appropriate timing, remove the facial mask.

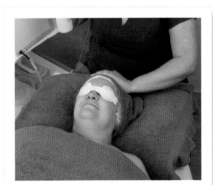

STEP 15 – Tone the entire face.

Lymph nodes

(Or **lymph glands**) These filter and clean lymph fluid before it is returned to the bloodstream. Help to prevent infection

HANDY HINT

Faster movements = lighter exfoliation

Slow movements = deeper exfoliation

INDUSTRY TIP

Clearly note on the client's record card the pressure settings or diamond heads used and the outcomes achieved.

HANDY HINT

Monitor the client's comfort and skin reaction throughout the treatment and adjust the level of exfoliation if needed.

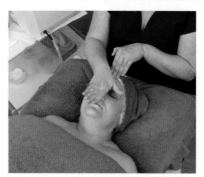

STEP 16 – Moisturise the entire face, using the correct product for the client's skin type.

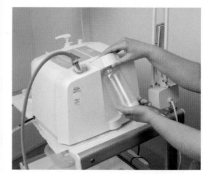

STEP 17 – Clear and clean the machine after the treatment is complete.

At the end of the treatment you should evaluate the treatment by checking that visible treatment outcomes have been achieved (eg that the skin texture is refined and smooth). Give any aftercare advice. Remind the client that certain outcomes (eg wrinkle reduction and pigmentation reduction) take time and might need further treatment.

INDUSTRY TIP

When carrying out exfoliation using microdermabrasion, use short movements from the centre of the face outwards. This will help you to make the speed and pressure more constant. Long sweeping movements often leave red lines on the client's skin.

INDUSTRY TIP

It is essential to use the correct pressure setting to get the best results. Your technique is equally as important. Practise as much as possible to improve your skills.

MAINTENANCE OF THE MACHINE

It is important to maintain the machine so that it remains in good working order:

- Empty the used crystal container after each client. Try to prevent the used crystals and dead skin cells from entering the atmosphere.
- After every treatment, clean the filters and lids according to the manufacturer's instructions.
- Dispose of the diamond head or clean the nozzle on a crystal machine.

ACTIVITY

Practise your movements on friends and family. Remember to overlap your movements and keep them short and at a constant speed. Begin by working on the backs of hands until your technique improves.

ACTIVITY

For each skin type, suggest a list of post-care products (from the range at your college or another range you are familiar with) that would be suitable for use by a client following a microdermabrasion treatment.

ADAPTING THE TREATMENT TO SUIT CLIENT NEEDS

- Wrinkles/scar tissue – work along the length of the wrinkle and from side to side within the borders of the wrinkle or scar. Continue to do this until red spots appear. This method works deeper and smoothes the area.
- Large areas (eg the back or tops of the arms) – treat the area in small sections. Take care to overlap each movement to avoid 'striping'. Keep the movements fluid and in the same direction across the area.
- Cellulite – repeat the lymphatic stimulation stage at least three times over each area.
- Contra-indications – on most microdermabrasion machines the vacuum suction stage can be done as a **stand-alone** treatment. This can be very useful for brightening and reviving skin where exfoliation is contra-indicated.

INDUSTRY TIP

To keep the microdermabrasion machine in good working order, it is vital to follow the manufacturer's instructions on cleaning and maintenance. Filters will need replacing regularly.

Stand-alone

Able to be done on its own

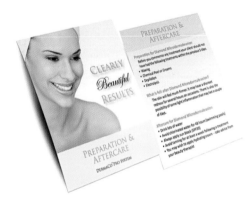

An aftercare leaflet

CONTRA-ACTIONS TO TREATMENT

A contra-action is an adverse reaction that can happen during or after a treatment. It is important to be aware of these reactions and provide advice to your client in case they do occur.

If contra-actions do occur during treatment, discontinue the treatment and provide appropriate action and advice.

Contra-action	Cause	Action to be taken
Erythema	■ Redness of the skin due to over-stimulation of the skin or an adverse reaction. ■ Usually occurs in first 24 hours but may be prolonged depending on the depth of treatment and skin sensitivity.	■ Avoid heat or further skin stimulation for at least 48 hours. ■ Protect skin from UV radiation. ■ Apply moisturising products. ■ Reduce pressure setting. ■ Increase speed of movements. ■ Avoid repeated movements over a specific area. ■ Avoid applying downward pressure on the hand piece.
Swelling (oedema)	■ Swelling due to fluid retention.	■ Make sure client has given you correct information about allergies. ■ Make sure that all products used in treatment were included in the sensitivity test. ■ Reduce pressure setting. ■ Increase speed of movements. ■ Avoid repeated movements over a specific area. ■ Avoid applying downward pressure on the hand piece.
Flaking or peeling of the skin	■ A natural reaction. ■ Shows that the skin is renewing itself.	■ Apply moisturising products.
Excessive bleeding	■ Removal of the epidermis to expose the dermis. ■ Treatment too deep.	■ Reduce pressure setting. ■ Increase speed of movements. ■ Avoid repeated movements over a specific area. ■ Avoid applying downward pressure on the hand piece.
Changes in pigmentation (hyper-pigmentation or hypo-pigmentation)	■ Dark patches on the skin (hyper-pigmentation which is caused by an increase in melanin in the skin). ■ Light patches of skin where the pigmentation has been lost (hypo-pigmentation which is caused by a decrease in melanin in the skin).	■ Protect skin from UV radiation. ■ Apply moisturising products. ■ Reduce pressure setting. ■ Increase speed of movements. ■ Avoid repeated movements over a specific area. ■ Avoid applying downward pressure on the hand piece.

Contra-action	Cause	Action to be taken
Red stripes on the skin	<ul><li>Too much downward pressure applied on hand piece.</li><li>Speed of hand piece was not constant.</li></ul>	<ul><li>Make sure speed of hand piece is constant.</li><li>Reduce pressure setting.</li><li>Increase speed of movements.</li><li>Avoid repeated movements over a specific area.</li><li>Avoid applying downward pressure on the hand piece.</li></ul>
Pin-point bruising	<ul><li>Flat, round red spots under the skin surface caused by bleeding between the epidermis and the dermis.</li></ul>	<ul><li>Reduce pressure setting.</li><li>Increase speed of movements.</li><li>Avoid repeated movements over a specific area.</li><li>Avoid applying downward pressure on the hand piece.</li></ul>

GENERAL CAUSES OF CONTRA-ACTIONS

The diagram below lists general contra-actions to microdermabrasion treatment.

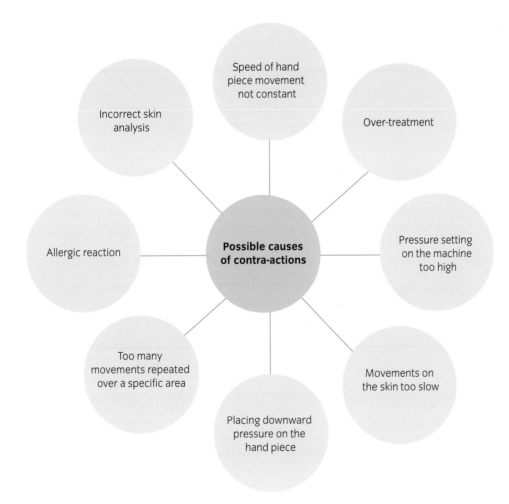

AHAs

Alpha hydroxy acids

HANDY HINT

Advise the client not to use 'dirty' moisturising creams (ie pots of cream which they have put their fingers into). These are likely to contain bacteria which can be transferred to their skin. Recommend that they purchase a new product and use a spatula for the duration of their microdermabrasion treatments.

HOME-CARE AND AFTERCARE ADVICE

Following a microdermabrasion treatment, you should give your client suitable aftercare advice to follow. This advice will help the client maximise the benefits of the treatment.

- Avoid alcohol, spicy foods, heat treatments and hard physical activity for 24 hours as these are stimulants and can contribute to the initial reddening of the skin.
- Do not use any products other than those recommended by your therapist. In particular, avoid perfumed products and those containing exfoliation ingredients such as **AHAs**.
- Avoid UV exposure and always use a sunscreen with an SPF 20 or above. Remember that you can't apply this for the first 24 hours.
- Avoid wearing make-up for 24 hours. If wearing make-up after this time, always use a clean applicator brush and try to use mineral make-ups.
- Use a gentle cleansing lotion and apply plenty of moisturising cream (after the first 24 hours).
- Avoid further skin treatments to the area to let the skin settle down.
- Follow the therapist's advice if any contra-actions occur.

TEST YOUR KNOWLEDGE

Use the questions below to test your knowledge of Chapter 321 to see how much information you have retained. These questions will help you revise what you have learnt in this chapter.

Turn to page 499 for the answers.

1 What type of treatment is microdermabrasion?
- **a** A muscle stimulation treatment
- **b** An exfoliating treatment
- **c** A high frequency treatment
- **d** A nourishing treatment

2 Which **one** of the following is **not** a material used in microdermabrasion machines?
- **a** Sodium bicarbonate (baking soda)
- **b** Fruit stones
- **c** Aluminium oxide
- **d** Sand

3 How long before a treatment should a sensitivity test be carried out?
- **a** 2 hours
- **b** 24 hours
- **c** 4 days
- **d** 2 weeks

4 Which **one** of the following would **not** be found on a diamond microdermabrasion machine?
- **a** Vacuum setting
- **b** Anti-clog button
- **c** Hand piece
- **d** Crystal flow button

5 Which **one** of the following needs to be replaced after every use of a microdermabrasion machine?
- **a** Crystals
- **b** Air pump
- **c** Filters
- **d** Nozzle

6 If changes in pigmentation (hyper-pigmentation or hypo-pigmentation) occur on a client's skin during a microdermabrasion treatment, which **one** of the following actions should be taken?
- **a** The crystal flow should be increased
- **b** The crystal flow should be reduced
- **c** Treatment should stop and aftercare advice should be given
- **d** The speed of the movements on the skin should be increased

7 Which **one** of the following is a contra-indication to microdermabrasion treatment?
- **a** Cancer
- **b** Pregnancy
- **c** Acid peels
- **d** Respiratory conditions

8 What level of sun protection factor (SPF) should a client use following a microdermabrasion treatment?
- **a** SPF 2
- **b** SPF 4
- **c** SPF 8
- **d** SPF 20 or above

9 How long should the exfoliation stage of a microdermabrasion treatment take?
- **a** 15 minutes
- **b** 30 minutes
- **c** 45 minutes
- **d** 60 minutes

10 Which **one** of the following would **not** result in red stripes being left on the skin following a microdermabrasion treatment?
- **a** The speed of the hand piece movement was not being consistent
- **b** Gaps left between hand piece movements
- **c** The pressure setting being too low but movements and pressure being consistent
- **d** Too much downward pressure was exerted on the hand piece

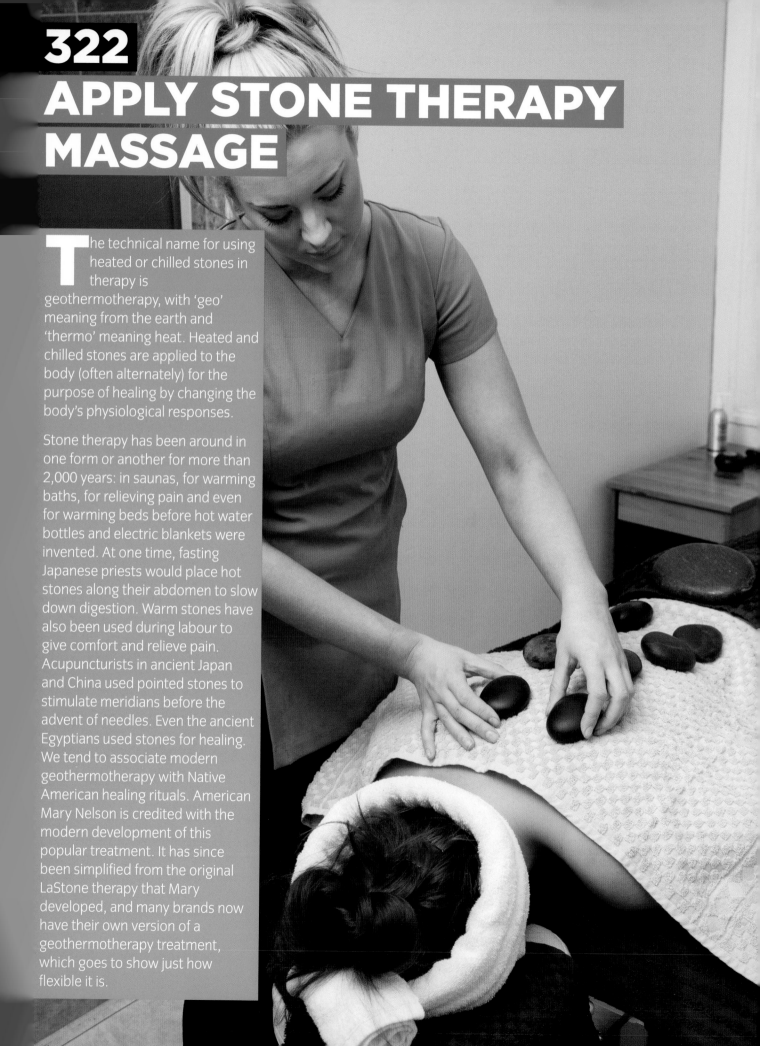

APPLY STONE THERAPY MASSAGE

The technical name for using heated or chilled stones in therapy is geothermotherapy, with 'geo' meaning from the earth and 'thermo' meaning heat. Heated and chilled stones are applied to the body (often alternately) for the purpose of healing by changing the body's physiological responses.

Stone therapy has been around in one form or another for more than 2,000 years: in saunas, for warming baths, for relieving pain and even for warming beds before hot water bottles and electric blankets were invented. At one time, fasting Japanese priests would place hot stones along their abdomen to slow down digestion. Warm stones have also been used during labour to give comfort and relieve pain. Acupuncturists in ancient Japan and China used pointed stones to stimulate meridians before the advent of needles. Even the ancient Egyptians used stones for healing. We tend to associate modern geothermotherapy with Native American healing rituals. American Mary Nelson is credited with the modern development of this popular treatment. It has since been simplified from the original LaStone therapy that Mary developed, and many brands now have their own version of a geothermotherapy treatment, which goes to show just how flexible it is.

In this chapter you will:

- be able to prepare for a stone therapy treatment
- be able to apply a stone therapy treatment.

You should make sure you are familiar with:

- the structure, function, position and action of the muscles of the body
- the location, function and structure of the bones of the body
- the location, function and structure of the circulatory and lymphatic systems.

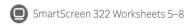 SmartScreen 322 Worksheets 5–8

PREPARE FOR STONE THERAPY MASSAGE

PREPARATION OF THE THERAPIST

As a therapist you will be working in close proximity to the client throughout this treatment. It is very important that you are dressed and presented in a professional manner. See Chapter 301 for more information.

Before you start any treatment you should make sure you are fully prepared physically by doing the hand exercises in Chapter 305/309, and that you are mentally focused. The client is paying for your time and attention and you should avoid any distractions.

INDUSTRY TIP

If you are aiming to entice the male market you should make sure that the reception area is neutral and includes male-oriented displays. Include current magazines for your male clients as well as ladies' magazines.

PREPARATION OF THE TREATMENT AREA

The treatment area should be fully prepared before the client arrives. You should make sure that all work surfaces have been cleaned and are tidy and organised. Any equipment that needs to be cleaned and sanitised, such as the heater and the stones, needs to be ready before you begin. Make sure that any equipment or products that you need are ready and easily accessible before you start, so that you do not have to interrupt the flow of your treatment to go and get anything.

INDUSTRY TIP

When choosing footwear, remember that flipflops can be noisy, and should also be avoided for safety reasons. Work shoes should be fully enclosed and secure on the feet.

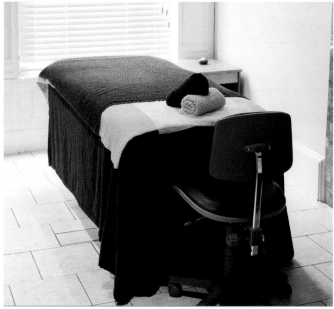

A prepared treatment area

THE TREATMENT ENVIRONMENT

The client needs to be comfortable during the treatment. Check and adjust the following so that the client can relax and enjoy their treatment.

- Aim for subtle lighting, with no glare in the client's eyes.
- Put on soft, gentle, relaxing music. However, some clients may prefer to have their treatment in silence.
- Make sure the room is warm, cosy and free from draughts.
- Make sure the room has a pleasing aroma – avoid the build-up of stale odours, pay attention to personal hygiene and use fragranced products.
- Remember to take into account the client's need for privacy.
- Avoid any unnecessary noise during your treatment – for example, when you remove the stones from the heater, do so with care.
- Make a quick check of the working area for hazards, and remove them or take steps to reduce any risks.

PREPARATION OF THE CLIENT

For full details on preparing a client for a massage treatment, see Chapter 305/309.

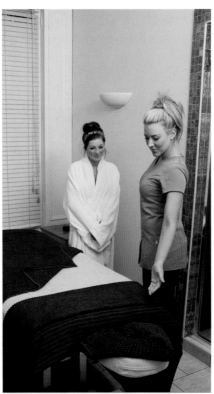

A therapist guiding a client to the treatment couch

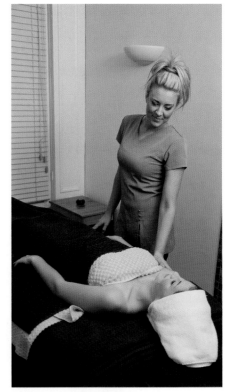

A client ready for treament

CONSULTATION

A detailed consultation to establish the client's priorities and needs must take place before every treatment. Further information on the consultation process can be found in Chapter 303. Stone therapy uses both hot and cold stones, and therefore an important part of the consultation is to carry out a thermal and tactile test (see Chapter 305/309 for information on thermal and tactile sensitivity testing). You can use a hot stone and a cold stone for thermal testing.

CONTRA-INDICATIONS

Chapter 305/309 gives an overview of contra-indications. You will need to make sure you are familiar with each condition. The following are contra-indications that you will need to be particularly aware of when offering stone therapy treatment.

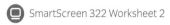 SmartScreen 322 Worksheet 2

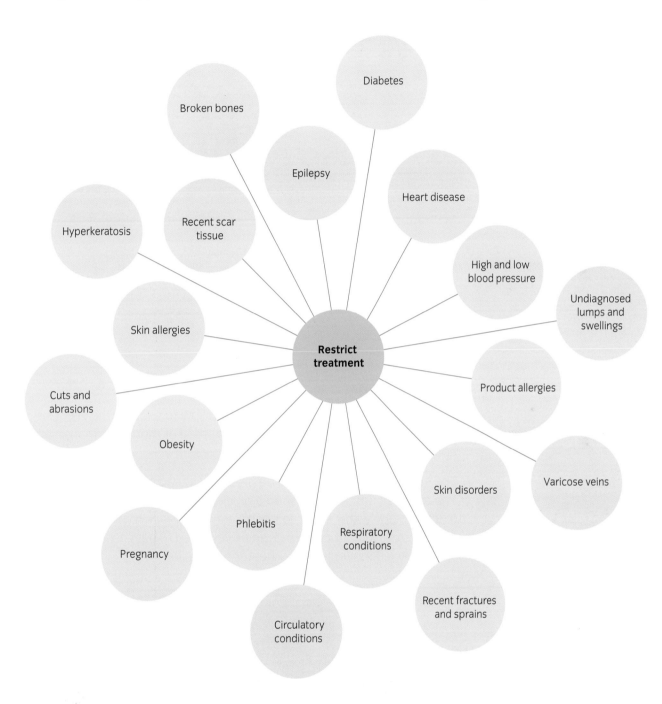

INDUSTRY TIP

A contradictory reaction to the application of heat is when erythema does not colour. The body reacts as if it is chilled and the skin has a blue-white appearance. This may be a sign of arteriosclerosis (remember, you cannot offer a diagnosis) and the treatment should be stopped immediately. Advise the client to consult their GP.

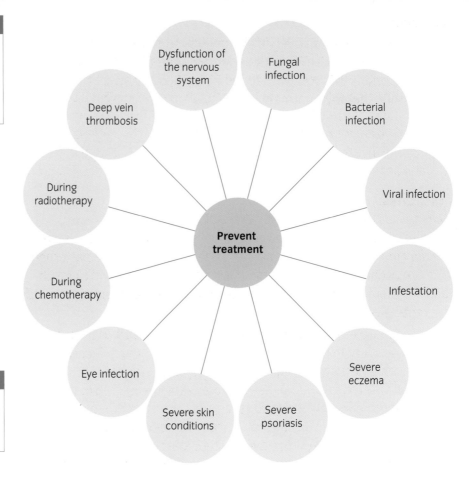

Center: **Prevent treatment**

- Dysfunction of the nervous system
- Fungal infection
- Bacterial infection
- Viral infection
- Infestation
- Severe eczema
- Severe psoriasis
- Severe skin conditions
- Eye infection
- During chemotherapy
- During radiotherapy
- Deep vein thrombosis

EQUIPMENT

You will need a treatment couch (with a pillow to support the client's neck), a trolley and a bin to dispose of waste. For more information on equipment, refer to Chapter 305/309.

The heater and stones should be prepared ahead of your client's arrival. The top shelf of the trolley should be cleansed and covered with a towel to absorb any water and also to give a quiet surface to place the stones on. The trolley can then be moved as you need to gain access to the stones. Avoid moving a heavy heater on a trolley.

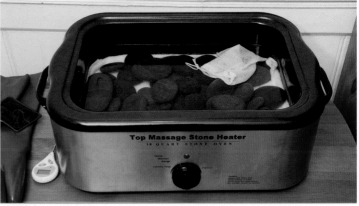

A stone heater

THE STONES

To perform a stone therapy treatment it is necessary to have a selection of stones. These vary in size, shape, colour and temperature.

Hot stones

- Basalt stones – these are made of fine-grained volcanic rock, created when the molten lava from a volcano is compressed. They are rich in iron and magnesium. Water from the sea or a river wears away the sharp edges, leaving a smooth, naturally shaped stone. Basalt stones appear darker once oil has been applied to them. They remain hot up to four times longer than other natural stones and release this heat slowly, making them ideal for hot massage. There are several different varieties of basalt stone.

Cool stones

- Marine – as the name suggests, these stones are found in water, specifically around volcanic islands. They are rich in minerals, as they are formed from the sediment on the ocean floor. They are patterned, and are usually a grey-green colour. Marine stones are cool to touch and are therefore used for cooling an area, reducing inflammation and promoting vasoconstriction.
- Marble – marble is an organic rock, which means it comes from living organisms. It contains calcite and limestone. In its original state, marble can feel rough to touch. It is a heavy stone which is also very cool. Marble stones are expensive as they are handcrafted to make them smooth enough for massage, and to fit small contours of the face. They are used to reduce inflammation and to cool areas of the body when the skin becomes overheated. Marble can be easily scratched and needs to be looked after carefully to prevent damage.

Massage stones vary in shape – they may be round, oblong or half-moon. They also come in various sizes, from large stones which are placed on the sacrum to more delicate stones which can be placed between the fingers and toes or over the eyes. A full body treatment will use around 55 different stones.

It is important to check stones before the treatment to see that they have no cracks or chips in them. Damaged stones can be felt by the client and may cause stretching of the skin or injury.

- Semi-precious – these are crystals or gemstones which vary in colour. They have properties which enable them to open the chakras and therefore help with rebalancing the mind, body and spirit. A set of seven different stones is used for stone therapy, with each relating to one of the colours of the chakras; it is placed on the corresponding chakra point during treatment.

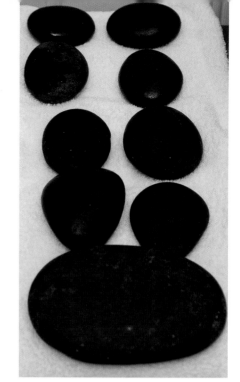

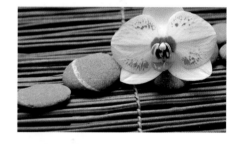

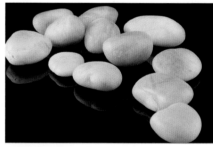

A selection of treatment stones

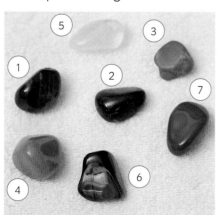

Seven semi-precious stones

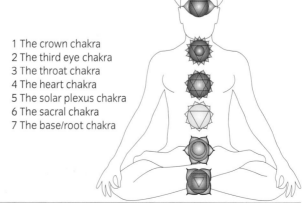

1 The crown chakra
2 The third eye chakra
3 The throat chakra
4 The heart chakra
5 The solar plexus chakra
6 The sacral chakra
7 The base/root chakra

Chakras

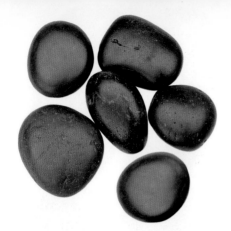

Thermotherapy (hot stones)

Hot stones can be used for placement, but they should always be covered with a towel or pillowcase. When they are applied as part of treatment they should be subtly introduced to the body with a flowing action. Effleurage with the hands first: hold the stone, effleurage with the side of the hand and then slide in the stone.

Stone shape/size	Image	Hot stone uses	Cold stone uses
Toe/finger stones, small and flat in appearance, approximately the size of a 10p		■ Between fingers and toes	■ Between fingers and toes ■ Can be placed over the eyes to reduce puffiness and inflammation
Small and round, 15–50mm in size		■ Placement stones on face ■ For massaging the body, by using the full surface area or the edge	■ Placement stones ■ Effleurage
Medium round, 60–75mm in size (palm size)		■ Placement stones ■ For massaging the hands, arms and deltoids	■ Placement stones ■ Effleurage ■ Bud technique
Large, thick and round, 75–100mm in size		■ For spinal layout ■ Placement stones ■ For massaging the larger muscle groups using the full surface area, or for deeper work using the edge only	■ Placement stones ■ For working large muscle groups
Oblong, pointy or trigger stone, 60–90mm in length		■ For deep tissue work – to apply pressure to areas of tension the pointy ends can be used, in the same way as thumbs	■ Oblong: pillow stone placed behind neck ■ Pointy: deep tissue work

Stone shape/size	Image	Hot stone uses	Cold stone uses
Contour stones (pillow and hand stones), 90–130mm in size		<ul><li>Placement stones</li><li>For use on the soles of the feet, held in the hands or behind the neck</li></ul>	
Extra-large stones (mother and father stones), too large to handle for massage, 110–130mm in size		<ul><li>Placement stones used on the sacrum or abdomen</li></ul>	<ul><li>Placement stones used on the sacrum or abdomen</li></ul>

Cryotherapy (cold stones)

When applying cold stones, hover the stone over the area first then slide the stone into place. If using a cold stone for deeper work ask the client to take a breath in and place the stone on to the body as the client breathes out.

INDUSTRY TIP

You may choose to display the stones in the salon as a talking point for clients.

ACTIVITY

Find a partner and blindfold them. Carefully practise placing different hot and cold stones on them. Ask your partner to give you feedback. If you apply the stones well, it should be hard for them to tell which is hot and which is cold.

ACTIVITY

Get to know your stones. Take a set of stones and put them into groups according to their use. You will need to know exactly what they all do, and in which area of the body. Check the results with your tutor to see if you are correct.

Preparation of the stones

After each use, the stones should be washed in hot soapy water, then placed on a clean surface or towel to air dry. Once dry they should be sprayed with a sanitising spray such as isopropyl alcohol. In the training environment the stones should be packed away to avoid damage. However the stones are stored, they need to be positioned somewhere they are not going to be moved to avoid cracks and chips.

Cleansing and re-energising the treatment stones

Stones absorb energy. They will fail to heat through and hold their heat when they have absorbed too much negative energy, and this is why it is necessary to energise them. This should be done on a regular basis depending on how often the stones are used. It is recommended that the stones are re-energised at least once a month. This does not include precious stones.

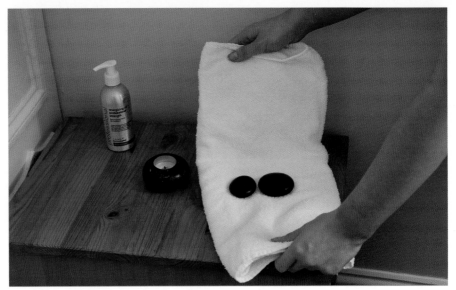
Cleaned stones being left to dry after use

1 Wash and scrub the stones in hot soapy water.
2 Leave the treatment stones out for a day in the sunlight, for example on a sunny windowsill, to absorb the sun's energy. (Do not leave precious stones in direct sunlight, as it can make the colours fade.)
3 Place the stones outside at new moon to absorb the Moon's energies; this is safe to do with all stones, including crystals.

In between treatments

- Store stones on a bed of natural sea salt, as this will draw out any impurities (with the exception of marble, as the salt may soften and split these stones).
- Hot stones can be recharged with a crystal called labradorite. Place it in the storage box with them or on top of the stones where they are on display.
- Cold stones can be recharged with moonstone.

HANDY HINT

When the stones are not holding their heat, it is a sign that they need energising.

> **INDUSTRY TIP**
>
> Thunderstorms re-energise stones, so if possible place them outside during a storm. While not very practical, returning the stones to the earth and covering them with soil is another way to re-energise them.

THE HEATER AND COOLER

The heater

The heater must be designed for the purpose of heating stones – no other device should be used, as you will not be covered by your insurance. The heater must be large enough to either hold a full set of stones for a full body treatment, or a set of back stones if carrying out a shorter treatment. You should also make sure you read the manufacturer's instructions on how to operate the heater safely. The heater should have a thermostatic control, so that the temperature of the water can be easily set and monitored. Before you turn the heater on, check for any damage to the equipment, flex or plug. Make sure the heater is placed on a stable work surface and can be accessed easily. Hot stone heaters generally take 45 minutes to heat a full set of stones.

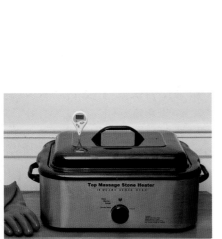
Stone heater

There are a couple of simple steps you need to take to maintain the heater ready for use.

- With the heater unplugged, wash it with hot soapy water, paying particular attention to the water line as this is where any residue will collect.
- Place a rubber mat at the bottom of the heater to prevent any noise the stones might make by knocking together.

The cooler

This is used to store marine and marble stones to ensure that they remain cool. There are two options for cooling stones:

- They can placed in a freezer bag and stored at the top of a fridge.
- They can be placed in a cooling container – an insulated container or a bowl or bucket filled with iced water. Alternatively, place them on freezer blocks, as these are less messy and can be reused.

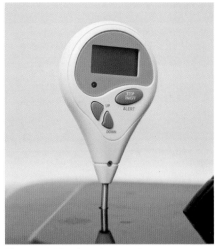

Thermostat to show temperature

> **INDUSTRY TIP**
>
> Never place cold stones in the freezer before use, as this might cause freezer burns to the skin.

ACCESSORIES

- Thermal gloves, for removing the stones from the heater – this will reduce the risk of burning or contact dermatitis.
- A slotted wooden spoon to help you lift the stones out of the heater.
- Net bags to place the stones in, to keep them organised in the tank.
- Thermometer – if the heater does not have a built-in thermostat, use a waterproof thermometer to check the water temperature, which should be 47–50°C.
- Props (rolled towels, cushions or pillows) to support the client's limbs during treatment.

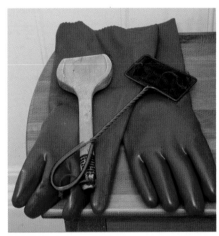

Stone therapy equipment

MASSAGE MEDIUMS

A massage medium is used during the treatment to allow the stones and hands to glide across the skin. This makes the treatment more comfortable and prevents dragging of the skin and excessive friction. The medium also leaves the skin feeling soft and supple. The oil used will also help to transfer the heat across the surface of the skin by conduction and convection. The oil is always applied to the client rather than the stones during treatment. See Chapter 305/309 for more about massage mediums. Essential oil blends should be avoided, as the heat will affect the blend and may also increase absorption, creating adverse contra-actions.

ACTIVITY

Ask your tutor if you can have a selection of different oils – try at least six and compare their texture and feel on the skin. Which oils did you prefer the feel of? Write down your reasons and discuss your findings with your colleagues.

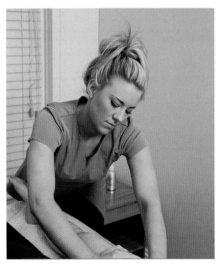

A therapist applying a massage medium prior to stone therapy

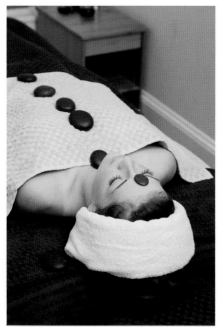

INDUSTRY TIP

Always use a light oil – a great oil to try is jojoba. This is good for all skin types and is more water-soluble than some other oils, making it easy to remove from the stones. Avoid heavy or rich oils, as these can be difficult to remove from the stones and are more likely to stain towels and sheets.

SKINCARE PRODUCTS

If the client is having their face treated, you will need cleansing products. Each company will have its own product range and training to support its use.

CONSUMABLES

You will also require some consumables:

- cotton wool to remove cleanser
- tissues
- couch roll to protect towels and maintain hygiene
- spatulas, to decant products hygienically.

APPLY A STONE THERAPY TREATMENT

PSYCHOLOGICAL AND PHYSIOLOGICAL EFFECTS OF TREATMENT

The physiological effects of stone therapy treatment are the same as those described in Chapter 305/309. However, using stones gives the following enhanced benefits.

Hot stones:

- vasodilation
- decreased blood pressure
- stimulation of digestion
- increased cellular metabolism
- relax muscle spasms
- increased muscle flexibility
- softening of muscle tissue
- increased range of joint movements
- increased activity of the parasympathetic nervous system.

Cold stones:

- vasoconstriction
- increased blood pressure
- increased activity of the sympathetic nervous system
- reduced pain
- decreased digestive function
- reduced inflammation
- reduced cellular activity
- reduced swelling and lymph congestion
- mental stimulation.

A relaxed client with stone placement

PSYCHOLOGICAL EFFECTS OF STONE THERAPY

Stone therapy has many psychological effects, similar to the psychological effects described in Chapter 305/309. It is fantastic for stress relief and is very relaxing.

Depending on the techniques used, the psychological effects of stone therapy include:

- induced state of relaxation
- reduced stress levels
- feeling of well-being
- uplifting effects.

MASSAGE TECHNIQUES

The techniques you use to apply the stones and your choice of hot or cold stones will enable you to achieve your client's treatment objectives. Most treatments combine hot and cold stones, and with correct technique and placement the client should not easily be able to tell the difference between the two.

The use of stones is not only beneficial to the client, but also to the therapist. You do not need to apply as much pressure as in a conventional massage, thereby preventing wear and tear to the joints and reducing the risk of repetitive strain injury. The philosophy of less is more is very true in this case: one stroke with a stone is equal to ten strokes with a hand.

In Chapter 305/309 you will have been introduced to the main massage techniques. You should familiarise yourself with these before studying the new techniques you will also use for stone therapy.

STONE THERAPY TREATMENT TECHNIQUES

Technique	Use with hot stones?	Use with cold stones?	Application
Effleurage 	Yes	Yes	Apply the massage medium with your hands to the client using slow effleurage. This will allow the client to become accustomed to your touch. Never just place the stones on to the body and start to massage with them. The stones should be introduced to the body in a subtle way. Hold the stone in your hand with the palm upwards. Slide the back of the hand onto the body and start to stroke, then slowly turn the hand over to introduce the edge of the stone. Check the heat before applying the flat surface on to the skin, and keep the stone moving.

Technique	Use with hot stones?	Use with cold stones?	Application
Petrissage	Yes	Yes	The stones are introduced to the body as above. Once contact is established, a range of petrissage movements can be carried out.
Frictions	Yes	Yes	Using the edge of the stone, rub it back and forth to create friction. Work across the fibres of the muscles.
Tapping (piesoelectric)	Yes	No	The effects created by this movement are similar to the vibrations used in Swedish massage, but they are much more profound and create an excellent rippling effect out across the muscle fibres. One stone is held and stays in contact with the body and the second stone is tapped on top of it. This technique is noisy but very therapeutic, creating vibrations deep into the muscle, and is ideal for tension nodules. It is also excellent for stimulating the lymphatic system.
Tucking	Yes	No	Once the stones have been used and have started to cool, they are tucked under the client's body to deliver warmth to an area. This prevents them losing too much contact with the body by being removed and placed on another surface. Tucking should be a smooth action, sliding the stone into place under the body once it is no longer required.

INDUSTRY TIP

While we tend to use heat for soothing and calming, cold can actually be better where there is pain. An example of this is menstruation pain – we would usually use a hot water bottle to soothe it, but cold can be more beneficial physically. (Heat is beneficial psychologically, though.)

Technique	Use with hot stones?	Use with cold stones?	Application
Placement	Yes	Yes	This can be used as a method of relaxation at the start of the treatment. This is a technique used to warm the muscles before the treatment begins. The stones are placed directly on to the client. The client may lie on the stones – with their skin protected by a sheet or pillowcase placed on the body, with a sheet or towel to protect the skin. When using hot stones, they may be placed directly in contact with the skin, such as in between the fingers and toes, or over the third eye.
Trigger points	Yes	Yes	By using the rounded point of a hot stone and pressing into an area of tension or a nodule within muscles, tension can be alleviated. The client should take a breath in, then the stone is pressed into the area of tension while they breathe out and held there for 30–90 seconds.

ADAPTING MASSAGE TECHNIQUES

The treatment objectives of stone therapy are:

- relaxation
- balance
- uplifting effect
- promoting a sense of well-being
- relief from muscular tension.

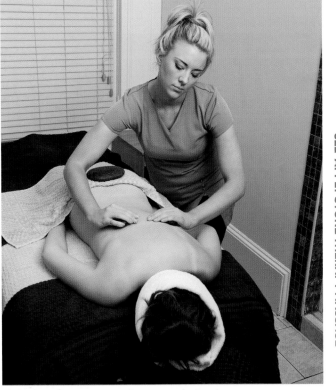

Therapist using stones to relieve muscular tension

It is important that massage movements are adapted to suit the client's treatment objectives, unless it is a signature treatment following a set routine. The selection and use of stones will depend on the client's requirements. Some general guidance is given below.

Client group	Suggested adaptations
Elderly	The client may have impaired senses and possibly poor circulation, so monitor the temperature of the stones carefully. Skin may be thin with a lack of subcutaneous tissue, so avoid deeper movements, and always use light pressure. Avoid tapping due to possible changes in the bone structure (joint stiffness, arthritis, osteoporosis).
Overweight	Use deeper pressure, more vigorous movements, petrissage and tapping. If the client is obese they should be advised against treatment, as the body may not be able to cope with the heat effectively. There may also be difficulty in locating trigger points.
Underweight	Use lighter pressure over bony areas. Avoid tapping and be cautious with trigger points; there may not be adequate muscle tissue to use this technique comfortably. Techniques will need to be fine-tuned and kept delicate due to lack of adipose tissue. Use extra covers to keep the client warm.
Good muscle tone	There will be firm, well-toned muscles and skin and the client will be within a normal weight range. All massage techniques can be used, in particular friction and trigger points. Use firm, deep movements. Alternating hot and cold stones will be very beneficial.
Poor muscle tone	Both muscles and skin tissue may be of poor tone. Try to gradually lead in to a state of relaxation, gently stretching the muscles with the stones. Avoid any wringing if there is loose skin. Use deeper movements over large areas and incorporate tapotement and petrissage. Gentle tapping will help to stimulate the muscles.

ACTIVITY

Imagine that a muscular male athlete, an elderly woman and an overweight client all wish to have a stone therapy massage. Think about how you would adapt your massage in order to meet the clients' needs and make sure that they remain comfortable throughout the treatment.

HANDY HINT

If the client is muscular, hot stones will relax the muscles – however, incorporating cold stones as well can help to reduce any inflammation around the joints or within the muscles. Consider alternating hot and cold stones, as this is thought to have therapeutic properties.

STONE THERAPY ROUTINE

Below is a suggested stone therapy routine. There are many different versions and you may be taught something different – this is only for guidance.

A stone therapy treatment will be flowing and will use a range of techniques. You should maintain contact between stone and skin as much as possible. Your treatment should be flowing and seamless while you adjust or arrange stones. Be aware of noise and keep movement of the stones to a minimum.

Suggested sequences

Client supine:

- spinal layout
- opening chakra
- right leg (1)
- left leg (2)
- right arm (3)
- left arm
- abdomen (4)
- face and scalp (5).

Client prone:

- left leg
- right leg
- back (6).

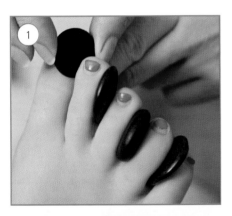
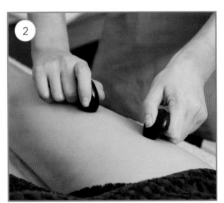
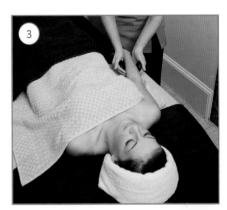
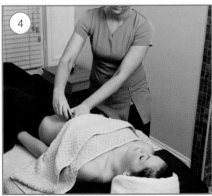
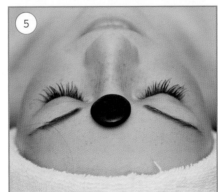
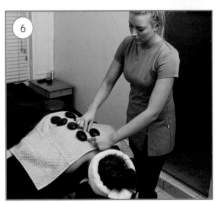

Treatment timing

A full stone therapy treatment will take between 75 and 90 minutes to carry out. A back treatment on its own will take 45 minutes.

STONE PLACEMENT

Stone placement is a popular way to relax the client. Seven stones are placed at the chakra points of the body, and semi-precious stones are placed in between them. As well as relaxing them, this also helps to rebalance the client.

Chakra name	Location	Colour
1 Crown	Top of the head	Purple
2 Third eye/Ajna	Middle of the forehead centred above the eyebrows	Indigo
3 Throat	Middle of the throat at the neck, above the collar bone	Blue/turquoise
4 Heart	Centre of the chest, by the heart	Green
5 Solar plexus	Below the sternum	Yellow
6 Sacral	Below the navel	Orange
7 Root/base	Base of spine/lower pelvic area	Red

Chakras

Chakras are emotional centres in the body that are linked to the physical body through the endocrine glands and organs situated in the same area. The energy that travels through the chakras can become unbalanced and disrupted due to emotional disturbance or stress. When this happens it is believed that illness may occur. Chakras are said to spin, and the speed at which they do so can either increase or decrease depending on the state of health. An increasing spin speed can lead to a feeling of agitation or stress, while a decrease can leave a person feeling tired and weary.

Chakras are said to resemble a blossom, the petals of which represent energy channels. Each different chakra has a different number of petals. Chakras react to light energy, which causes them to vibrate at certain frequencies. These frequencies relate to specific sounds and colours.

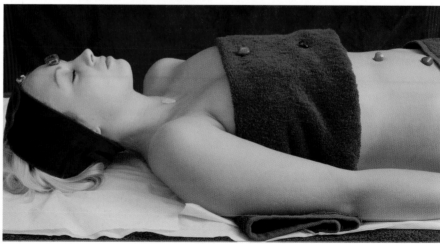

A client with chakra stones positioned on them

SPINAL LAYOUT

Ask the client to lie on the couch in a supine position. Wrap the client in a sheet and cover with an additional towel or cover if required.

Tell the client that they must tell you during treatment if any of the stones you are using are too hot or uncomfortable in their placement or application. Collect the spinal layout stones from the heater and place on a towel.

Place the 16 spinal layout stones in position, tucking the butterfly stones that will sit under the sacrum into the pillowcase.

The spinal stones consist of:

- four narrow stones which sit in a butterfly shape under the sacral lower back area
- four round, thick stones which sit under the lumbar regions (latissimus dorsi muscle) of the back
- four smaller, round stones that are a bit flatter in shape and sit under the ribs (top of the latissimus dorsi)
- four narrow, more oblong-shaped stones which sit under the upper back (under the rhomboid muscles)
- one oblong stone which can be placed behind the neck, inside a sock for comfort if desired.

Help the client down on to the couch and on to the stones, where they should lie for between ten and 30 minutes. Reassure the client that this should be a pleasant sensation. Adjust any stones as required so that the client is lying comfortably.

Offer the client the hand stones to hold – you may also like to place stones between the toes and fingers.

You can now either place chakra stones, or treat an area on the front of the body. For a back treatment the client may be left to relax on the stones and benefit from the deep tissue warmth before turning them over to massage the back.

CHAKRA PLACEMENT

Stand on the left-hand side of the couch. You can use either precious stones for the placement, or hot or cold stones. It is recommended that cold stones are not used on their own for this treatment, but are mixed with hot stones.

Start with the first chakra and work in a clockwise direction, creating a semicircle in between each chakra point and the next. Think of each chakra flower opening and envisage the correct chakra colour (see page 451), then slowly slide the stone into place. Lift the hand with a semicircular movement in a clockwise direction to the next chakra point.

You can leave your client to relax for a few minutes if you are doing a relaxation treatment. If you are doing a back treatment you can begin to massage around the neck and décolletage.

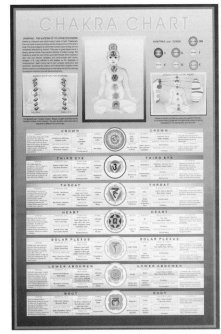

An example of a chakra chart

If you are doing a full-body stone therapy treatment, you will start the treatment on the client's right leg (the one on your left as you stand at the foot of the couch). Once the spinal placement treatment and/or treatment of the front of the body is complete, you should always remember to close the chakras to keep the energy in. This is done by simply reversing the sequence you performed to open the chakras. Start with the crown chakras and take your hand in an anticlockwise direction, while picturing the chakra flow closing. As you work down the rest of the chakras, place your hand on top for a moment and then slide and slowly lift the stone from the body. You should finish with the heart chakra.

On completion of the treatment, gather up any tucked stones and remove them to the trolley. Remove any placement stones. Let the client know that the treatment is complete.

HOME-CARE AND AFTERCARE ADVICE

Following the treatment you should give the client suitable aftercare advice to follow. This will help to maximise the benefits the client gets from the treatment. You can find out more about aftercare advice in Chapter 305/309.

ACTIVITY

Review any lifestyle changes that you might discuss with the client as part of aftercare advice. Make a list of the benefits that the client might gain from following the advice you give.

CONTRA-ACTIONS

For detailed information about contra-actions, refer to Chapter 305/309.

BURNS

Burns are a particular consideration when offering stone therapy. They should never occur, but can happen if you:

- fail to check and monitor the temperature of the heater or do not use one with a thermostat
- apply placement stones directly to the skin without protection
- don't check the temperature of the stones before application.

Make sure to consider all of the above when offering a professional treatment to avoid injury to your client.

For information on client feedback and evaluation, see Chapter 305/309.

Use the questions below to test your knowledge of Chapter 322 to see how much information you have retained. These questions will help you revise what you have learnt in this chapter.

Turn to page 499 for the answers.

1 Marble stones are made of which **one** of the following?
  a Calcium carbonate
  b Calcium silicate
  c Calcium phosphate
  d Calcium nitrate

2 What colour are basalt stones?
  a Grey-blue
  b Grey-brown
  c Grey-green
  d Grey-yellow

3 A cool box is used for which of the following stones?
  a Basalt and marble
  b Semi-precious and basalt
  c Marine and basalt
  d Marine and marble

4 Which **one** of the following describes a trigger point?
  a An area of tension knots
  b The crown chakra
  c The largest stone
  d The heater on/off switch

5 What is the maximum temperature a stone heater should reach?
  a 25°C
  b 37°C
  c 45°C
  d 60°C

6 Which of the following can be used to carry out a thermal sensitivity test?
  a Hot and cold stones
  b Cotton bud and cold stone
  c Orange stick and cotton bud
  d Orange stick and hot stone

7 Where is the third eye located?
  a The feet
  b The chest
  c The stomach
  d The head

8 Which **one** of the following stones will remain cold the longest?
  a Basalt
  b Marble
  c Jade
  d Slate

9 How long does a full stone therapy treatment take?
  a 60 minutes
  b 75 minutes
  c 80 minutes
  d 95 minutes

10 Which **one** of the following stones holds heat the longest?
  a Basalt
  b Marble
  c Jade
  d Marine

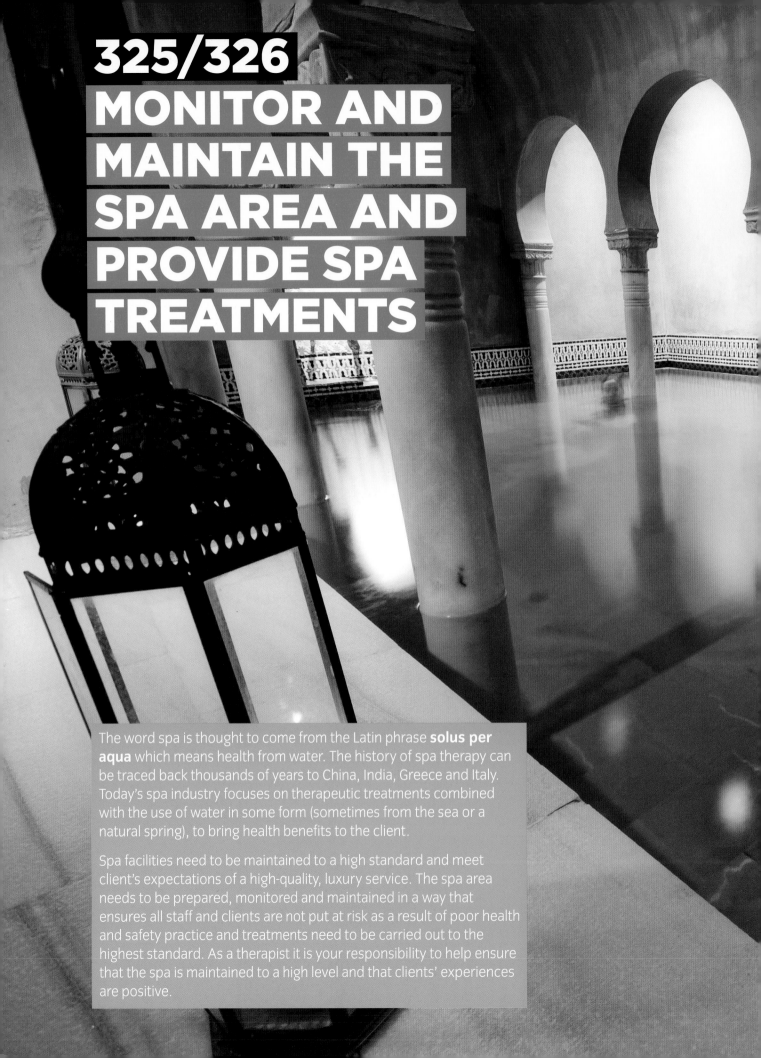

MONITOR AND MAINTAIN THE SPA AREA AND PROVIDE SPA TREATMENTS

The word spa is thought to come from the Latin phrase **solus per aqua** which means health from water. The history of spa therapy can be traced back thousands of years to China, India, Greece and Italy. Today's spa industry focuses on therapeutic treatments combined with the use of water in some form (sometimes from the sea or a natural spring), to bring health benefits to the client.

Spa facilities need to be maintained to a high standard and meet client's expectations of a high-quality, luxury service. The spa area needs to be prepared, monitored and maintained in a way that ensures all staff and clients are not put at risk as a result of poor health and safety practice and treatments need to be carried out to the highest standard. As a therapist it is your responsibility to help ensure that the spa is maintained to a high level and that clients' experiences are positive.

In this chapter you will learn how to:

- prepare, monitor and maintain the spa area
- prepare for and provide spa treatments.

PREPARE, MONITOR AND MAINTAIN THE SPA TREATMENT AREA

In this part of the chapter you will learn about:

- environmental conditions
- health and safety working practices
- preparation of equipment.

ENVIRONMENTAL CONDITIONS

For most clients a spa treatment is a memorable experience that should start as soon as they enter the spa environment. The decor, lighting, music and **aroma** should set the scene and prepare clients for their experience. This memorable experience should continue into the treatment areas (including the changing rooms, which should have secure lockers so that clients feel happy leaving their belongings there). You should also:

- provide disposable footwear and large fluffy robes
- make sure that the area is at the right temperature (ie it is warm enough so that the client feels comfortable when they have undressed).

The spa's relaxation area needs to be an area of calm with:

- comfortable furnishings
- relaxing music
- relaxing lighting
- a good supply of drinking water and refreshments.

HEALTH AND SAFETY WORKING PRACTICES

The spa environment needs to be kept clean at all times. Areas for showering need to:

- follow all health and safety guidelines for cleanliness
- have a regular supply of clean laundered towels and robes
- have a regular supply of complimentary toiletries for the client to try (that reflect the products and brand used in the spa).

The wet area in a spa is an ideal breeding ground for harmful **micro-organisms** due to the use of warm temperatures and water within treatments. It is therefore essential that the area is sterilised, **disinfected** and that standards of health and safety are maintained on a daily basis:

- Disinfect the duck boards (the wooden boards people stand on) and check for damage.
- Wipe down floors and surfaces with an appropriate disinfectant cleaner.
- In between clients make sure any product residue is removed from shower plugholes as it looks unprofessional.

Solus per aqua

Health from water

HANDY HINT

You should refresh your knowledge of anatomy and physiology for this chapter.

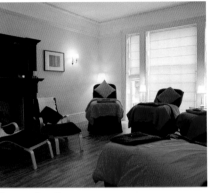

A spa relaxation area

Aroma

Smell

INDUSTRY TIP

Broken duck boards should be replaced. Cracks in duck boards provide an ideal breeding ground for germs.

HANDY HINT

You can maximise retail opportunities by providing complimentary toiletries.

Micro-organisms

Very small living things (bacteria or viruses) that can only be seen through a microscope

Disinfect

To inhibit the growth of micro-organisms

PREPARATION OF EQUIPMENT

To reduce the risk of **cross-infection**, you need to follow the manufacturers' instructions for cleaning equipment. When preparing the equipment and work area you also need to carry out the following tasks:

- Sauna/steam room:
  - Air personal sauna/steam cabinets in between clients.
  - Disinfect sauna pods after each client – make sure it is disinfected at least once every day.
  - Remove any water and leave the door open overnight to allow the cabinet to dry out.
  - Disinfect larger communal saunas every day and leave the door open to air dry overnight.
- Check and change water filters on spa pools regularly according to the manufacturer's instructions.
- Disinfect the edge of the spa bath daily.
- Clean hydrotherapy bath jets and shower heads daily.

Other best practice tips

- For each piece of equipment, make sure notices are displayed that explain:
  - how to use each piece of equipment
  - what the effects of the equipment are
  - when the equipment should not be used.
- Only use towels and gowns once. They should be washed after each use.
- Provide shower caps for clients, especially if they have recently coloured their hair to prevent the colour from contaminating the spa water.
- Use disposable tissue where possible.
- Provide the client with flip-flops which can be washed after use, or disposable spa footwear.

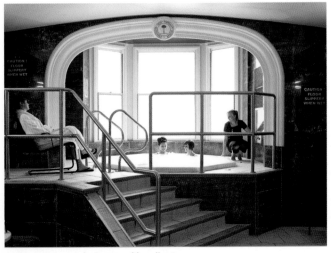

A clean spa area being used by clients

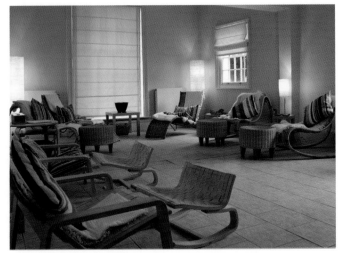

A clean and tidy relaxation area

ACTIVITY

Carry out a risk assessment of the spa area in your college or workplace.

In this part of the chapter you will learn about:

- preparation for spa treatments
- consultation
- contra-indications.

WHY DON'T YOU...
make a list of all the personal protective equipment (PPE) that a spa therapist might need.

PREPARATION FOR SPA TREATMENTS

In addition to the steps already discussed on page 468 to reduce the risk of cross-infection and cross-contamination, the following measures should also be taken:

- Clients need to shower before and after each treatment to remove any products and degrease their skin to reduce the risk of any oils contaminating the water.
- Clients with long hair should tie it up so that it is not in the water. Long hair may become trapped in filters.
- Clients need to remove plasters before they use the spa so that they do not become loose and end up in the water.

CONSULTATION

Prior to treatment you should always carry out a consultation. This not only assesses the client's needs and objectives but also assesses whether the treatment is suitable for the client. By identifying any potential contra-indications during the treatment you can assess whether or not it is safe to proceed with the treatment. More detailed information on the consultation process and communication techniques can be found in Chapter 303 Client care and communication in beauty-related industries (pages 212–215 and 206–211).

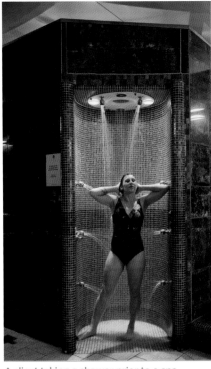

A client taking a shower prior to a spa treatment

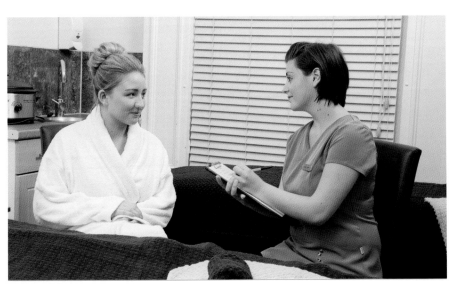

Carrying out a consultation prior to a treatment

CONTRA-INDICATIONS

In addition to the general contra-indications listed in Chapter 303 (page 215), there are a number of contra-indications that are specific to spa treatments:

Contra-indication	Treatment	Restricts/prevents treatment	Reason
Recent botox	Massage	Restricts treatment	Avoid massage treatments for 24 hours to prevent movement of the injected product.
Body piercing	Massage	Restricts treatment	Avoid the pierced area until it is fully healed.
Claustrophobia	Wet flotation	Restricts treatment	It might cause the client to have a panic attack if they are in an enclosed space.
Alcohol use within the last six hours	Sauna, steam room, hot tubs	Restricts treatment	It might impair sweating and cause overheating of the body through dehydration.
High or low blood pressure	Sauna, steam room, hot tubs, cold treatments	Prevents treatment	Can cause fainting and nausea. Client should seek medical advice before use.
Heart conditions	Sauna, steam room, hot tubs, cold treatments	Prevents treatment	Can cause fainting and nausea. Client should seek medical advice before use.
High fever	Sauna, steam room, hot tubs, cold treatments	Prevents treatment	Might increase the client's already high temperature.

INDUSTRY TIP

Make sure that both you and the client sign the consultation form to show that you have discussed the above contra-indications.

You should not carry out spa treatments on a client:

- after they have had a heavy meal
- if they are under the influence of drugs
- during the first two days of their menstrual cycle (due to bleeding and tenderness in the abdominal area).

ACTIVITY

Design a consultation checklist for use during consultations for spa treatments. Be sure to include everything.

HANDY HINT

Even if the client has no contra-indications, make a note on the consultation card saying that they have none. Don't leave it blank as this just looks like it hasn't been filled in.

TEMPERATURES, TIMINGS AND FREQUENCY OF SPA TREATMENTS

Some suggested, timings, frequency and temperatures of treatments are suggested below.

Treatment	Temperature	Length of treatment	Frequency of treatment	Humidity levels
Heat treatments				
Finnish sauna	70–100°C	15–20 minutes	2–3 times a week	10–15%
Laconium	55–65°C	15–20 minutes	2–3 times a week	15–20%
Sauna pod	Depends on chosen setting	20–30 minutes	2–3 times a week	5%
Steam pod/cabinet	45–50°C	10–20 minutes	2–3 times a week	n/a
Steam room	40–43°C	15–20 minutes	2–3 times a week	n/a
Caldarium	40–45°C	15–20 minutes	2–3 times a week	n/a
Hydrotherapy treatments				
Spa pool	37–40°C	10–15 minutes	Daily	n/a
Hydrotherapy bath	37–40°C	15–20 minutes	2–3 times a week	n/a
Wet flotation	35°C	30–60 minutes	1–2 times a week	n/a
Dry flotation	35–40°C	30–40 minutes	1–2 times a week	n/a

> **HANDY HINT**
>
> The table above contains suggestions. You should always refer to the manufacturers' instructions for specific information.

PROVIDE SPA TREATMENTS

In this part of the chapter you will learn about:

- heat treatments
- hydrotherapy treatments
- other treatments (including body wraps)
- home-care and aftercare advice
- contra-actions to treatment.

There are a variety of treatments used within the spa environment. It is essential that you are aware of:

- how each treatment works
- the benefits/treatment objectives of each treatment
- how to use the equipment within a spa safely and correctly
- how to carry out safety checks/tests on each piece of equipment
- the guidance you need to provide clients on using the equipment.

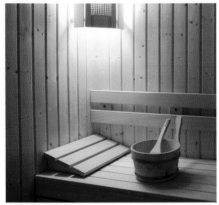

A sauna room

Humidity

The amount of water vapour in the air

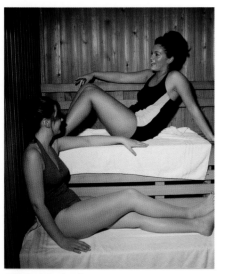

Clients relaxing in a sauna

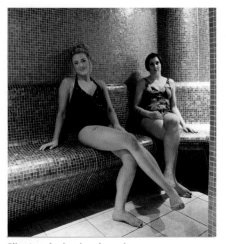

Clients relaxing in a laconium

Aromatic essences

Pleasant-smelling plant extracts used for scent

HEAT TREATMENTS

SAUNA

A sauna is a room or pod that is heated to provide a dry heat with low **humidity**.

There are three main types of sauna:

- Finnish sauna (Tyrolean)
- laconium
- sauna pod.

Finnish sauna (or Tyrolean sauna)

This is a traditional wood-lined sauna cabin made from pine. It usually has two tiers of seating. An electric stove heats up specially made stones. Water is poured onto the stones and it evaporates quickly with the heat rising to the top of the sauna. It is necessary for clients to shower before entering the sauna as this will start them sweating. As the heat rises, the upper tier of seating gets the hottest so advise new clients to sit on the lower level.

Laconium

This type of sauna is based on a form of dry sauna used by the Romans. It has heated tiles on the floor, walls and seating. The heating usually comes from underfloor heating rather than a stove. **Aromatic essences** (eg lavender or eucalyptus), lighting and water features can be added to create a relaxing atmosphere. It gives a gentler heat than the traditional Finnish sauna. It allows the body to heat up gradually and is used for gentle cleansing and purifying of the skin because of the gentle heat. As the heat is not as intense, this type of sauna is quite sociable as most people can tolerate the heat.

HANDY HINT

Humidity is low in saunas and high in steam rooms.

Sauna pod

A sauna pod is used for an individual treatment. It is suitable for those clients who do not feel comfortable sharing a sauna with other people. The client's body is enclosed in the pod with a hole for the head. The pod is then heated up to a temperature that suits the client.

Health and safety checks on saunas

At the start of each day or 30–45 minutes before use, you need to switch on the sauna to allow it to heat up to the required temperature.

During this time, you will need to check the sauna to make sure that:

- there is no damage to seats/benches and walls
- the stove guard is in place and secure
- the sauna stones are in place
- the thermostat is in working order
- the door opens and closes properly
- all the lights are working correctly
- the emergency call button is working
- the directions for use, explanation of the benefits and list of precautions are on display
- there are no slip or trip hazards
- the water bucket is free from mould, has distilled water in it and that there is a ladle for pouring the water on the stones (Finnish sauna)
- the air vents are open and unobstructed.

Client guidance on using a sauna

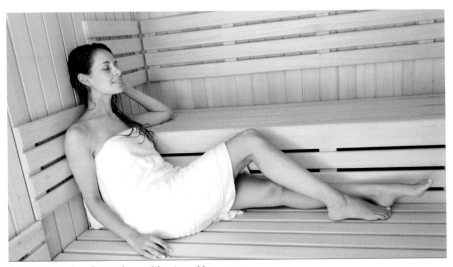

A client covering themselves with a towel in a sauna

Clients should:

- have had a thorough consultation to make sure that no contra-indications are present
- read the guidance notice on how to use the sauna safely
- remove all jewellery and metal piercings as the metal may heat up and cause a burn
- remove contact lenses and glasses
- remove all make-up
- sit on a towel if they are not wearing a bathing suit

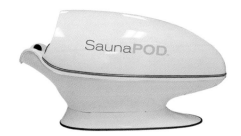

- maintain modesty
- sit on the lower bench when they first enter and make a note of the time
- use the sauna for a maximum of 10 minutes
- take a shower after leaving the sauna to lower the body temperature (and if desired return to the sauna for a further 10 minutes).
- shower and relax for 20 minutes to allow the body temperature to return to normal
- drink plenty of water to rehydrate the body after use.

ACTIVITY

Make a checklist of everything that the therapist needs to do when preparing the sauna and steam room area for use by a client.

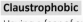
Claustrophobic
Having a fear of enclosed spaces

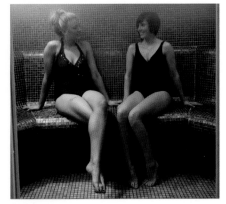
A steam room

STEAM ROOM

Steam rooms originate from Turkish baths which have been in use for thousands of years. The inside of a steam room (including the seats) is completely tiled. Water is heated in a boiler and the steam is piped into the room. The whole room, and therefore the whole of the client's body (including their head), is covered in steam. Some people find steam rooms **claustrophobic**. There is a higher level of humidity so this is a wet heat treatment.

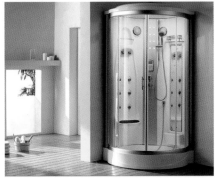
A steam cabinet

STEAM CABINET/BATH

There are a number of different types of steam baths/cabinets available. They are often made of fibreglass, with a hinged door or a sealable plastic covering. The client sits on an adjustable seat inside and places their head through an opening at the top. You will need to place a towel around the neck area to help seal the unit and prevent steam from leaking out. Water is heated in a small tank inside the pod to create the steam. The steam reaches a temperature of between 45–50°C.

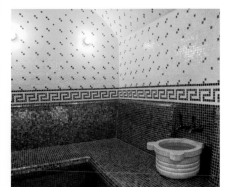
Caldarium

CALDARIUM

A caldarium is a steam room that has aromatherapy essential oils added to the steam. The heat does not become as intense as in an ordinary steam room. There may be a Kneipp hose within the caldarium that allows clients to apply cold water to their body to cool down during the treatment.

HAMMAM

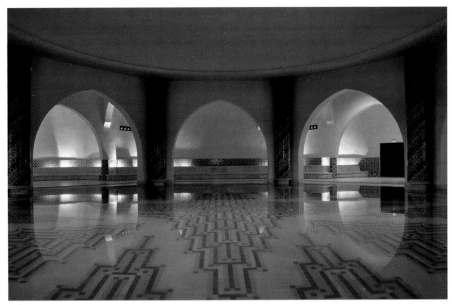

A hammam

This is another type of steam room that originates from Turkey/the Middle East. It is also found in North Africa. It is often decorated in mosaics with a blue, gold or brown colour scheme to reflect its eastern origins. It produces a hot, steamy aromatic effect. A traditional hammam would be made up of a series of rooms:

- the caldarium: the hot room
- a tepidarium: a relaxation room usually heated to body temperature
- a frigidarium: a cool room.

Traditionally the hammam treatment would involve going from the hottest room to the coolest room.

Health and safety checks on steam rooms

At the start of each day, the steam room needs to be switched on to allow it to heat up to the required temperature. This time will vary according to the size of the room.

During this time you should check the steam room to make sure that:

- there is no damage to the seats and walls
- the ventilation is working and the warning notice on steam room usage is in place
- the thermostat is in working order
- the door opens and closes properly
- all lights are working correctly
- the emergency call button is working
- the directions for use, explanation of the benefits and list of precautions are on display
- there are no slip or trip hazards.

> **WHY DON'T YOU...**
> have a look on the Internet and research the types of products that can be used on the body in a hammam.

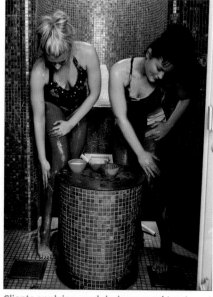

Client guidance on using a steam room

Clients should:

- have had a thorough consultation to make sure that no contra-indications are present
- read the guidance notice on how to use the steam room safely
- remove all jewellery and metal piercings as the metal may heat up and cause a burn
- remove contact lenses and glasses
- remove all make-up
- sit on a towel if they are not wearing a bathing suit
- maintain modesty
- stay in the steam room for a maximum of 20 minutes
- shower and relax for 20 minutes after leaving the steam room to allow the body temperature to return to normal
- drink plenty of water to rehydrate the body.

ACTIVITY

Make a list of different spa treatments that could be combined with a sauna or steam room session to form a treatment package.

RASUL

A rasul (also known as serail) is a heated mud treatment that comes from the Middle East. Traditionally, it was performed within a traditional ceremony based on social cleansing. The treatment takes place in a steam room (or a series of steam rooms) with a temperature of 42–60°C. The steam room may have two or more tiled seats which are often very decorative in their design. **Mood rocks** and twinkle lights are also commonly used to improve the experience.

Warm mud that is rich in minerals is applied all over the body by a therapist or the client. The client then relaxes in the warm, herbal-scented steam room or chamber. Sea salt may also be placed in the rasul chamber for the therapist or client to apply at the beginning of the treatment to provide additional exfoliation. After a short time, either the therapist showers the client with cool water or the client showers themself with cool water to rinse away the mud.

> **HANDY HINT**
>
> The mud applied during the treatment has exfoliating and cleansing actions. The particular mud used may be local to the area or sourced for its health-promoting, medicinal and mineral properties.

Health and safety checks on a rasul chamber

You need to carry out health and safety checks on a daily basis. You need to check to make sure that:

- there is no damage to any surfaces
- all the lights are working correctly
- the emergency call button is working
- the directions for use, explanation of the benefits and list of precautions are on display
- there are no slip or trip hazards.

> **HANDY HINT**
>
> In addition to the general benefits of heat treatments, rasul treatments help to exfoliate and cleanse the skin and improve skin texture.

Mood rocks

Glowing crystals

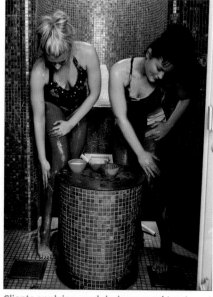

Clients applying mud during a rasul treatment

> **INDUSTRY TIP**
>
> When adding products to the rasul mud (eg grapeseed oil for ease of mud application), always make sure that the client does not have any allergies.

> **WHY DON'T YOU...**
>
> do some research into the different kinds of mud that are used in a rasul treatment and find out the properties of each mud.

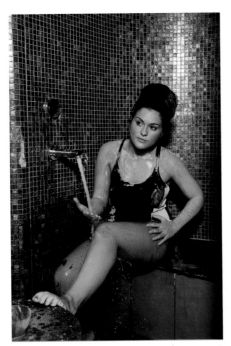

Client removing mud during a rasul treatment

HANDY HINT

Chill treatments that reduce body temperature, such as plunge pools or ice rooms, will stimulate sensory nerve endings. As with heat treatments, this creates an analgesic effect which gives temporary pain relief.

HANDY HINT

A rasul treatment can be used prior to a body massage to warm the muscles. It will make the massage more effective as it makes it easier for the therapist to get deep into the warmed muscles.

EFFECTS AND BENEFITS/TREATMENT OBJECTIVES OF HEAT TREATMENTS

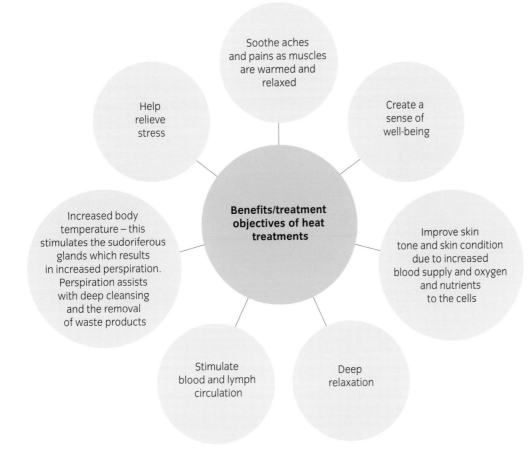

Soothe aches and pains as muscles are warmed and relaxed

Help relieve stress

Create a sense of well-being

Increased body temperature – this stimulates the sudoriferous glands which results in increased perspiration. Perspiration assists with deep cleansing and the removal of waste products

Benefits/treatment objectives of heat treatments

Improve skin tone and skin condition due to increased blood supply and oxygen and nutrients to the cells

Stimulate blood and lymph circulation

Deep relaxation

HYDROTHERAPY TREATMENTS

Hydrotherapy is the use of water for healing and well-being. It has greater benefit if hot and cold water are alternated during a treatment as this stimulates the circulation and leaves the client feeling **invigorated**.

Hydrotherapy is a long-established method of treatment. It has been used for the treatment of disease and injury by the ancient Romans, the Chinese and the Japanese.

The main types of hydrotherapy equipment are:

- spa pool/bath/Jacuzzi/whirlpool
- hydrotherapy baths
- blitz showers
- Swiss/Vichy shower.

> **HANDY HINT**
>
> The nineteenth-century Bavarian monk, Father Sebastian Kneipp, reintroduced hydrotherapy as he believed that disease could be cured by using water to get rid of waste from the body.

SPA POOL

Also known as a Jacuzzi or a whirlpool, a spa pool can seat up to ten people (depending on the size of the pool). Heated water is forced through jets. This causes the water to bubble and creates a gentle massaging effect on the body. The water from the spa bath is filtered and recirculated meaning that it is not changed after each client. Every week the spa attendant should carry out a full service on the spa pool equipment. The spa pool should be cleaned thoroughly every day to remove any residue.

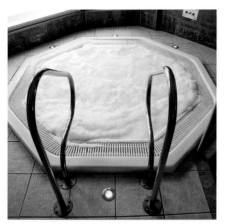

A spa pool

You will need to carry out the following specific tests on the spa pool a couple of times a day to test the quality of the water and to make sure that it is safe:

- **pH balance** (acidity/alkalinity) – the pH needs to be balanced to make sure that the water is neither too acidic nor too alkaline. If it is too acidic, the water can become cloudy. If it is too alkaline, this may cause a build-up of limescale in the equipment.
- Water hardness (ie calcium content) – water contains calcium which may make it hard or soft. If there is too much calcium this may cause a build-up of limescale on the equipment.
- Water temperature – this needs to be tested to make sure that the spa pool isn't too cold or too hot.

PH balance
A measure of the acidity or alkalinity of the water. If the water is acidic, the pH is less than 7 and if it is alkaline, the pH is greater than 7

> **HANDY HINT**
>
> Chlorine is the most widely used disinfectant used in swimming pools. Bromine, like chlorine, can be used in the maintenance of swimming pools and also spa pools (hot tubs).

> **INDUSTRY TIP**
>
> Make sure that spa guests/clients always shower before any water treatment to prevent the spread of water-borne infections.
>
> Legionnaires' disease is caused by bacteria that grow in warm water that is recirculated (eg in a spa pool). Good hygiene in the spa wet areas is essential to prevent these bacteria from growing. Symptoms of the disease include tiredness, aching muscles, headaches, cough and fever.

The results of the water quality tests need to be recorded for the **environmental health officer** to review on their visit. By keeping records of these it shows that the spa is following health and safety requirements.

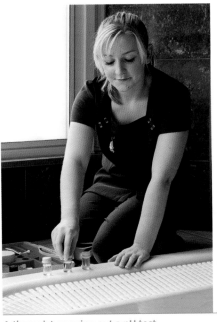 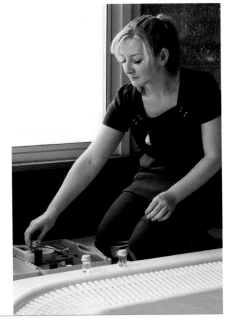

A therapist carrying out a pH test

INDUSTRY TIP

The Langelier Saturation Index is a calculation that is used to show whether water is corrosive or likely to form limescale.

INDUSTRY TIP

As a guide, the pH of a spa pool should be between 7.2 and 7.6.

INDUSTRY TIP

As a guide, the water temperature in a:

- spa pool should be between 34–37ºC
- swimming pool should be between 27–30˚C.

pH testing

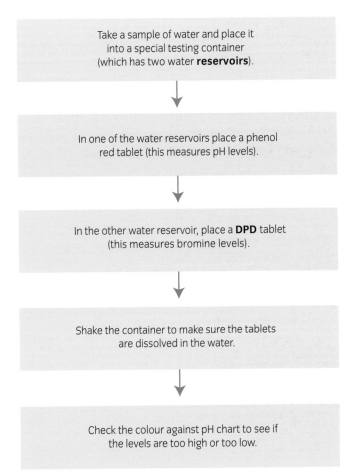

Take a sample of water and place it into a special testing container (which has two water **reservoirs**).

↓

In one of the water reservoirs place a phenol red tablet (this measures pH levels).

↓

In the other water reservoir, place a **DPD** tablet (this measures bromine levels).

↓

Shake the container to make sure the tablets are dissolved in the water.

↓

Check the colour against pH chart to see if the levels are too high or too low.

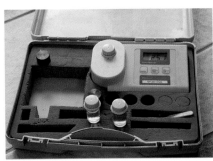

A Palintest® kit

Reservoir

Part of a container that holds a liquid

DPD

Diethyl-p-phenylenediamine

INDUSTRY TIP

The test for pH is often referred to as the Palintest®.

INDUSTRY TIP

The swimming pool is also a piece of hydrotherapy equipment. This also needs to be tested in the same way as the spa pool.

ACTIVITY

Design a water treatment checklist for use in a spa.

HANDY HINT

When placing the tablets in the water reservoir do not let them touch your skin because this will affect the pH reading, as the tablet will register the pH reading of your skin.

HANDY HINT

It is very important that the spa pool water and swimming pool water are tested and that the levels are within those recommended by the manufacturer.

INDUSTRY TIP

A thermal suite within a spa has a range of hot and cold experiences to cleanse the body, relax the muscles and invigorate the client.

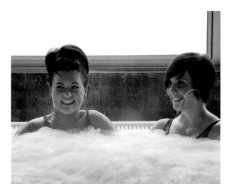

Clients using a spa pool

Client guidance on using a spa pool

Clients should:

- have had a thorough consultation to make sure that no contra-indications are present
- read the guidance notice on how to use the spa pool safely
- remove all jewellery and metal piercings
- shower and remove all make-up before entering the pool
- tie up long hair and use a shower/bathing cap if their hair has been coloured recently
- only enter the pool when it is not bubbling so the steps and floor of the pool are fully visible
- stay in the pool for a maximum of 20 minutes
- hold onto the rails for additional support when the water jets are massaging the skin
- take a shower and relax for 20 minutes after leaving the pool to allow the body temperature to return to normal
- drink plenty of water to rehydrate the body.

Health and safety checks on hydrotherapy equipment

You will need to carry out the following general health and safety checks on hydrotherapy equipment. You need to make sure:

- there is no damage to any surfaces
- the water is at the correct temperature
- there is a handrail in place and that it is secure
- all lights are working correctly
- the emergency call button is working
- the directions for use, explanation of the benefits and list of precautions are on display
- there are no slip or trip hazards
- the spa pool water is tested at the start of each day for temperature, water hardness and pH balance
- the spa pool water is monitored regularly throughout the day.

HYDROTHERAPY BATH

A hydrotherapy bath is designed for individual use. It has water jets positioned around the inside of the bath. These jets force water against the body, giving a gentle massage. Sometimes these baths have a water hose which can be used to direct water onto specific parts of the body. The water temperature in the hydrotherapy bath is usually preset to approximately 37–40°C. The bath may be used for relaxation or a preset programme can be used to target the jets at a specific part of the body. Products may be added to the bath to further enhance the treatment:

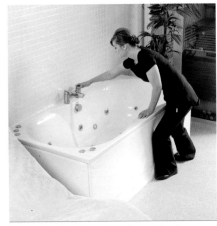

A therapist filling a hydrotherapy bath

Product	Example	Use/benefit
Algae	**Marine** minerals (eg seaweed)	■ Helps to stimulate the circulation. ■ Helps to detoxify the body. ■ Has a general toning effect.
Salt	Mineral salts (eg potassium, magnesium, calcium)	■ Helps to stimulate circulation. ■ Helps to detoxify the body. ■ Has a relaxing effect on tired and aching muscles.
Pre-blended aromatherapy oils	Essential oils – lemon and juniper or lavender and camomile	■ Depends on the blend used. ■ The aroma will have an immediate effect on the senses. ■ Relaxing and calming.
Milk		■ Ideal for a mature or dehydrated skin. ■ Very soothing and nourishing.

Marine

From the sea

INDUSTRY TIP

If a client has severe varicose veins, avoid using the manual hose on the hydrotherapy bath on the affected area.

INDUSTRY TIP

When adding products such as milk, algae or pre-blended aromatherapy oils to the hydrotherapy bath, always check first that the client does not have an allergy to the product.

BLITZ SHOWER

A blitz shower uses powerful water jets to invigorate the circulation and revitalise tired muscles. The temperature can be varied from hot to cold for a more stimulating experience.

SWISS/VICHY SHOWER

The client lies down on a cushioned treatment table. Above the table is a row of five to seven shower heads. While the client is lying down they are sprayed with water. It is used during spa treatments to remove products and as a form of hydro-massage.

HANDY HINT

Thalassotherapy

The word comes from the Greek – 'thalassa' meaning sea and 'therapia' meaning treatment. All treatments use some form of sea water, seaweed or algae to help moisturise and revitalise the body and skin.

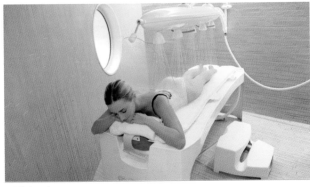

A Vichy shower

BENEFITS/TREATMENT OBJECTIVES OF HYDROTHERAPY TREATMENTS

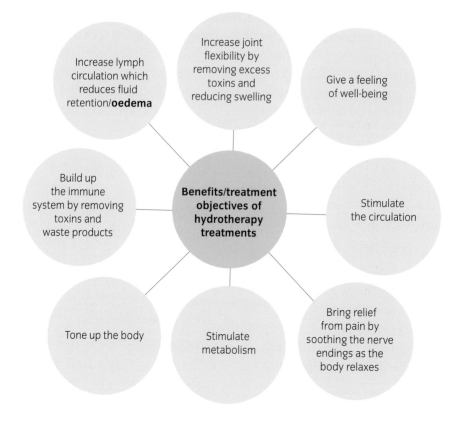

Increase lymph circulation which reduces fluid retention/**oedema**

Increase joint flexibility by removing excess toxins and reducing swelling

Give a feeling of well-being

Build up the immune system by removing toxins and waste products

Benefits/treatment objectives of hydrotherapy treatments

Stimulate the circulation

Tone up the body

Stimulate metabolism

Bring relief from pain by soothing the nerve endings as the body relaxes

Oedema

A condition where excess fluid collects in the tissues of the body

HANDY HINT

Kneipp therapy is the use of alternate hot and cold herbal baths by a client to stimulate the circulation and create a feeling of well-being.

OTHER SPA TREATMENTS

FLOTATION

There are two different types of flotation used in the spa:

- dry flotation
- wet flotation.

DRY FLOTATION

As the name suggests this is a dry treatment. Unlike wet flotation (where the client is placed into a tank of water) the client lies on a board on the surface of the water. This board is protected with a thick vinyl covering which also protects the client. The board is then lowered onto the water so that the client is floating on it. It is similar to lying on a water bed.

HANDY HINT

Dry flotation is often used alongside a body wrap treatment.

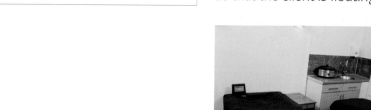

A dry flotation bed

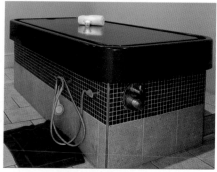

A heated hammam bed

325/326 MONITOR AND MAINTAIN THE SPA AREA AND PROVIDE SPA TREATMENTS

Health and safety checks for dry flotation treatments

You need to carry out the following health and safety checks prior to treatments:

- Check the vinyl covering for any splits or tears.
- Make sure that the mechanism for raising/lowering the board is working.
- Check the temperature of the water in the bed (refer to manufacturer instructions).

Client guidance – dry flotation treatments

Clients should:

- have had a thorough consultation to make sure that no contra-indications are present
- shower and remove all make-up prior to treatment
- be aware that the bench will be lowered so that flotation can take place
- be comfortable and warm
- float for approximately 20 minutes
- shower after treatment and relax for 15 minutes to allow the body temperature to return to normal
- drink plenty of water to rehydrate the body.

HANDY HINT

During a dry flotation treatment, you could provide other spa treatments to clients (eg a body mask).

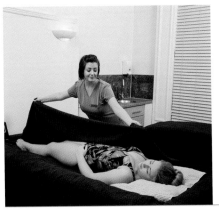 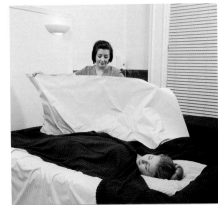 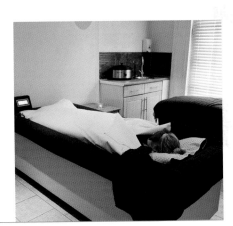

Dry flotation treatments

WET FLOTATION

A specially made bath or tank is filled with about 25cm of salt- and mineral-rich warm water (between 34°C and 36°C). The client floats on the water. As the water contains so much salt it is impossible to sink. This gives a feeling of weightlessness. This feeling of floating helps the muscles to relax and therefore reduces back pain and other muscular aches and pains. As the water won't allow the client sink, they don't have to concentrate on supporting or moving the body which allows their brain to relax.

Client preparation for wet flotation treatments

The flotation tank is soundproofed to help clients to relax. You should also provide clients with earplugs to make sure that they aren't disturbed by any noise. You need to make sure the room is in darkness as this slows the electrical activity of the brain. Darkness also helps balance the brain's activity so that the creative side of the brain becomes more dominant than the logical side of the brain.

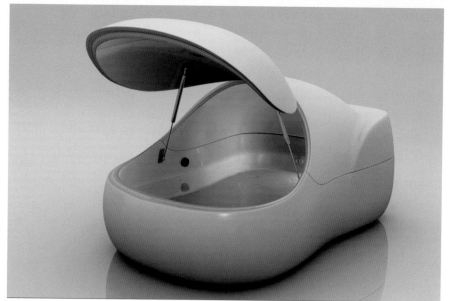
A wet flotation tank

Health and safety checks for wet flotation treatments

You need to carry out health and safety checks twice a day. You need to check to make sure that:

- there is no damage to any surfaces
- the water is at the correct temperature (between 34°C and 36°C)
- the lights are working correctly
- the emergency call button is working
- the directions for use, explanation of the benefits and list of precautions are on display
- there are no slip or trip hazards.

In addition to the general checks, you should also check at the start of each day and during the day that:

- the water is at the correct temperature (approximately 34–36°C)
- the water is at the correct level and has no debris in it
- that the pH balance is 7.2–7.4
- the filters aren't blocked (and any other checks in line with the manufacturer's instructions)
- the intercom is working.

Client guidance – wet flotation treatments

Clients should:

- have had a thorough consultation to make sure that no contra-indications are present
- shower and remove all make-up before entering the flotation tank
- read the guidance notice on how to use the flotation tank safely
- have had a demonstration and explanation by the therapist on how the tank works (eg lighting, audio levels and opening and closing of the pod)
- wear ear plugs to prevent water getting into their ears
- relax
- be aware that the therapist will use the intercom to check the client is comfortable

- shower at the end of the treatment to remove salt and toxins from the skin
- relax for 20 minutes after the treatment
- drink plenty of water to rehydrate the body.

BENEFITS/TREATMENT OBJECTIVES OF FLOTATION TREATMENTS

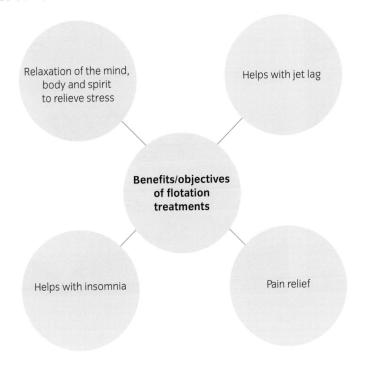

HANDY HINT

Soundproofing and lighting are optional for a wet flotation. Some people may not like the feeling of darkness and silence. If a client doesn't like darkness or silence, then you should dim the lights and play some gentle music instead. Recommend total darkness as this helps the body and mind to switch off completely.

INDUSTRY TIP

Research has shown that flotation can help pain relief (eg pain caused by rheumatoid arthritis).

INDUSTRY TIP

Flotation can be used by clients who are pregnant.

ACTIVITY

Research two spas that include flotation as part of a pre- or post-treatment package.

BODY WRAP TREATMENTS

Body wrapping is another popular treatment offered by many spas. Body wrap treatments help with **detoxification**, relaxation, improving the skin's appearance or can be used as part of a slimming programme. A mask or body wrap product is applied to the skin and the client is wrapped in plastic, foil or bandages (if it is a treatment to aid slimming).

Depending on the manufacturer's instructions the client may have a heated blanket applied or use the dry flotation bed. The wrap and heat from the blanket causes the body's temperature to increase. This then increases the circulation and encourages the body to sweat which gets rid of any impurities.

Body wrapping can also be used as part of a weight loss and toning programme. Body wrap treatments for this purpose often use bandages that are pre-soaked in a product that improves skin tone and that are wrapped around the area where the client wants to achieve weight loss. The objective of the wrap is to improve the skin tone which will help to give the skin a firmer and tighter appearance.

Detoxification

The process of removing toxins from the body

HANDY HINT

Dry skin brushing is recommended before any body treatment to stimulate blood and lymph circulation and remove toxins.

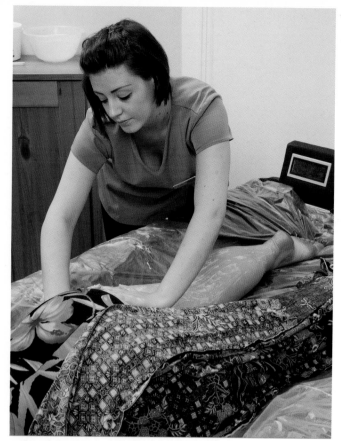

Body exfoliation as part of a body wrap treatment

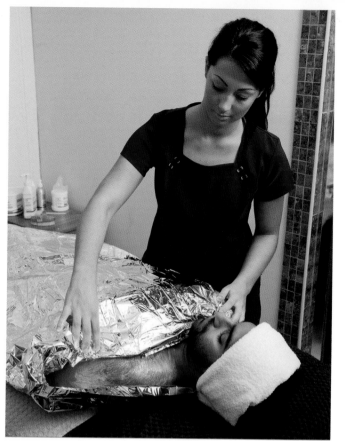

Therapist completing a body wrap treatment

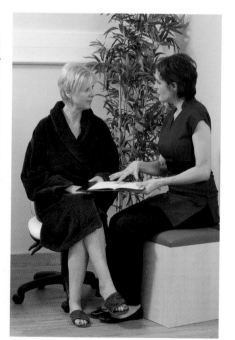

Consultation for body wrap treatments

Before carrying out a body wrap treatment, you need to carry out a thorough consultation by:

- using open questions to establish the treatment objectives and identify any possible contra-indications
- referring to clients' record cards to review previous treatments
- using visual aids to explain the treatment to clients.

You should also record the results of any patch/sensitivity tests that have been carried out. These tests will need to be carried out a minimum of 24 hours prior to treatment by applying a small amount of the product to the client's skin. Thermal testing can be carried out immediately before heat treatments to check the client's sensitivity to heat.

As part of your consultation it is important to establish which treatment objective is most appropriate for your client:

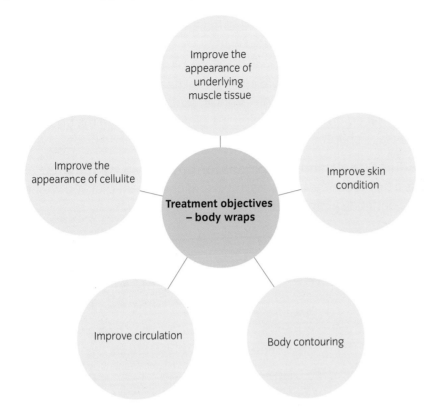

Improve the appearance of underlying muscle tissue

Improve skin condition

Treatment objectives – body wraps

Improve the appearance of cellulite

Improve circulation

Body contouring

ACTIVITY

Working in pairs, carry out a thermal sensitivity test on each other using hot and cold test tubes. Fill one test tube with cold water and one with warm water. Ask your partner to close their eyes and then place each of the test tubes onto their skin. Ask them to tell you which one is cold and which one is warm.

Body wrap treatment objectives

Body assessment

As part of the consultation for a body wrap treatment, you will need to carry out an assessment of the client's body. You will need to discuss with the client any specific conditions that they may want to try to improve with the treatment:

- Cellulite – this is usually found on the bottom, thighs and hips and has a dimpled appearance on the skin. It is a build-up of fat cells that slows down the removal of toxins. It quite often feels cold and can be the result of:
  - poor diet
  - lack of exercise
  - a slow metabolism
  - poor circulation.
- Fluid retention – this usually occurs around the ankles, in the lower limbs and in the abdominal area. It can be due to standing for long periods of time or hormone changes, particularly around menstruation.

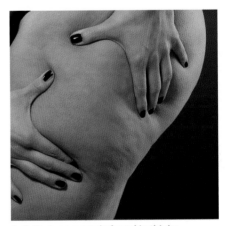

Cellulite is commonly found in thighs

325/326 MONITOR AND MAINTAIN THE SPA AREA AND PROVIDE SPA TREATMENTS

HANDY HINT

All women and men, whatever their shape and size, can suffer from cellulite.

- Adipose tissue – commonly referred to as excess fat. It forms the subcutaneous layer below the skin and its main purpose is to store fat and release it as energy when needed by cells in the body. Women tend to store excess weight around the hips and thighs whilst men store it on the abdomen and waist.
- Postural faults – a client's posture can be affected by their occupation, muscle condition, lifestyle and general health. Postural faults that you should be aware of include lordosis, scoliosis and kyphosis. For further information on postural faults, see pages 254–255 in the body massage chapter.

Products, tools and equipment for body wrap treatments

Listed below are the products, tools and equipment that you will need to carry out body wrap treatments.

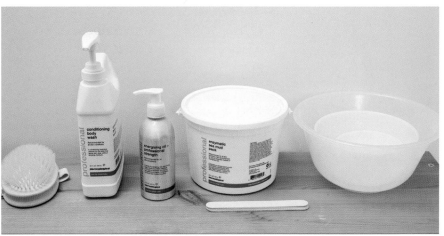

A range of products, tools and equipment used in a body wrap treatment

Products/tools/equipment	Description	Use/benefit
Cleanser	■ Body cleanser – sprays	■ Removes surface debris, oils and barriers. ■ Cleansing makes sure that the body wrap product/mask can penetrate into the skin.
Exfoliator	■ A cream/liquid containing small man-made abrasive beads or abrasive natural products (eg sea salt or fruit and nut kernels).	■ Gives a deeper cleanse.
Body wrap products	■ Body wrap products can be applied directly to the skin or via bandages applied to the limbs or body. ■ Products can include seaweed, thermal products and cryo-based products.	■ Help to achieve the treatment objective.

Products/tools/equipment	Description	Use/benefit
Body masks	■ Mud-based, seaweed or milk-based products applied prior to wrapping the client.	■ Help to achieve the treatment objective. ■ Improve the appearance of the skin. ■ Improve skin tone. ■ Detoxification.
Materials for wrapping the body (after applying mask or body wrap products)	■ Plastic wrap. ■ Bandages. ■ Linen strips. ■ Foil blanket.	■ Used to help the product penetrate into the skin. ■ Assist with body contouring.
Heated blanket/wrap	■ Electric blanket that produces heat. ■ Often broken down into zoned areas of heat so the client can choose which area to have heated. ■ Manually controlled **thermostat**.	■ Helps to maintain body temperature throughout the treatment. ■ Encourages body's temperature and therefore circulation to increase. ■ Causes the body to sweat which gets rid of any impurities.
Couch	■ Adjustable therapy couch. ■ Protected with couch roll.	For the client to lie on during the treatment.
Trolley	■ Clean trolley. ■ Set up in an organised way for treatment. ■ Trolley should have sufficient space for all your tools and equipment.	To hold the necessary equipment and products for the treatment.
Bowls	■ For body wrap products. ■ Flexible (ie bendy) bowls in varying sizes.	For **decanting** products. For mixing products. Need to be flexible and bend to break up mud that might have set in the bowl. Can be used to pour products directly onto the skin.
Spatulas	■ Usually made of wood. ■ Can be plastic or metal.	■ For dispensing products to avoid cross-contamination. ■ Used for mixing products.
Body brush	■ A natural bristle brush.	■ Used to brush the body when dry in long alternate strokes working in the direction of the lymphatic system. ■ Aids **desquamation** of the skin. ■ Helps with the removal of waste products. ■ Increases circulation. ■ Improves the appearance of cellulite. ■ Improves skin colour and tone.

Products/tools/ equipment	Description	Use/benefit
Sauna	▪ Dry heat room.	▪ Used before treatment. ▪ Increases body temperature to relax the client and allow for better penetration of the products.
Steam	▪ Wet heat room.	▪ Used before treatment. ▪ Increases body temperature to relax the client and allow for better penetration of the products.
Plastic wrap	▪ Fine plastic disposable wrap.	▪ To protect the therapy couch. ▪ To wrap the client in after they have had a body mask applied.

Thermostat

A device that controls temperature

Desquamation

Shedding of the skin

Decanting

Pouring from one container to another

INDUSTRY TIP

If you are using dry flotation as part of the treatment to help with relaxation and absorption of products, you will need to make sure that all the necessary equipment is set up – see pages 482–483.

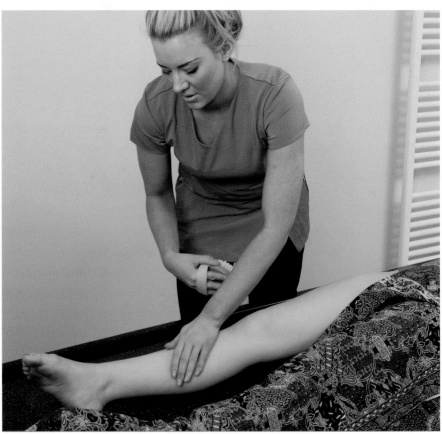

Body brushing is an ideal way to prepare the body for a body wrap

Other equipment that you may need:

▪ a tape measure – to measure improved skin tone on the client
▪ disposable paper underwear – for use by the client to avoid any damage to their own underwear
▪ couch roll – to protect the couch and for the client to stand on.

Body masks

During the consultation you will have agreed the client's treatment objectives. You will therefore need to select the right type of body mask to achieve these objectives.

Body masks are used to improve the appearance of the skin, improve tone and for detoxification. As with face masks, body masks can be setting or non-setting masks. You should be able to remove the mask from the client whilst they are on the therapy couch by using hot towels or mitts. However, it is better to have a shower cubicle so that the client can remove the product thoroughly. This method of removal is less messy and the shower cubicle can be cleaned easily to remove all traces of the product.

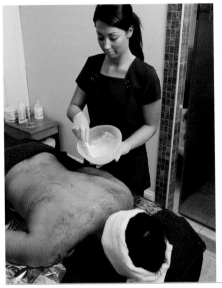 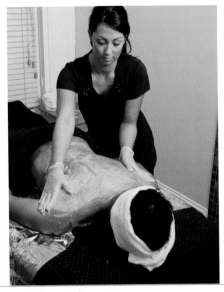 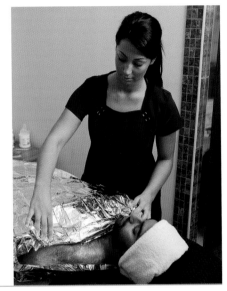

A client undergoing a body mask treatment

The main types of body mask are:

- Mud masks – these are made of mud and clay from the sea bed. They are rich in active minerals and are used to detoxify, firm and cleanse the skin. Their smell is sometimes unpleasant so they may have essential oils added to make them smell better.
- Algae/seaweed masks – this type of mask contains a rich source of trace elements, minerals and salts. A variety of seaweeds are used:
  - *fucus vesiculosus* – detoxifies, firms, tones and hydrates
  - *laminaria digitata* – high in iodine with diuretic properties
  - *ascophyllum nodosum* – balancing and relaxing.
  - *spirulina* – firms, antioxidant and anti-inflammatory.
- Milk masks – these are rich in vitamins. Milk masks contain milk whey which contains calcium, magnesium, potassium and sodium. They are used to improve dry, sensitive skin and various skin conditions.

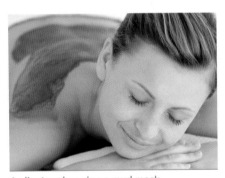

A client undergoing a mud mask

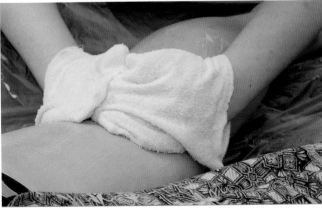

Using mitts to remove body products is good practice

HANDY HINT

Laminara digitata is great for stimulating the lymphatic system and improving the appearance of cellulite because of its diuretic properties.

HANDY HINT

A Swiss/Vichy shower could be used to remove the body mask.

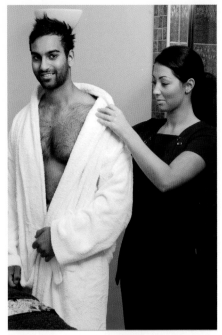

Body wraps are popular treatments for male clients

Body contouring/slimming wraps

The aim of body contouring/slimming wraps is to help the client lose inches by improving muscle tone and aiding detoxification. These can be applied as a standalone treatment or can also be applied after the client has used the spa facilities. There are two main types of wrap:

- Cryowraps – these are cold wraps. A cold wrap treatment reduces excess fluid in the hips, thighs and legs and improves the appearance of cellulite. The coldness of the wrap stimulates the circulation so this is an ideal treatment for someone who is just starting out on a weight-loss programme.
- Thermal wraps – these are self heating. The heat encourages perspiration which assists with the removal of waste products and toxins from the body.

Effects and benefits of a body wrap treatment

Specific benefits and effects of a body wrap will depend on the products that are used.

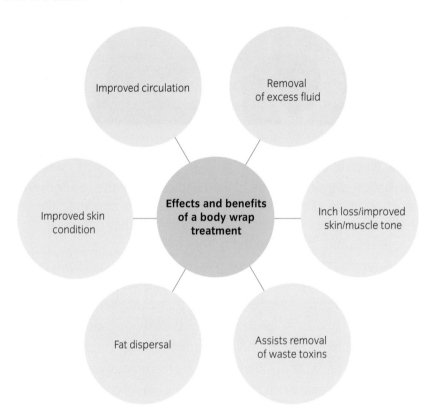

Improved circulation

Removal of excess fluid

Improved skin condition

Effects and benefits of a body wrap treatment

Inch loss/improved skin/muscle tone

Fat dispersal

Assists removal of waste toxins

WHY DON'T YOU...
research a well-known brand of products used in spas. Write down the body treatments that their products can be used in and the key ingredients that they use in their products. What are the benefits of these ingredients? Discuss your findings with the rest of the group.

INDUSTRY TIP

Some spas use grape extract, coconut, herbs, flowers, hay and even peat in their body wrap treatments. Grape extract stimulates the circulation and improves the lymph system. Coconut is good for cleansing and moisturising. Flowers add a nice fragrance and hay and peat cleanse the skin and help to regenerate it.

Application of a body mask

- Carry out a consultation and agree the treatment objectives with the client.
- Prepare the treatment area. Make sure that a heated blanket and plastic or foil sheets are placed on the therapy couch and that all the necessary products are on the trolley.
- Mix the body mask in a bowl using warm water and a spatula. Make sure you follow the manufacturer's instructions.

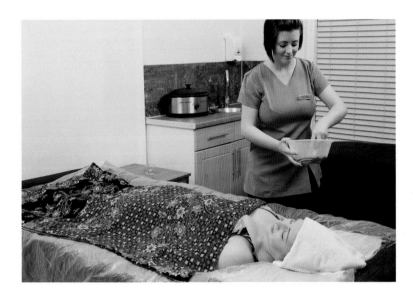

- Ask the client to lie face up on the couch and cover them with blankets for warmth.
- If you are using an exfoliation or body brushing treatment apply it at this point.
- Apply the mask using either a soft brush or your hands. Ask the client to lie on their side so you can apply it to their back. Then apply the mask to the front of the body.

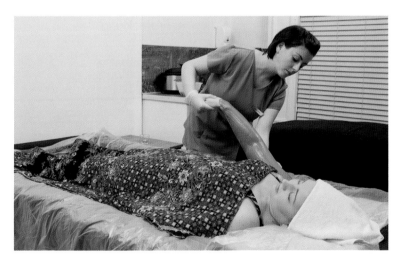

INDUSTRY TIP

A head or foot massage can be given at this part of the treatment if appropriate.

HANDY HINT

Heat increases the body's temperature which affects hydration levels. Make sure that the client has a good supply of water during the treatments.

- Work quickly to keep the product warm and avoid the client getting too cold.
- Wrap the plastic or foil blanket around the client and place a heated blanket placed over the top. This traps the heat next to the skin and improves the circulation. If you are using dry flotation, you do not

need to place the heat blanket on the client as the warmth from the dry flotation will help to maintain the body temperature.

- Let the client relax for 15–20 minutes depending upon the manufacturer's instructions. Then either remove the product using hot towels/mitts or take the client to the shower to remove the body mask. Depending on the type of mask used, moisturiser or cream can be applied at this stage of the treatment. A milk wrap leaves the skin very soft so no moisturising product is needed.

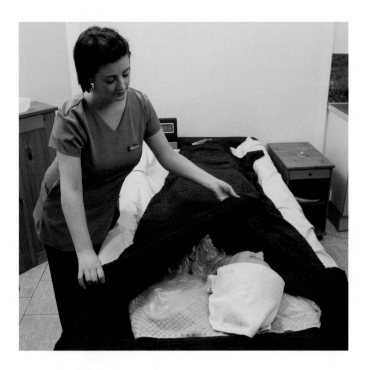

- Once the client has removed the body mask, give them five minutes to relax before providing home-care/aftercare advice.
- Give the client a glass of water for rehydration and take them back to the reception area. Ask them if they would like to rebook and show them any retail products that you have recommended.

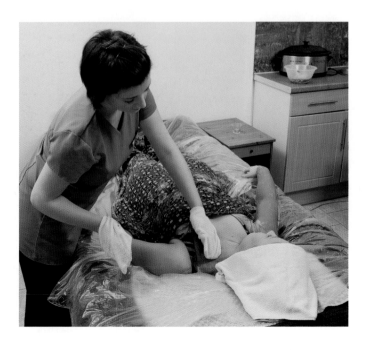

Application of slimming wraps

The following routine can be used when carrying out a slimming wrap treatment on a client.

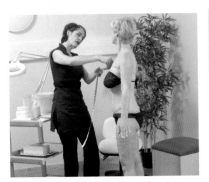

STEP 1 – Measure the client before the treatment so you can give them details of its effects afterwards.

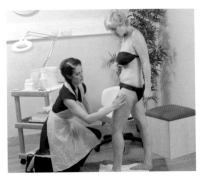

STEP 2 – Apply the product to the client.

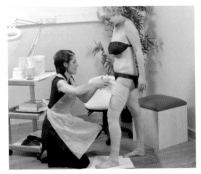

STEP 3 – Starting from the ankle, apply the slimming wrap bandages to the client's leg making sure that they are snug but not too tight. Apply to both legs.

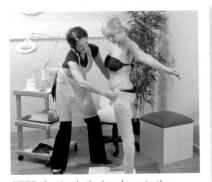

STEP 4 – Apply the bandages to the client's waist. Make sure that there are no gaps in the bandages.

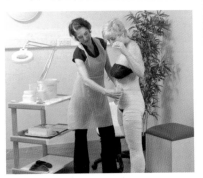

STEP 5 – Apply the bandages to the client's abdomen.

> **INDUSTRY TIP**
>
> Wraps may be combined with other treatments (eg a facial or a manicure). Remember to offer these additional treatments to the client.

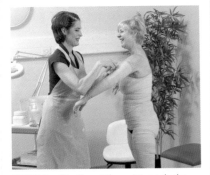

STEP 6 – Starting at the wrist, apply the slimming wrap bandages to one arm and then apply the bandage to the other arm.

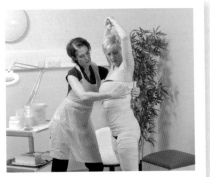

STEP 7 – Apply the bandage to the client's bust area. You will have to ask the client to raise their arms.

325/326 MONITOR AND MAINTAIN THE SPA AREA AND PROVIDE SPA TREATMENTS

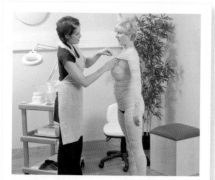

STEP 8 – Make sure that the bandages are secure before you commence the treatment.

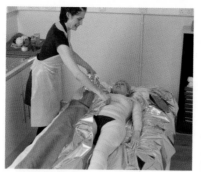

STEP 9 – Allow the client to relax on the dry flotation bed and apply the wrapping materials.

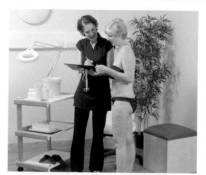

STEP 10 – Once the treatment has finished, allow the client to shower. Remember to measure them again and provide details of the inches they have lost on their body as a result of the treatment.

ACTIVITY

Make a list of everything you could do as a spa therapist to make sure a client's visit to the spa is a memorable treatment and experience.

HOME-CARE AND AFTERCARE ADVICE

Following a spa treatment, you should give your client suitable aftercare advice to follow. This advice will help the client maximise the benefits of the treatment. Suggest that the client:

- drinks plenty of water as this will help to flush out the toxins that have been released and rehydrate the body
- rests for at least 20 minutes following a heat treatment to allow their heart rate to return to normal
- avoids alcohol, caffeine, nicotine and drugs (unless prescribed) for 24 hours
- eats a light diet, avoiding processed foods and very spicy foods for 24 hours
- returns for a programme of treatments (for *all* spa treatments) – a minimum of six should be recommended for them to see any real benefits
- looks at their lifestyle to see if they can make any healthy changes
- uses recommended home-care products to achieve the most effective results.

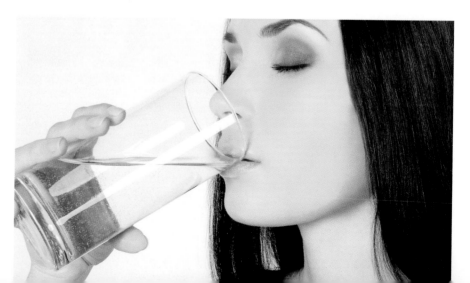

CONTRA-ACTIONS

A contra-action is an adverse reaction that can happen during or after a treatment. The table below lists some contra-actions that might occur and the actions to take if they do.

Contra-action	Cause	Action to be taken
Dehydration (causing fainting, sickness, dizziness and breathing difficulties)	■ Overheating causing excessive sweating and loss of body salts.	■ Client should rest and lie down. ■ Drink plenty of water. ■ Apply a cool compress to the forehead.
Cramps	■ Overheating causing excessive perspiration and loss of body salts.	■ Client should drink plenty of water. ■ Stretch muscles.
Heat exhaustion (causing dizziness, sickness, headaches and fainting)	■ Loss of fluids. ■ Loss of salts.	■ Client should rest and lie down. ■ Drink plenty of water or fluids containing salts and minerals (eg sports drinks) to replace lost salts. ■ Apply a cool compress to the forehead.
Severe erythema (including irritation and swelling)	■ Allergy to a product. ■ Over-stimulation of the circulatory system due to heat.	■ Suggest that client takes a cool shower to remove products and lower the skin temperature. ■ If irritation continues for more than 24 hours, client should seek medical advice.
Respiratory disorder (eg asthma attack)	■ Dry heat can affect the airways and cause an asthma attack.	■ Get the client to take their medication. ■ If they are panicking get them to focus on controlling their breathing. ■ If severe, seek medical advice.
Burning/scalding	■ Client didn't remove metal jewellery before treatment. ■ Client has touched a heating source. ■ Client has sat in front of the steam inlet in the steam room.	■ Apply cold water to burns. ■ Cover burns with a dry dressing. ■ If no dressing is immediately available, a sterile plastic wrap will protect the area from infection. ■ If severe, seek medical help.

TEST YOUR KNOWLEDGE

Use the questions below to test your knowledge of Chapter 325/326 to see how much information you have retained. These questions will help you to revise what you have learnt in this chapter.

Turn to page 499 for the answers.

1 A Palintest® is used to check:
   a For product allergies
   b The temperature of the spa pool
   c The pH balance of the spa water
   d The humidity of the steam room

2 What is a caldarium?
   a Sauna
   b Spa pool
   c Body wrap
   d Steam room

3 Why is milk added to a hydrotherapy bath?
   a To detoxify
   b To soothe and nourish
   c To stimulate the circulation
   d To stimulate lymphatic drainage

4 What is erythema?
   a Redness of the skin
   b Severe swelling
   c A severe headache
   d Sweating/perspiration

5 Which **one** of the following is a contra-action to spa treatments?
   a Increased pulse rate
   b Increased perspiration
   c Fainting
   d Ingrown hairs

6 What was the name of the monk who believed that disease could be cured by using water to get rid of waste from the body?
   a Kneipp
   b Algae
   c Hammam
   d Galen

7 What does 'hydro' mean?
   a Hot
   b Cold
   c Water
   d Temperature

8 Which **one** of the following is a specific effect of a seaweed body wrap?
   a Detoxifying
   b Moisturising
   c Desquamation
   d Nourishment

9 What should the temp of a Finnish sauna be?
   a 70–100°c
   b 60–80°c
   c 45–60°c
   d 40–45°c

10 Which **one** of the following treatments can a client have if they are pregnant?
   a Sauna
   b Rasul
   c Flotation
   d Seaweed wrap

TEST YOUR KNOWLEDGE ANSWERS

Anatomy and physiology
1 a, **2** a, **3** b, **4** c, **5** d, **6** a, **7** c, **8** d, **9** d, **10** d, **11** a, **12** d, **13** a, **14** c, **15** a, **16** c, **17** a, **18** a, **19** b, **20** c, **21** d, **22** c, **23** c, **24** c, **25** c

301 Working with colleagues within beauty-related industries
1 b, **2** c, **3** d, **4** c, **5** a, **6** a, **7** a, **8** d, **9** d, **10** b

302 Carry out and monitor health and safety practice in the salon
1 d, **2** b, **3** d, **4** c, **5** a, **6** d, **7** a, **8** c, **9** b, **10** d

303 Client care and communication in beauty-related industries
1 b, **2** d, **3** d, **4** c, **5** a, **6** a, **7** b, **8** a, **9** c, **10** a

304 Promote and sell products and services to clients
1 d, **2** b, **3** d, **4** c, **5** d, **6** c, **7** c, **8** b, **9** b, **10** a

305/309 Provide body massage and provide massage using pre-blended aromatherapy oils
1 c, **2** d, **3** c, **4** b, **5** b, **6** d, **7** b, **8** d, **9** b, **10** a

306/307 Provide facial and body electrotherapy treatments
1 b, **2** c, **3** a, **4** b, **5** c, **6** d, **7** c, **8** c, **9** c, **10** d

308 Provide electrical epilation
1 d, **2** d, **3** a, **4** a, **5** c, **6** b, **7** a, **8** d, **9** a, **10** c

311 Provide Indian head massage
1 d, **2** c, **3** d, **4** d, **5** c, **6** a, **7** c, **8** a, **9** c, **10** d

313 Provide self-tanning
1 c, **2** d, **3** b, **4** b, **5** c, **6** d, **7** c, **8** b, **9** c, **10** b

317 Apply individual permanent lashes
1 c, **2** a, **3** b, **4** b, **5** c, **6** c, **7** c, **8** a, **9** c, **10** c

321 Apply microdermabrasion
1 b, **2** d, **3** b, **4** b, **5** a, **6** b, **7** c, **8** d, **9** a, **10** c

322 Apply stone therapy massage
1 a, **2** a, **3** d, **4** a, **5** c, **6** a, **7** d, **8** b, **9** b, **10** a

325/326 Monitor and maintain the spa area and provide spa treatments
1 c, **2** d, **3** b, **4** a, **5** c, **6** a, **7** c, **8** a, **9** a, **10** c